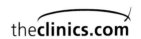

GASTROENTEROLOGY CLINICS OF NORTH AMERICA

Nutrition in Gastrointestinal Illness

GUEST EDITOR
Alan L. Buchman, MD, MSPH

March 2007 • Volume 36 • Number 1

SAUNDERS

An Imprint of Elsevier, Inc.
PHILADELPHIA   LONDON   TORONTO   MONTREAL   SYDNEY   TOKYO

W.B. SAUNDERS COMPANY
A Division of Elsevier Inc.

Elsevier Inc. • 1600 John F. Kennedy Blvd., Suite 1800 • Philadelphia, Pennsylvania 19103-2899

http://www.theclinics.com

GASTROENTEROLOGY CLINICS
OF NORTH AMERICA   Volume 36, Number 1
March 2007   ISSN 0889-8553
Editor: Kerry Holland   ISBN-13: 978-1-4160-3911-2
ISBN-10: 1-4160-3911-2

Reprints. For copies of 100 or more, of articles in this publication, please contact the Commercial Reprints Department, Elsevier Inc., 360 Part Avenue South, New York, New York 10010-1710. Tel. (212) 633-3813 Fax: (212) 462-1935 e-mail: reprints@elsevier.com.

The ideas and opinions expressed in *Gastroenterology Clinics of North America* do not necessarily reflect those of the Publisher. The Publisher does not assume any responsibility for any injury and/or damage to persons or property arising out of or related to any use of the material contained in this periodical. The reader is advised to check the appropriate medical literature and the product information currently provided by the manufacturer of each drug to be administered to verify the dosage, the method and duration of administration, or contraindications. It is the responsibility of the treating physician or other health care professional, relying on independent experience and knowledge of the patient, to determine drug dosages and the best treatment for the patient. Mention of any product in this issue should not be construed as endorsement by the contributors, editors, or the Publisher of the product or manufacturers' claims.

Gastroenterology Clinics of North America (ISSN 0889-8553) is published quarterly by Elsevier Inc., 360 Park Avenue South, New York, NY 10010-1710. Months of issue are March, June, September, and December. Business and Editorial Offices: 1600 John F. Kennedy Blvd., Suite 1800, Philadelphia, PA 19103-2899. Customer Service Office: 6277 Sea Harbor Drive, Orlando, FL 32887-4800. Periodicals postage paid at New York, NY and additional mailing offices. Subscription prices are $215.00 per year (US individuals), $110.00 per year (US students), $313.00 per year (US institutions), $237.00 per year (Canadian individuals), $373.00 per year (Canadian institutions), $281.00 per year (international individuals), $143.00 per year (international students), and $373.00 per year (international institutions). Foreign air speed delivery is included in all *Clinics* subscription prices. All prices are subject to change without notice. POSTMASTER: Send address changes to *Gastroenterology Clinics of North America*, Elsevier Periodicals Customer Service 6277 Sea Harbor Drive, Orlando, FL 32887-4800. **Customer Service: 1-800-654-2452 (US). From outside of the US, call 1-407-345-4000. E-mail: hhspcs@harcourt.com**

Gastroenterology Clinics of North America is also published in Italian by II Pensiero Scientifico Editore, Rome, Italy; and in Portuguese by Interlivros Edicoes Ltda., Rua Commandante Coelho 1085, 21250 Cordovil, Rio de Janeiro, Brazil.

Gastroenterology Clinics of North America is covered in *Index Medicus, Excerpta Medica, Current Contents/ Clinical Medicine, Science Citation Index, ISI/BIOMED*, and *BIOSIS*.

Printed in the United States of America.

GASTROENTEROLOGY CLINICS
OF NORTH AMERICA

Nutrition in Gastrointestinal Illness

GUEST EDITOR

ALAN L. BUCHMAN, MD, MSPH, FACP, FACN, AGAF, Associate Professor of Medicine, Division of Gastroenterology, Northwestern University Medical School, Feinberg School of Medicine, Chicago, Illinois

CONTRIBUTORS

SUSAN H. BARTON, MD, Instructor of Medicine, Division of Gastroenterology and Hepatology, Mayo Clinic, Rochester, Minnesota

MARK H. DELEGGE, MD, FACG, AGAF, FASGE, Professor of Medicine, Digestive Disease Center, Medical University of South Carolina, Charleston, South Carolina

JOHN K. DIBAISE, MD, Associate Professor of Medicine, Division of Gastroenterology and Hepatology, Mayo Clinic, Scottsdale, Arizona

LUKE M. DRAKE, MD, Department of Medicine, Medical University of South Carolina, Charleston, South Carolina

MARTIN H. FLOCH, MD, MACG, AGAF, Digestive Disease Section, Yale University School of Medicine, New Haven, Connecticut

JONATHAN P. FRYER, MD, Associate Professor of Surgery, Division of Transplantation, Department of Surgery, Feinberg School of Medicine, Northwestern University, Chicago, Illinois

NIRMALA GONSALVES, MD, Instructor of Medicine, Division of Gastroenterology, Northwestern University, The Feinberg School of Medicine, Chicago, Illinois

PALLE BEKKER JEPPESEN, MD, PhD, Department of Medical Gastroenterology, Rigshospitalet, Copenhagen, Denmark

DARLENE G. KELLY, MD, PhD, Associate Professor, Division of Gastroenterology and Hepatology, Mayo Clinic, Rochester, Minnesota

ROBERT F. KUSHNER, MD, Professor, Department of Medicine, Northwestern University Feinberg School of Medicine, Wellness Institute, Chicago, Illinois

STEPHEN A. McCLAVE, MD, Professor of Medicine, Director of Clinical Nutrition, Division of Gastroenterology/Hepatology, Department of Medicine, University of Louisville School of Medicine, Louisville, Kentucky

JOSEPH A. MURRAY, MD, Professor, Division of Gastroenterology and Hepatology, Mayo Clinic, Rochester, Minnesota

JACQUELINE PARK, MD, Digestive Disease Section, Yale University School of Medicine, New Haven, Connecticut

MICHELLE M. ROMANO, RD, LD, CNSD, Assistant Professor of Nutrition, Mayo Clinic College of Medicine; and Clinical Dietitian, Home Enteral Coordinator, Jacksonville, Florida

JAMES S. SCOLAPIO, MD, Professor of Medicine, Division of Gastroenterology and Hepatology, Mayo Clinic, Jacksonville, Florida

DOUGLAS L. SEIDNER, MD, FACG, Director, Nutrition Support Team, Department of Gastroenterology and Hepatology, Cleveland Clinic Foundation, Cleveland, Ohio

ANDREW UKLEJA, MD, Assistant Professor of Medicine, Director of Nutrition Support Team, University of South Florida, Tampa, Florida

SUSAN E. WILLIAMS, MD, MS, RD, CNS, Fellow, Clinical Nutrition and Metabolism, Department of Gastroenterology and Hepatology, Cleveland Clinic Foundation, Cleveland, Ohio

GASTROENTEROLOGY CLINICS
OF NORTH AMERICA

Nutrition in Gastrointestinal Illness

CONTENTS VOLUME 36 • NUMBER 1 • MARCH 2007

Hospital-based malnutrition continues to be an important comorbidity affecting clinical outcomes. Knowledge of performing an appropriate nutrition assessment and implementing a rational nutrition therapy should be part of any patient's hospital plan of care. Familiarity with nutrition assessment scoring systems and nutrition assessment tools should be part of any gastroenterologist's expertise. Assessment of a patient's caloric and protein needs should be part of any hospital patient's clinical evaluation.

Parenteral nutrition plays a vital role for patients with intestinal failure and those who are unable to maintain oral or enteral nutrition alone. Parenteral nutrition has been shown to improve clinical outcome in patients with malnutrition and intestinal tract dysfunction. The use of parenteral nutrition is not without risk of serious complications. Parenteral nutrition complications can be divided into mechanical related to vascular access, septic, and metabolic. This article provides a review on the short- and long-term complications of parenteral nutrition and their management.

Microecology of the gastrointestinal tract is the physiologic basis for the effect of dietary fiber, prebiotics and probiotics on the host. The ecology consists of the gastrointestinal tract, primarily the intestines, the foods that are fed into the tract, and the flora living within. Within this ecology, normal flora and probiotics, ferment dietary fiber and prebiotics to produce short chain fatty acids and substances that are absorbed and effect the host at the intestinal level and systemically. In this review, we will discuss the effects of prebiotics, probiotics and dietary fiber in gastrointestinal disorders and diseases.

The benefit of early enteral nutrition (EN) for the disease process and for patient outcome in severe acute pancreatitis is dramatic. A narrow window of opportunity exists during which there is potential for EN to decrease disease severity and reduce overall complications. Most patients with severe pancreatitis tolerate enteral feeds. Any signs of symptom exacerbation or increasing inflammation in response to EN may be ameliorated by subtle adjustments in the feeding strategy. In this manner, provision of EN represents primary therapy in the management of the patient with acute pancreatitis and is emerging as the gold standard of therapy in nutrition support for this disease process.

Eosinophilic gastrointestinal disorders are characterized by eosinophilic infiltration and inflammation of the gastrointestinal tract in the absence of previously identified causes of eosinophilia, such as parasitic infections, malignancy, collagen vascular diseases, drug sensitivities, and inflammatory bowel disease. These disorders include eosinophilic esophagitis, eosinophilic gastroenteritis, eosinophilic enteritis, and eosinophilic colitis. This article focuses mainly on eosinophilic esophagitis and eosinophilic gastroenteritis.

Celiac disease is characterized by small bowel enteropathy, precipitated in genetically susceptible individuals by the ingestion of "gluten," which is a term used to encompass the storage proteins of wheat, rye, and barley. Although the intestine heals with removal of gluten from the diet, the intolerance is permanent and the damage recurs if gluten is reintroduced. This damage causes a wide variety of consequence including maldigestion and malabsorption, resulting in the characteristic, although not universal, features of malnutrition. This article examines recent advances in the understanding of the spectrum of celiac disease, illustrates the impact of celiac disease on nutrition, and describes approaches to the management of the disease.

Growth Factors in Short-Bowel Syndrome Patients 109
Palle Bekker Jeppesen

Malabsorption is a key finding in patients with short-bowel syndrome. Malabsorption of nonessential and essential nutrients, fluids, and electrolytes, if not compensated for by increased intake, leads to diminished body stores and subclinical and (eventually) clinical deficiencies. After intestinal resection, adaptation (a spontaneous progressive recovery from the malabsorptive disorder) may be evident. This article describes selected factors responsible for the morphologic and functional changes in the adaptive processes and presents results of clinical trials that use either growth hormone or glucagon-like peptide-2 to facilitate a condition of hyperadaptation in short-bowel patients.

Home Parenteral and Enteral Nutrition 123
John K. DiBaise and James S. Scolapio

Home parenteral and enteral nutrition (HPEN) has evolved to become a very successful, lifesaving treatment in the management of patients with intestinal and oral failure, respectively. Nevertheless, the provision of HPEN remains intrusive, expensive, and continues to be associated with significant morbidity. The management of HPEN by a nutrition support team that optimally includes an experienced clinician, nurse specialist, dietitian, and pharmacist reduces HPEN-related morbidity and may reduce costs associated with its use. Because clinical expertise in the management of patients receiving HPEN is not widely available, the referral of these patients to experienced centers for periodic assessment should be encouraged.

Intestinal Transplantation: Current Status 145
Jonathan P. Fryer

Intestine transplant is indicated for patients with intestinal failure who are unable to be weaned from parenteral nutrition (PN). Long-term PN, although life sustaining in many patients, can be associated with life-threatening complications including PN-associated liver disease (PNALD). Most patients are not considered for intestine transplant until they have developed severe PNALD and also need a liver transplant. Overall outcomes with intestinal transplantation are steadily improving, and current 1-year patient survivals for intestine-only transplants are now similar to those for liver transplant. Intestinal transplantation should be considered earlier in intestinal failure patients who are at high risk for developing PNALD and other life-threatening complications.

Metabolic bone disease is often silent, often undiagnosed, and occurs frequently in patients with chronic gastrointestinal illnesses. Potentially modifiable risk factors, such as malnutrition, malabsorption, prolonged use of glucocorticoids, and a sedentary lifestyle, can lead to low bone mass, an increased rate of bone loss, and debilitating bone disease. This article explores common gastrointestinal illnesses that place patients at risk for developing metabolic bone disease. Concepts are presented to assist the practitioner in identifying patients at risk; clinical evaluation and diagnostic test selection are discussed, and therapeutic options for the prevention and treatment of metabolic bone disease in gastrointestinal illness are presented.

Because obesity is associated with an increased risk of multiple health problems, it is important for gastroenterologists and all health care providers routinely to identify, evaluate, and treat patients for obesity in the course of daily practice. Therapy for obesity always begins with lifestyle management and may include pharmacotherapy or surgery. Setting an initial weight loss goal of 10% over 6 months is a realistic target, followed by long-term management.

GASTROENTEROLOGY CLINICS
OF NORTH AMERICA

Gastroenterol Clin N Am 36 (2007) xi–xiii

GASTROENTEROLOGY CLINICS
OF NORTH AMERICA

Preface

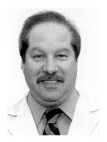

Alan L. Buchman, MD, MSPH, FACP, FACN, AGAF

Guest Editor

Nutrition is a significant part of gastroenterology. Nutrient assimilation involves all aspects of the gastrointestinal tract. Salivary glands are involved in digestion. The esophagus acts as a food conduit. The stomach serves as a temporary food storage depot from which numerous physiologic responses are elicited. The pancreas secretes enzymes that are required for nutrient digestion. The gallbladder secretes bile that is required for fat digestion. Nutrient, electrolyte, and fluid absorption occurs in the small and large bowel, and the liver is primary organ for nutrient metabolism. In essence, the primary function of the gastrointestinal tract and biliary system is that related to nutrient intake, absorption, and metabolism; sufficient for survival. It is incumbent on the gastroenterologist to understand the role of the gastrointestinal tract in nutrient assimilation and to understand when and how to intervene when it is compromised, to prevent the development of systemic nutrient disorders.

In this issue of *Gastroenterology Clinics of North America*, devoted to nutrition, Dr. DeLegee describes the nutrition assessment. At a minimum, a brief nutritional assessment should be performed on every patient seen by a gastroenterologist. Patients with moderate to severe malnutrition are at increased risk for inpatient and periprocedural morbidity and mortality. A brief nutritional assessment and nutritional risk calculation may be performed by history and physical examination with review of clinical laboratory tests during an office visit or even while waiting for the nurse to hook up the endoscope for a variceal bleeder, and the nutritional risk can be determined. One must first determine which patients are particularly at risk before determination of whether, what type, what amount, and by what route (the four WWWs) nutritional intervention is required.

0889-8553/07/$ – see front matter © 2007 Published by Elsevier Inc.
doi:10.1016/j.gtc.2007.01.010 gastro.theclinics.com

All medical therapy is provided following a cost-benefit analysis that weighs in favor of therapy. Nutritional support is no exception, and may be associated with numerous complications. To achieve maximal efficacy and minimal risk/cost, patients must be monitored appropriately. Drs. Ukleja and Romano discuss the various mechanical, metabolic, gastrointestinal, and hepatobiliary complications of parenteral nutrition, and suggest methods for their mitigation. One must avoid rapid repletion of undernourished patients to avoid development of potentially life-threatening refeeding syndrome.

Drs. Park and Floch define prebiotics, probiotics, and dietary fiber, and then discuss contemporary data on their use as disease-modifying agents in colonic neoplasia, diverticular disease, irritable bowel syndrome, inflammatory bowel disease, diarrhea, constipation, and hepatic encephalopathy. Dr. McClave addresses the development of a systemic inflammatory response during acute pancreatitis and its modification using parenteral or enteral nutritional support.

Dr. Gonsalves discusses a more recently recognized disorder, eosinophilic esophagitis, which may be associated with environmental toxins, including food or allergies. A disease found not only in the pediatric population, but also in adults, it is increasingly recognized in the community. The pathophysiology underlying eosinophilic esophagitis, its endoscopic and histologic findings, and currently recommended therapy are discussed by Dr. Gonsalves. Just as the prevalence of what may be a food-mediated disorder seems to be increasing in prevalence, celiac sprue is also much more prevalent in the community than once suspected. Drs. Barton, Kelly, and Murray review recent advances in the understanding of this disorder, its presentation, its pathophysiology, and its sequelae.

Patients with short-bowel syndrome undergo intestinal "adaptation" postenterectomy, during which segmental nutrient absorption improves, presumably related to a hormonally mediated increase in mucosal absorptive surface. Dr. Jeppesen discusses this process and the currently available data on the use of exogenous growth factor therapy with growth hormone and glucagon-like peptide II. Many of these patients are destined for long-term home parenteral nutrition. Drs. DiBase and Scolapio discuss the appropriate indications for this therapy, and the indications for home enteral nutritional therapy. Patients who receive the latter are often overlooked and are not seen by the gastroenterologist once the feeding tube has been placed until tube-related complications develop. Drs. DiBase and Scolapio discuss the proper assessment of the patient and their environment necessary to avoid many complications. Optimal feeding routes are discussed, along with the indications for each route. Complications, outcomes, and cost are also discussed.

For patients who have failed home parenteral nutrition and appropriate medical management including intestinal rehabilitation, and are on their way to development of potentially life-threatening complications, such as loss of vascular access or irreversible liver disease, intestinal transplantation is an increasingly viable option. Dr. Fryer discusses the appropriate indications for this surgery and the pretransplant evaluation. Postoperative management and surveillance and treatment of graft rejection and infection, the complications of greatest concern, are discussed.

The gastroenterologist must be cognizant of nongastrointestinal manifestations of gastrointestinal disease. Patients with gastrointestinal disease, such as inflammatory bowel disease, celiac sprue, and other malabsorptive disorders including short-bowel syndrome, may develop metabolic bone disease. Drs. Williams and Seidner discuss the recognition of metabolic bone disease and risk factors of which gastroenterologists should be aware.

The largest nutritional problem facing America is the obesity epidemic. Although many of the reviews in this issue focus largely on the patient with a nutritional deficit, an overabundance of nutrition, specifically energy, may also result in both direct and indirect morbidity. It must be recognized, however, that even the obese individual may develop malnutrition. Dr. Kushner describes the nutritional assessment of the overweight patient and the initial medical management, which should include lifestyle modifications, dietary therapy, physical activity, and behavioral modification. Pharmacotherapy may be an important adjunctive therapy in some individuals. Surgery is generally reserved for individuals with severe obesity or moderate obesity who have developed obesity-related complications.

It is hoped that this edition of *Gastroenterology Clinics of North America* stimulates the reader to incorporate nutritional diagnosis and intervention into their everyday clinical practice and to seek out additional education to provide appropriate services for their patients from a nutritional perspective.

Alan L. Buchman, MD, MSPH, FACP, FACN, AGAF
Division of Gastroenterology
Northwestern University Medical School
Feinberg School of Medicine
676 North St Clair Street, Suite 1400
Chicago, IL 60611, USA

E-mail address: a-buchman@northwestern.edu

Gastroenterol Clin N Am 36 (2007) 1–22

GASTROENTEROLOGY CLINICS
OF NORTH AMERICA

Nutritional Assessment

Mark H. DeLegge, MD, FACG, AGAF, FASGE*, Luke M. Drake, MD

Digestive Disease Center, Medical University of South Carolina,
96 Jonathan Lucas Street, 210 Clinical Science Building, Charleston, SC 29425, USA

Thirty years ago, hospital malnutrition was described as being very prevalent, yet poorly identified by medical teams [1]. Unfortunately, this situation has not changed significantly. Protein-calorie malnutrition is still very common in hospitalized patients, and remains poorly recognized by many clinicians [2]. In a recent study of Brazilian hospitalized patients, 48% of the patients were deemed to be malnourished. Despite this alarming number, most physicians in this study did not assess their patient's nutritional status or make nutritional therapy a major component of their patient's hospital medical plan [3].

Protein-calorie malnutrition is important clinically when it is severe enough to impact one's physiologic function, inhibit their response to medical therapies, or prolong time to recovery. The physiologic devastation seen with protein-calorie malnutrition is secondary to loss of total body protein and muscle function [4]. When more than 20% of one's usual body weight is lost, most physiologic body functions become significantly impaired [5]. Studies evaluating the relationship of loss of body weight to loss of body protein have shown a strong correlation [6].

Protein malnutrition can be divided into two generalized categories: marasmus and kwashiorkor. Patients with marasmus have a significant deficit of total body fat and body protein with a slight increase in extracellular water. Clinically, this presents as obvious body wasting. The eyes may be sunken and the skull and cheekbones may be prominent [7]. The plasma albumin is often in the low normal range. Resting energy expenditure (REE) in these individuals is not increased despite severe physiologic dysfunction. In contrast, whereas patients with kwashiorkor have similar deficits of body protein and fat, they also have markedly increased extracellular fluid and low plasma albumin levels [7]. To the casual observer, this increase in extracellular fluid may mask underlying weight loss. Patients with kwashiorkor typically have an accelerated metabolic rate, and if measured, their physiologic function is also significantly impaired.

End-organ function is adversely affected by malnutrition. Muscle strength decreases over time. Respiratory function, including forced expiratory volume,

*Corresponding author. E-mail address: deleggem@musc.edu (M.H. DeLegge).

0889-8553/07/$ – see front matter
doi:10.1016/j.gtc.2007.02.001

vital capacity, and peak expiratory flow, declines. An association between impaired respiratory gas exchange and malnutrition in chronic obstructive respiratory disease patients has been described [8]. Malnutrition can also reduce cardiac output, impair wound healing, and depress immune function [9]. Nutritional repletion, however, can often reverse these degenerative processes and significantly improve patient outcomes. The difficulty lies not only in the treatment of such conditions, but also in identifying individuals at risk so that appropriate interventions can be made.

NUTRITION ASSESSMENT

Research in nutrition assessment continues to develop. Early research in assessing patients for the presence of malnutrition resulted in tools and markers being developed for surveying large populations over a short period of time. Many of these tools and markers were then brought to the hospitalized setting and used on individual patients. Jones and colleagues [10] reported on 44 separate tools published in the past 25 years for determining nutritional status. Most of the perceived traditional markers of protein-calorie malnutrition, such as serum albumin, have such poor sensitivity and large variance that their use on individual patients is of limited value.

A traditional nutrition assessment often includes a dietary, medical, and body weight history. Measurements of current body weight and height are recorded. Serum protein levels, body anthropometric measurements, immune competence efficacy, and functional measurements of muscle strength may be incorporated into the overall final assessment. Individually, these measurements often have limited value in accurately determining a patient's nutrition risk. For example, dietary history as recalled by patients can be overestimated by an average of 22% [11]. Most physicians and nurses rely on a patient's recall of their own weight, rather than a direct measurement (a very unreliable practice) [12].

Studies have consistently revealed the inadequacy of any single assessment method or tool to assess a patient's nutritional state. As a result, combinations of diverse measurements have been developed into "scoring systems" designed to increase the sensitivity and specificity in determining nutritional status [13]. In general, a global approach to nutrition assessment in hospitalized patients provides a more definitive picture of a patient's true nutritional risk. Care must be taken, however, to ensure the validity of the nutritional screening or assessment tool. For example, Green and Watson [14] reported on 71 nutrition screening and assessment tools available for use by nurses, and found that most had not been subjected to any validity or reliability testing. Despite this fact, all are currently being used in clinical practice.

Weight History

Recent weight loss is a very sensitive marker of a patient's nutritional status [15]. Weight loss of more than 5% in 1 month or 10% in 6 months before hospitalization has been shown to be clinically significant [16]. When 20% of usual body weight has been lost in 6 months or less, severe physiologic dysfunction occurs. In one studied surgical population, weight loss of more than 5% in the month before hospital admission correlated with both an increased length of hospital stay and time of rehabilitation [17].

It is not always possible to diagnose malnutrition based on body habitus visualization alone. For example, patient's who are obese, or those with edema, may be very difficult to assess nutritionally solely relying on their body size or body weight.

Even though measured weights are usually an accurate, easily trackable, and reliable assessment of one's nutritional status, recalled weights are much less precise. Although theoretically simple to obtain, some individuals as a result of neurologic impairment have great difficulty recalling their usual body weight or recent weight history. Numerous studies have documented huge variances in reported weights when a patient's own weight recall is used as the sole determining factor, with sensitivities as low as 65%. A recent randomized study from Europe noted that in 500 patient admissions, a weight was recorded only 67% of the time [18]. In a separate study of 4000 patients, weights were only recorded 15% of the time even though a scale was available within 150 ft of the patient's bed in 75% of the cases [2].

Anthropometrics

Interest in body composition methodology has grown over the past decades. Anthropometrics is the scientific study of measurements of the human body. Estimates of body energy stores can be estimated by measurement of body compartments. Anthropometrics is used as a bedside method of estimating body fat and protein stores using two bedside instruments: a Lange caliper and tape measure (Fig. 1). These tools allow direct linear measurement of body fat and protein stores. The measurements obtained from anthropometrics are compared with reference study normals and then followed in the same patient over time. A drawback of anthropometrics is its reliance on age-, sex-, and race-matched reference values. Additionally, because muscle mass is somewhat dependent on exercise, bedridden patients can have decreased muscle mass without a corresponding reduction in body protein stores.

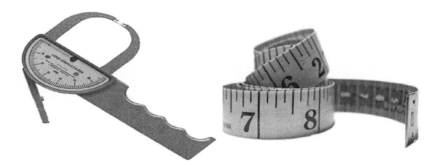

Fig. 1. Bedside anthropometric tools: Lange calipers and tape measure.

Inaccurate measurements of body protein and fat stores using anthropometric methods are common in certain patient populations. For example, critically ill patients and patients with liver disease or renal disease often present with total body water increase and significant edema. Furthermore, there is significant variance among clinicians measuring anthropometrics in the same patient, reported to range from 5% to 23% [2].

The measurement of the triceps skinfold with a Lange caliper has been recognized as an indirect marker of body fat stores. Body fat stores can be tracked over time to provide an estimate of the chronicity of a weight loss process. The measurement of the circumference of the midpoint of the upper arm using a tape measure or midarm muscle circumference has also been recognized as an indirect marker of body protein stores [19]. The minimum midarm muscle circumference known to be compatible with survival is between 900 and 1200 mm^2 [9], Lastly, a widely accepted definition of malnutrition is body mass index (BMI) less than 20 kg/m^2 and midarm muscle circumference less than the fifteenth percentile.

PLASMA PROTEINS

Plasma proteins, such as albumin, prealbumin, transferrin, ferritin, and retinol-binding protein, have all been used as nutritional markers (Table 1). In the past 30 years, there have been over 20,000 citations on albumin [20]. One third of albumin is maintained in the intravascular compartment and two thirds in the extravascular compartment. Serum albumin levels are a representation of both liver albumin synthesis and albumin degradation or losses. The serum concentrations of albumin and other plasma proteins are affected by a patient's total body water status, liver function, and renal losses. Although purported as reliable nutritional markers, serum proteins are best considered markers of a patient's overall health status rather than a true nutritional marker. Reinhardt and associates [21] demonstrated a linear correlation between the degree of hypoalbuminemia and the 30-day mortality rate in hospitalized patients. An increase in hospital mortality was also seen in geriatric patients with low serum albumins undergoing cardiovascular surgery [22]. Careful studies have shown serum albumin to be a less sensitive indicator of a patient's nutritional status as compared with clinical judgment based on a patient's medical history and physical examination [23].

Table 1	
Serum protein half-lives	
Protein	Half-life
Albumin	18 d
Transferrin	8 d
Prealbumin	2–3 d
Retinol-binding protein	2 d
Ferritin	30 h

DIRECT MEASUREMENTS OF BODY PHYSIOLOGIC FUNCTION

Direct measurements of body functions can be used as markers of the degree and significance of malnutrition. For example, skeletal muscle function can be rapidly affected by malnutrition regardless of other major disease processes, such as sepsis, trauma, or renal failure [24].

In critically ill patients who are not able to follow commands, bedside muscle function can still be tested. Stimulation of the ulnar nerve at the wrist with measurement of contraction of the abductor pollicus longus has been standardized [25]. Force-frequency curves have been recorded in controls and standardized.

In the patient who is able to follow commands, muscle mass can be determined from handgrip strength by the use of a bedside tool known as a "handgrip dynamometer" (Fig. 2). Hospitalized patients with poor grip strength have been shown to have an increase in hospital length of stay, reduced ability to return home, and increased mortality [26].

CLINICAL SCORING SYSTEMS

Overall nutritional status is best estimated through the evaluation of a combination of variables including historical, physical, and laboratory data. Although many such tools exist, not all are equally validated. Additionally, concern remains regarding the degree of correlation between different screening tools currently in use. To complicate matters further, despite using different data, various scoring systems are discussed more or less interchangeably when mentioned in the literature. Other limitations of these tools include lack of generalizability (ie, developed for specific patient populations); complex and time-consuming methodology; requirement for specialists (eg, dietitians) to complete the tool scoring; and usage of parameters that are not routinely or readily available [27].

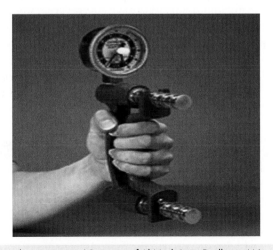

Fig. 2. Handgrip dynamometer. (*Courtesy of* AliMed, Inc., Dedham, MA; with permission.)

Even though it is evident that nutritional assessment using clinical scoring systems is imperfect, they remain the best nutrition assessment tool available to clinicians. There are efforts underway to evaluate better the efficacy of the current nutrition assessment tools available [28,29]. Clinical correlation does exist between some screening tools and more complex and sophisticated techniques assessing body composition and function [29,30]. The following clinical scoring systems incorporate the most widely used and accepted scoring systems available today.

Subjective Global Assessment

The subjective global assessment (SGA) is a tool used to recognize and document nutritional problems in patients. It includes a dietary and medical history, a functional assessment, and a physical examination (Fig. 3) [31]. Fiaccadori and colleagues [32] validated the SGA system by both anthropometry and serum albumin measurements and predicted morbidity and mortality in patients with acute renal failure. More recently, the SGA has been shown to have good correlation with the nutrition risk index (NRI) and other anthropometric and laboratory data in hospitalized patients [29]. Additionally, nutritional status or risk as defined by the SGA and the malnutrition universal screening tool, nutrition risk score (NRS), and NRI were shown to correlate significantly with length of hospital stay [33].

SGA (A) level is designated as a minimal change in food intake, a minimal change in body function, and a steady body weight. SGA (B) level consists of clear evidence of decreased food intake with some physiologic functional changes, but no significant change in body weight. SGA (C) level consists of a significant decrease in body weight and food intake along with a reduction in physiologic function. In a study by Hasse and colleagues [34], the SGA scoring system was shown accurately to detect the nutritional status in liver transplant patients with a significant degree of intraobserver agreement. Detsky and colleagues [31] demonstrated that the SGA model could be easily taught to practitioners with good reproducibility from clinician to clinician.

In should be noted, however, that despite its ability accurately to assess one's nutritional state, critics have found the SGA to be both time consuming and complex in methodology [27]. Additionally, the requirement for patients subjectively to recall data inevitably leads to some degree of inaccuracy.

Mini Nutritional Assessment

The mini nutritional assessment is a rapid and reliable tool for evaluating the nutritional status of the elderly (Fig. 4). It is composed of 18 items and takes approximately 15 minutes to complete [35]. The assessment includes an evaluation of a patient's health, mobility, diet, anthropometrics, and a subject self-assessment. A developmental study demonstrated that the mini nutritional assessment was as accurate as a nutrition assessment by two expert nutrition physicians [35]. A second validation study determined that the mini nutritional assessment was as accurate as a physician-performed nutrition assessment combined with the addition

Scored Patient-Generated Subjective Global Assessment (PG-SGA)

Patient ID Information

History (Boxes 1-4 are designed to be completed by the patient.)

1. Weight *(See Worksheet 1)*

In summary of my current and recent weight:

I currently weigh about _____ pounds
I am about _____ feet _____ tall

One month ago I weighed about _____ pounds
Six months ago I weighed about _____ pounds

During the past two weeks my weight has:
☐ decreased (1) ☐ not changed (0) ☐ increased (0)

Box 1 ☐

2. Food Intake: As compared to my normal intake, I would rate my food intake during the past month as:
☐ unchanged (0)
☐ more than usual (0)
☐ less than usual (1)
I am now taking:
☐ *normal food* but less than normal amount (1)
☐ little solid food (2)
☐ only liquids (3)
☐ only nutritonal supplements (3)
☐ very little of anything (4)
☐ only tube feedings or only nutrition by vein (0)

Box 2 ☐

3. Symptoms: I have had the following problems that have kept me from eating enough during the past two weeks (check all that apply):
☐ no problems eating (0)
☐ no appetite, just did not feel like eating (3)
☐ nausea (1)   ☐ vomiting (3)
☐ constipation (1)   ☐ diarrhea (3)
☐ mouth sores (2)   ☐ dry mouth (1)
☐ things taste funny or have no taste (1) ☐ smells bother me (1)
☐ problems swallowing (2)   ☐ feel full quickly (1)
☐ pain; where? (3) _____
☐ other** (1) _____
** Examples: depression, money, or dental problems

Box 3 ☐

4. Activities and Function: Over the past month, I would generally rate my activity as:
☐ normal with no limitations (0)
☐ not my normal self, but able to be up and about with fairly normal activities (1)
☐ not feeling up to most things, but in bed or chair less than half the day (2)
☐ able to do little activity and spend most of the day in bed or chair (3)
☐ pretty much bedridden, rarely out of bed (3)

Box 4 ☐

Additive Score of the Boxes 1-4 ☐ A

The remainder of this form will be completed by your doctor, nurse, or therapist. Thank you.

5. Disease and its relation to nutritional requirements *(See Worksheet 2)*

All relevant diagnoses (specify) _____
Primary disease stage (circle if known or appropriate)   I   II   III   IV   Other _____
Age _____

Numerical score from Worksheet 2 ☐ B

6. Metabolic Demand *(See Worksheet 3)*

Numerical score from Worksheet 3 ☐ C

7. Physical *(See Worksheet 4)*

Numerical score from Worksheet 4 ☐ D

Global Assessment *(See Worksheet 5)*
☐ Well-nourished or anabolic (SGA-A)
☐ Moderate or suspected malnutrition (SGA-B)
☐ Severely malnourished (SGA-C)

Total PG-SGA score
(Total numerical score of A+B+C+D above) ☐
(See triage recommendations below)

Clinician Signature _____ RD RN PA MD DO Other __ Date _____

Nutritional Triage Recommendations: Additive score is used to define specific nutritional interventions including patient & family education, symptom management including pharmacologic intervention, and appropriate nutrient intervention (food, nutritional supplements, enteral, or parenteral triage). First line nutrition intervention includes optimal symptom management.

0-1	No intervention required at this time. Re-assessment on routine and regular basis during treatment.
2-3	Patient & family education by dietitian, nurse, or other clinician with pharmacologic intervention as indicated by symptom survey (Box 3) and laboratory values as appropriate.
4-8	Requires intervention by dietitian, in conjunction with nurse or physician as indicated by symptoms survey (Box 3).
≥ 9	Indicates a critical need for improved symptom management and/or nutrient intervention options.

© FD Ottery, 2001

Fig. 3. Subjective global analysis. (*Courtesy of* Faith D. Ottery, MD, Philadelphia, PA; with permission.)

of biochemical markers [36]. Most recently, the mini nutritional assessment has been shown to be a good predictor of nutritional imbalance in institutionalized patients [37]. A mini nutritional assessment score of more than 24 indicates no nutritional risk, whereas a score of 17 to 23 indicates a potential risk of malnutrition and a score less than 17 indicates definitive malnutrition.

MINI NUTRITIONAL ASSESSMENT
MNA®

ID# _____

Last Name: _____ First Name: _____ M.I. ____ Sex: ____ Date: _____

Age: ____ Weight, kg: _____ Height, cm: _____ Knee Height, cm: _____

Complete the form by writing the numbers in the boxes. Add the numbers in the boxes and compare the total assessment to the Malnutrition Indicator Score.

ANTHROPOMETRIC ASSESSMENT

	Points
1. Body Mass Index (BMI) (weight in kg) / (height in m)² a. BMI < 19 = 0 points b. BMI 19 to < 21 = 1 point c. BMI 21 to < 23 = 2 points d. BMI ≥ 23 = 3 points	☐
2. Mid-arm circumference (MAC) in cm a. MAC < 21 = 0.0 points b. MAC 21 ≤ 22 = 0.5 points c. MAC > 22 = 1.0 points	☐.☐
3. Calf circumference (CC) in cm a. CC < 31 = 0 points b. CC ≥ 31 = 1 point	☐
4. Weight loss during last 3 months a. weight loss greater than 3kg (6.6 lbs) = 0 points b. does not know = 1 point c. weight loss between 1 and 3 kg (2.2 and 6.6 lbs) = 2 points d. no weight loss = 3 points	☐

GENERAL ASSESSMENT

5. Lives independently (not in a nursing home or hospital) a. no = 0 points b. yes = 1 point	☐
6. Takes more than 3 prescription drugs per day a. yes = 0 points b. no = 1 point	☐
7. Has suffered psychological stress or acute disease in the past 3 months a. yes = 0 points b. no = 2 points	☐
8. Mobility a. bed or chair bound = 0 points b. able to get out of bed/chair but does not go out = 1 point c. goes out = 2 points	☐
9. Neuropsychological problems a. severe dementia or depression = 0 points b. mild dementia = 1 point c. no psychological problems = 2 points	☐
10. Pressure sores or skin ulcers a. yes = 0 points b. no = 1 point	☐

DIETARY ASSESSMENT

11. How many full meals does the patient eat daily? a. 1 meal = 0 points b. 2 meals = 1 point c. 3 meals = 2 points	☐

Ref.: Guigoz Y, Vellas B and Garry PJ. 1994. Mini Nutritional Assessment: A practical assessment tool for grading the nutritional state of elderly patients. Facts and Research in Gerontology. Supplement #2: 15-59.

©1994 Nestec Ltd (Nestlé Research Center)/Nestlé Clinical Nutrition

	Points
12. Selected consumption markers for protein intake • At least one serving of dairy products (milk, cheese, yogurt) per day? yes ☐ no ☐ • Two or more servings of legumes or eggs per week? yes ☐ no ☐ • Meat, fish or poultry every day? yes ☐ no ☐ a. if 0 or 1 yes = 0.0 points b. if 2 yes = 0.5 points c. if 3 yes = 1.0 points	☐.☐
13. Consumes two or more servings of fruits or vegetables per day? a. no = 0 points b. yes = 1 point	☐
14. Has food intake declined over the past three months due to loss of appetite, digestive problems, chewing or swallowing difficulties? a. severe loss of appetite = 0 points b. moderate loss of appetite = 1 point c. no loss of appetite = 2 points	☐
15. How much fluid (water, juice, coffee, tea, milk,...) is consumed per day? (1 cup = 8 oz.) a. less than 3 cups = 0.0 points b. 3 to 5 cups = 0.5 points c. more than 5 cups = 1.0 points	☐.☐
16. Mode of feeding a. Unable to eat without assistance = 0 points b. self-fed with some difficulty = 1 point c. self-fed without any problem = 2 points	☐

SELF ASSESSMENT

17. Do they view themselves as having nutritional problems? a. major malnutrition = 0 points b. does not know or moderate malnutrition = 1 point c. no nutritional problem = 2 points	☐
18. In comparison with other people of the same age, how do they consider their health status? a. not as good = 0.0 points b. does not know = 0.5 points c. as good = 1.0 points d. better = 2.0 points	☐.☐

ASSESSMENT TOTAL (max. 30 points): ☐☐.☐

MALNUTRITION INDICATOR SCORE		
≥ 24 points	well-nourished	☐
17 to 23.5 points	at risk of malnutrition	☐
< 17 points	malnourished	☐

Fig. 4. Mini nutritional assessment. (*Courtesy of* the Nestle Nutrition Institute, Glendale, CA; with permission. ©1994 Nestec Ltd.)

Nutrition Risk Score

The NRS was developed in 1992 to assess a patient's nutritional risk at hospital admission [38]. The NRS contains variables of weight loss, BMI, food intake, and physiologic stress (Box 1). The NRS is obtained on hospital admission and reassessed weekly. In one validation study, the NRS correlated well with the

Box 1: Nutrition risk score

NUTRITION RISK SCORE

Patient's Name: Ward:

Date of Birth: Date:

Weight: Height/Length:

Please circle relevant score. Only select **one** score from each section.

1.	PEDIATRICS (0-17 years) PRESENT WEIGHT	SCORE	ADULTS (≥ 18 years) WEIGHT LOSS IN LAST 3 MONTHS (Unintentional)	SCORE
	Expected weight for length	0	No weight loss	0
	90-99% of expected weight for length	2	0-3 kg weight loss	1
	80-89% of expected weight for length	4	>3-6 kg weight loss	2
	≤79% of expected weight for length	6	6 kg or more	3

			BMI (Body Mass Index)	
			20 or more	0
2.	Omit Question 2		18 or 19	1
	For Pediatrics		15-17	2
			Less than 15	3

3. APPETITE

- Good appetite, manages most of 3 meals/day (or equivalent) 0
- Poor appetite, poor intake – leaving > half of meals provided (or equivalent) 2
- Appetite nil or virtually nil, unable to eat, NBM (for > 4 meals) 3

4. ABILITY TO EAT/RETAIN FOOD

- No difficulties eating, able to eat independently. 0
- No diarrhea or vomiting.

- Problems handling food, e.g., needs special cutlery. 1
  Vomiting/frequent regurgitation, or diarrhea).

- Difficulty swallowing, requiring modified consistency. 2
  Problems with dentures, affecting food intake. Problems with chewing, affecting food intake.
  Slow to feed. Moderate vomiting and/or diarrhea (1-2/day for children).
  Needs help with feeding (e.g. physical handicap).

- Unable to take food orally. Unable to swallow (complete dysphagia). 3
  Severe vomiting and/or diarrhea (>2/day for children). Malabsorption.

5. STRESS FACTOR

- **No Stress Factor:** (Includes admission for investigation only). 0

- **Mild**   Minor surgery. Minor infection. 1

- **Moderate**   Chronic disease. Major Surgery. Infections. 2
  Fractures. Pressure sores/ulcers. CVA.
  Inflammatory bowel disease. Other gastrointestinal disease.

- **Severe**   Multiple injuries. Multiple fractures/burns. 3
  Multiple deep pressure sores/ulcers. Severe sepsis.
  Carcinoma/malignant disease.

TOTAL_____

Adapted from Reilly HM, Martineau JK, Moran A, et al. Nutritional screening: evaluation and implementation of a simple nutrition risk score. Clinical Nutrition 1995;14:271; with permission.

16-item NRI [39]. There was little variance in scores between dietitians or between dietitians and nurses when evaluating the same patient. The NRS has been adopted as the national nutrition assessment standard in the United Kingdom [40].

Nutritional Risk Index

The NRI was developed by the Veteran's Affairs Total Parenteral Nutrition group [41] in 1991 for use in the evaluation of the efficacy of perioperative total parenteral nutrition in patients undergoing thoracic or abdominal surgery. The NRI relies on serum albumin measurements and differences in a patient's current and previous body weight (Box 2). It has been used in clinical studies with reasonable reliability [42]. In a mixed group of Irish medical and surgical patients, the NRI identified patients with a prolonged length of stay in the hospital, or a reduced ability to return home, and a higher patient mortality [17].

Geriatric Nutritional Risk Index

The geriatric nutrition risk index (GNRI) is an adaptation to the NRI. The GNRI is specifically designed to predict the risk of morbidity and mortality in hospitalized elderly patients (Box 3) [43]. Because the normal weight of elderly patients is often difficult to determine, this tool substitutes "ideal weight" in place of "usual weight" used by the NRI. The GNRI is calculated using a special formula incorporating both serum albumin and weight loss. Ideal body weight is calculated using the Lorentz formula based on the patient's height and gender [43]. After determining the GNRI score, patients are categorized into four grades of nutrition-related risk: (1) major, (2) moderate, (3) low, and (4) no risk. Finally, the GNRI scores are correlated with a severity score that takes into account nutritional status–related complications.

The GNRI is not an index of malnutrition, but rather a nutrition-related risk index. Two independent predictors of mortality in the elderly, weight loss and serum albumin, are used to calculate the GNRI. Interestingly, studies have shown that by measuring these two variables, the GNRI is a more reliable prognostic indicator of morbidity and mortality in hospitalized elderly patients than are other techniques using albumin or BMI alone [44].

Box 2: Nutritional risk index

$$NRI = 1.519 \times \text{serum albumin (g/L)} + 0.417 \times (\text{current weight/usual weight}) \times 100$$

No nutrition risk: NRI > 100
Borderline nutrition risk: NRI > 97.5
Mild nutrition risk: NRI 83.5–97.5
Severe nutrition risk: NRI < 83.5

Box 3: Geriatric nutrition risk index

$$GNRI = [1.489 \times albumin\ (g/L)] + [41.7 \times (weight/WLo)]$$

The GNRI results from replacement of ideal weight in the NRI formula by usual weight as calculated from the Lorentz formula (WLo). Four grades of nutrition-related risk: major risk (GNRI <82); moderate risk (GNRI 82–91); low risk (GNRI 92 to ≤98); and no risk (GNRI >98).

Malnutrition Universal Screening Tool

The malnutrition universal screening tool is designed to detect protein-energy malnutrition and those individuals at risk of developing malnutrition by using three independent criteria: (1) current weight status, (2) unintentional weight loss, and (3) acute disease effect [45]. The patient's current body weight is determined by calculating BMI (kilograms per square meter). Weight loss (over past 3–6 months) is determined by looking at the individual's medical record. An acute disease factor is then included if the patient is currently affected by a pathophysiologic condition and there has been no nutritional intake for more than 5 days. A total score is calculated, placing the patients in a low-, medium-, or high-risk category for malnutrition (Box 4). A major advantage of this screening tool is its applicability to adults of all ages across all health care settings. Additionally, this method provides the user with management guidelines once an overall risk score has been determined. Studies have shown that malnutrition universal screening tool is quick and easy to use and has good concurrent validity with most other nutrition assessment tools tested [45].

Instant Nutritional Assessment

The most rapid and simplest measure of nutritional status is the instant nutritional assessment (Table 2). A serum albumin and the total lymphocyte count form the basis of this evaluation [46]. Significant correlations between depressed levels of these parameters and morbidity and mortality have been previously noted. Not surprisingly, abnormalities of these same parameters are even more significant in critically ill patients [47]. Although not designed to replace more extensive assessment measures, this technique allows for quick identification and early intervention in those individuals in greatest danger of developing complications of malnutrition. Additionally, some studies have suggested that serum albumin levels can be used as markers of length of stay in hospitalized patients [48]. The lower the serum albumin, the longer the lengths of hospital stay.

OTHER BEDSIDE TECHNOLOGIES

Bioelectric Impedence

Bioelectric impedence (BIA) is a noninvasive method to determine body composition. It is based on the resistance of a fat-free mass to administration of

Box 4: Malnutrition universal screening tool (MUST)

BMI score	Weight loss score (unplanned weight loss in 3–6 months)	Acute disease effect
BMI >20 (>30 obese) = 0	Wt loss <5% = 0	Add a score of 2 if there
BMI 18.5–20 = 1	Wt loss 5%–10% = 1	has been or is likely to
BMI <18.5 = 2	Wt loss >10% = 2	be no nutritional intake For >5 days

Add all scores
↓

Overall risk of malnutrition and management guidelines

0 Low risk Routine clinical care	1 Medium risk Observe	≥2 High risk Treat
Repeat screening Hospital: Weekly Care homes: Monthly Community: annually for special groups (>75 y)	Document dietary intake for third if subject in hospital or care home If improved or adequate intake, little clinical concern; if no Improvement, clinical concern: Follow local policy Repeat screening Hospital: weekly Care home: at least monthly Community: at least every 2–3 months	Refer to dietitian, nutrition support team, or implement local policy Improve and increase overall nutritional intake Monitor and review care plan Hospital: weekly Care home: monthly Community: month

a high-frequency, alternating, low-amplitude (50 kHz) electrical current. It is inexpensive, easy to perform, and reproducible [49]. BIA has been validated against both underwater weighing and isotope dilution, two bench research gold standards used for determining body composition [50]. One drawback of BIA is its assumption of a normal body water status being approximately

Table 2
Instant nutritional assessment parameters

Parameter		Abnormal if
Serum albumin	– – – – – – →	<3.5 g%
Total lymphocyte count	– – – – – – →	<1500/mm^3

72% to 74%. In clinical cases of body edema or body dehydration, BIA may be inaccurate [51]. A study in patients with renal failure found BIA to be inaccurate secondary to abnormal volume status [52]. In contrast, BIA was found to be accurate in determining muscle mass in a group of patients with cystic fibrosis when compared with isotope dilution methods [53].

RESEARCH LABORATORY METHODS OF NUTRITIONAL ASSESSMENT

Because of their ease of use, practicality, and cost effectiveness, bedside tools to assess body composition are the most widely used. A basic understanding of the underlying principles used to determine body makeup is crucial to appreciate fully the nature of these devices. The following describes both age-old gold standards against which other tests are compared, and more newly developed laboratory methods of nutritional assessment [7].

Hydrodensitometry

For years, hydrodensitometry, or underwater weighing, has been regarded as a gold standard for body composition analysis. This laboratory technique is based on Archimedes' principle, which states that the volume of an object submerged in water is equal to the volume of water the object displaces. Additionally, it assumes that the density and specific gravity of lean tissue (muscle and bone) is greater than that of fat tissue. Lean tissue sinks and fat tissue floats.

To perform hydrodensitometry the subject is first placed in a temperature-regulated tank or pool and submerged. After complete exhalation, the subject is weighed underwater on a suspended chair or frame for approximately 10 to 15 seconds. Archimedes' principle is applied by comparing the mass of the subject in air with the mass of the subject in water. Of note, corrections for the density of water corresponding to the water temperature are made. Because body density is simply a ratio of body mass to body volume, it can easily be calculated from these measurements. Once body density is known, percent body fat can be easily estimated by one of two different equations [54]. Because the density of fat-free mass is known to differ with age, gender, ethnicity, level of body fitness, and activity level, population-specific formulas for the conversion of body density to percent body fat have been developed [55]. Overall test-retest reliability for hydrodensitometry has been reported to be very good ($r = .99$) [56].

Whole-Body Counting and Nuclear Activation

Shielded whole-body counters can measure the radiographic decay of various, naturally occurring minerals and substances, such as ^{40}K [57]. The ^{40}K count can be used to determine total body potassium. Total body potassium can then be used to calculate body cell mass and fat-free mass. Whole-body counting and nuclear activation is considered a gold standard for determining body composition.

Dual Energy X-ray Absorptiometry

Dual energy x-ray absorptiometry was originally designed for the determination of bone density and mass. It was subsequently found to be effective for quantifying fat and muscle mass of the human body. A typical scan takes approximately 30 minutes and exposes the patient to 1 mrad of radiation (Fig. 5) [57]. Dual energy x-ray absorptiometry has been documented to be a more sensitive determinant of fat-free mass as compared with anthropometric measurements of triceps skinfold thickness measurements or BIA [58].

CT and MRI

CT and MRI are imaging modalities capable of measuring body composition including muscle mass and visceral tissue [57]. CT measures radiographic scatter of tissue based on density, whereas MRI measures nuclear relaxation times from the nuclei of atoms within a magnetic field.

Near-Infrared Interactance

Near-infrared interactance, although originally designed by the agriculture industry to assess the composition of grains and seeds, is used today by nutritionists and exercise scientists alike to provide estimates of body fat in patients and athletes [59]. This field technique operates on the principles of light absorption and reflection. By comparing the light absorption of two different wavelengths in combination with anthropometric data (weight and height), and the use of appropriate regression equations, body fat is estimated.

Some of the main advantages of this device are its speed, ease of use, high degree of portability, and low cost. The test is performed in a matter of minutes (~3 minutes) by placing an infrared probe over the biceps muscle and measuring optical densities of the underlying tissue. To standardize testing, two specific wavelengths based on the absorption of fat and water are used and the instrument is calibrated by measuring a signal from a reference block made of Teflon [60]. Additionally, specific equations catered to individual patient populations can be used to help reduce variance [61].

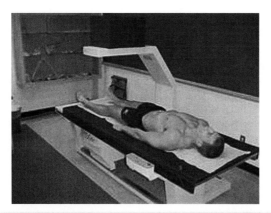

Fig. 5. DEXA scanner. (*Courtesy of* Wichita State University, Department of Kinesiology and Sports Studies, Wichita, KS; with permission.)

Despite the appeal of this method, controversy exists regarding its validity. Although some studies have claimed good reliability and validity in young athletes, others have shown poor correlation in specific patient populations, such as the obese [54]. Research consistently shows that near-infrared interactance underestimates body fat, and this error is accentuated with increasing body fatness [62].

CALORIMETRY IN NUTRITION

The roots of nutrition science are based on the principles of calorimetry, or heat measurement. Although direct calorimetry, or the measure of total heat loss from the body, was first studied and served as the gold standard for studying human metabolism, it is indirect calorimetry (IC), or the measure of total energy production by the body, that is used more extensively today.

Indirect Calorimetry

IC is able to quantify energy expenditure based on the physiologic relationship between oxygen intake and carbon dioxide release and heat and energy production. More simply, IC measures O_2 consumption and CO_2 production (Fig. 6) [63]. Calculation of the REE is the end result of IC and is estimated to be approximately 10% greater than the basal energy expenditure (BEE), which can only be measured in deep sleep [64,65]. REE is thought to account for 75% to 90% of total energy expenditure. The remainder of total energy expenditure is made up of thermogenesis resulting from nutritional intake (diet-induced thermogenesis); environment (shivering and nonshivering thermogenesis); and physical activity [66]. It should be noted that IC is unable to differentiate nonprotein calories from total calories. Although protein requirements are not measured by IC, they can be easily determined by several different methods (see later).

In addition to determining the 24-hour caloric requirements as reflected by the REE, IC also provides the investigator with a measure of substrate use

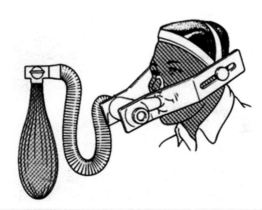

Fig. 6. Indirect calorimetry. (*Courtesy of* the Nestle Nutrition Institute, Glendale, CA, with permission. © 1994 Nestec Ltd.)

by calculation of the respiratory quotient (RQ) [66]. Defined by the ratio VCO_2/VO_2, the RQ is purported to be a measurement of substrate use in vivo. An RQ greater than 1 is generally considered to be consistent with overfeeding, and an RQ less than 0.80 is considered to be consistent with underfeeding. Notably, there is an associated physiologic range for the RQ (0.67–1.3), and values outside this range can only be generated by error. In practice, these extreme values are used as a determinant of test validity [66–68].

The necessary duration of IC to provide accurate and valid results is not known. At present, most procedures continue for predetermined intervals or until a steady state is reached [69]. Before testing, patients should be maintained on bed rest for 30 minutes and kept in a thermoneutral environment [70]. Patients on oral diets should fast overnight, whereas patients on total parenteral nutrition or enteral tube feeds should be placed on a continuous infusion rate up until the point of testing. Analgesics and anxiolytics should be administered appropriately if clinically required [69].

The two instruments currently available for conducting IC include the "classic" metabolic cart and hand-held instruments (Fig. 7) [71]. The classic metabolic cart measures both oxygen consumption and carbon dioxide production and automatically calculates EE and the RQ. Most predictive calorie equations in use today were derived from the use of this device. Unfortunately, classic carts are expensive; difficult to mobilize and calibrate; and require additional staffing (ie, respiratory therapists) to perform the testing.

Recently, small hand-held IC devices have been developed. These devices calculate REE by measuring only oxygen consumption; no RQ is determined [71]. So far, these devices have only been validated in healthy individuals. Conversely, these hand-held devices are highly portable, self-calibrating, require minimal operator training, and cost considerably less than classic carts. Nutrition enthusiasts are optimistic that the reduced cost and ease of operation of these new devices will make IC more commonplace in the monitoring of energy metabolism in the hospital and outpatient setting.

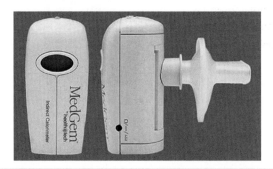

Fig. 7. MEDGEM hand-held oximeter for basal energy assessment. (*Courtesy of* Microlife USA, Dunedin, FL; with permission.)

Whole-Room Calorimetry

The most precise measurements of energy expenditure are obtained through the practice of whole-room indirect calorimetry. This technique provides extremely accurate measurements (>98%) of oxygen consumption and carbon dioxide production over long periods of time in individuals moving freely about a room [72]. Whole-room calorimetry uses the same principles and equations as IC and helps bridge the gap between laboratory research and the free living environment. Whereas IC uses the metabolic cart to measure energy expenditure, whole-room indirect calorimetry measures changes in oxygen and carbon dioxide inside an airtight room to obtain the same result. Whole-room indirect calorimetry is not only able to measure the subject's energy expenditure, but also his or her usage of energy fuels including fats, protein, and carbohydrate. The individual being studied is held in a closed room and gas exchange is measured through analyzers attached to the unit. Subjects are instructed to follow strict study protocols, dividing their time between reading, sleeping, sitting, and exercising over a period of 24 to 72 hours. Although precise, this technique of measuring energy expenditure is not practical, considering few individuals are willing to submit themselves to such a lengthy test.

NUTRITIONAL INTERVENTION

Calorie-Protein-Water Requirements

After determination of an individual's nutritional status or degree of malnutrition, appropriate intervention can be initiated. Nutritional intervention can include dietary advice, enteral supplementation, appetite stimulation, enteral tube feeding, and parenteral nutrition. Specialized nutritional intervention may include the use of anabolic agents, immune-stimulating enteral formulations, medium-chain triglycerides, probiotics, or other novel approaches. To begin intervention, clinicians must first determine the patient's caloric, protein, and water requirements.

Calorie Needs

There are multiple formulations used to determine a patient's caloric needs. The most commonly used formula is the Harris-Benedict [73] equation. This equation estimates a patient's BEE using the following formulas:

$$\text{Men} : 66 + \{13.7 \times \text{weight (kg)}\} + \{5.0 \times \text{height (cm)}\} - \{(6.8 \times \text{age})\}$$
$$= \text{kcal/day}$$
$$\text{Women} : 655 + \{(9.6 \times \text{weight (kg)})\} + \{1.8 \times \text{height (cm)}\} - \{(4.7 \times \text{age})\}$$
$$= \text{kcal/day}$$

One must determine the weight to use in this calculation. If a patent is less than 80% or greater than 120% of their ideal body weight, an adjusted body weight should be calculated. If their body weight is between 80% and

120% of their ideal body weight, their actual body weight is their dosing weight.

$$\text{Ideal body weight for men} = 130 \text{ lb for first 5 ft of height and 3 lb for each additional in;}$$

$$\text{for women} = 120 \text{ lb for first 5 ft of height and 3 lb for each additional in}$$

$$\text{Adjusted body weight (if needed)} = \{(\text{current body weight} - \text{ideal body weight}) \times 25\%\} + \text{ideal body weight}$$

Using the patient's actual body weight or adjusted body weight, the patient's BEE is calculated using the Harris-Benedict equation. The patient's BEE is multiplied by a physiologic stress factor to arrive at their actual daily calorie needs:

Maintenance–mild stress (1–1.2)
Moderate stress (1.3–1.4)
Severe stress (1.5)
BEE × stress factor = daily caloric needs

Protein-Nitrogen Needs

A patient's daily nitrogen balance is a measure of their daily intake of nitrogen minus their daily excretion of nitrogen. The intake is nutritional nitrogen intake and the excretion is measured urinary nitrogen losses plus 2 to 4 g of nitrogen losses through skin and stool. Daily nitrogen balance can be calculated as follows:

Collect 24-hour urinary urea nitrogen and obtain total grams of nitrogen
Add 4 g of nitrogen for insensible losses (stool and skin)
24-hour urinary urea nitrogen + 4 g = daily nitrogen needs to maintain a stable nitrogen balance

Nitrogen balance

A positive nitrogen balance is known as "anabolism" and is important for wound healing, recovery from illness, and growth. A positive nitrogen balance consists of a greater daily nitrogen intake as compared with nitrogen excretion. On the contrary, a negative nitrogen balance is known as "catabolism." This is commonly seen in critically ill patients and is the result of a greater daily nitrogen excretion as compared with nitrogen intake.

Daily nitrogen needs can be converted to daily protein needs by using the following formula:

Total grams in nitrogen × 6.25 = total grams of protein required/day

Table 3
Quick formulas for protein and calorie need

	Protein needs	Calorie needs
Minimal severity of illness	0.8 g/kg/d	20–25 kcal/kg/d
Moderate severity of illness	1.0–1.5 g/kg/d	25–30 kcal/kg/d
Severe severity of Illness	1.5–2.5 g/kg/d	30–35 kcal/kg/d

Quickie Formulas for Protein and Calorie Need

There are more rapid methods available to determine a patient's daily calorie and protein needs (Table 3). These quick formulas have been shown to be reliable in most patients.

Daily Water Needs

Daily water needs for patients are based on maintenance needs plus losses through urine, stool, emesis, and wound output. There are quick methods for determining water needs, however, that are reliable for most patients: 30 mL H_2O/kg body weight/d, or 1 mL H_2O/kcal delivered of tube feeding/day. Add 300 mL for every average degree of centigrade temperature elevation in 24 hours. Patients with significant stool, emesis, wound, or urine output may require more volume. Patients on fluid restriction may require less volume.

SUMMARY

The existence of malnutrition in hospitalized patients is both well documented and alarming. There is currently no universally accepted or validated approach comprehensively to evaluate one's nutritional state. Furthermore, good clinical studies have repeatedly shown that no single body or laboratory measurement is capable of adequately predicting one's nutritional risk. It is important for physicians to have familiarity with both objective and subjective measures of one's basic body needs and functional capacity.

Because of their ability globally to assess nutritional needs, clinical scoring systems have gained popularity in clinical practice. Nevertheless, each has its own limitations, underscoring the importance of the need for further evaluation of the efficacy of these tools [28]. When appropriately used, these tools lead to early identification of at-risk patients and allow for speedy intervention, which not only provides better care but leads to decreased costs [74–76].

Malnutrition is surprisingly pervasive and detrimental. When equipped with the proper clinical tools, however, the physician is more likely to provide safe, efficacious nutritional intervention and ultimately lead to improved clinical outcomes.

References

[1] Butterworth CE. The skeleton in the closet. Nutr Today 1974;1:4–8.
[2] Waitzberg DL, Caiffia WT, Correia MTD. Hospital malnutrition: the Brazilian national survey (IBRANUTR): a study of 4000 patients. Nutrition 2001;17:575–80.

[3] Correia MITD, Waltzberg DL. The impact of malnutrition on morbidity, mortality, length of hospital stay and costs evaluated through a multivariate model analysis. Nutrition 2003; 22:235-9.

[4] Windsor JA, Hill GL. Weight loss with physiologic impairment: a basic indicator of surgical risk. Ann Surg 1988;207:290-9.

[5] Jeejeebhoy KN, Detsky AS, Baker JP. Assessment of nutritional status. JPEN J Parenter Enteral Nutr 1990;14:193S-9S.

[6] Arora NS, Rochester DF. Effect of body weight and muscularity on human diaphragm muscle mass, thickness and area. J Appl Physiol 1992;52:64-70.

[7] Hill GL, Jonathan E. Rhoads lecture. Body composition research: implications for the practice of clinical nutrition. JPEN J Parenter Enteral Nutr 1992;16:197-218.

[8] Rogers RM, Donahue M, Constantino J. Physiologic effects of oral supplementation feeding in patients with chronic obstructive pulmonary disease. Am Rev Respir Dis 1992;146: 1511-7.

[9] Heymsfield SB, McMannus C, Stevens V, et al. Muscle mass: reliable indicator of protein-energy malnutrition severity and outcome. Am J Clin Nutr 1982;35:1192-9.

[10] Jones JM. The methodology of nutritional screening and assessment tools. J Hum Nutr Diet 2002;15:59-71.

[11] Simmons SF, Reuben D. National intake monitoring for nursing home residents: a comparison of staff documentation, direct observation and photography models. J Am Geriatr Soc 2000;48:209-13.

[12] Leonard Jones JE, Arrowsmith H, Davidons C, et al. Screening by nurses and junior doctors to direct malnutrition when patients are first assessed in the hospital. Clin Nutr 1995;14: 336-40.

[13] Schnedier SM, Hebuterne X. Use of nutritional scores to predict clinical outcomes in chronic diseases. Nutr Rev 2000;1:31-8.

[14] Green SM, Watson R. Nutrition screening and assessment for use by nurses: literature review. J Adv Nurs 2005;50:69-83.

[15] Morgan DB, Hill GL, Baker JP. The assessment of weight loss from a single measurement of body weight: problems and limitations. Am J Clin Nutr 1980;33:2101-10.

[16] Blackburn GL, Bistrian BR, Maini BS, et al. Nutritional and metabolic assessment of the hospitalized patient. JPEN J Parenter Enteral Nutr 1977;1:11-22.

[17] Corish CA. Pre-operative nutritional assessment. Proc Nutr Soc 1999;58:821-9.

[18] Campbell SE, Avenell A, Walker AE. Assessment of nutritional status in hospital in-patients. QJM 2002;95:63-7.

[19] Hall JCH, O'Quigley J, Giles GR, et al. Upper limb anthropometry: the value of measurement variance studies. Am J Clin Nutr 1980;33:1846-8.

[20] Jeejeebuoy KN. Nutritional assessment. Gastroenterol Clin North Am 1998;27: 347-69.

[21] Reinhardt GF, Myscofski RD, Wilkens D, et al. Incidence and mortality of hypoalbuminemic patients in hospitalized veterans. JPEN J Parenter Enteral Nutr 1980;4:357-9.

[22] Redy MY, Ryan T, Starr NJ. Perioperative determinants of morbidity and mortality in elderly patients undergoing cardiac surgery. Crit Care Med 1996;26:196-7.

[23] Klein S. The myth of serum albumin as a measure of nutritional status. Gastroenterology 1990;99:1845-50.

[24] Brough W, Horne G, Blount A, et al. Effects of nutrient intake, surgery, sepsis and long-term administration of steroids on muscle function. BMJ 1986;293:983-8.

[25] Menton PA. Voluntary strength and disease. J Physiol 1954;123:533-64.

[26] Webb AR, Newman LA, Taylor M, et al. Handgrip dynamometry as a predictor of postoperative complications reappraisal using age standardized grip strengths. JPEN J Parenter Enteral Nutr 1989;13:30-3.

[27] Ferguson M, Capra S, Bauer J, et al. Development of valid and reliable malnutrition screening tool for adult acute hospital patients. Nutrition 1999;15:458-64.

[28] Corish CA, Flood P, Kennedy NP. Comparison of nutritional risk screening tools in patients on admission to hospital. J Hum Nutr Diet 2004;17:133–9, 141–3.
[29] Sungurtekin H, Sungurtekin U, Hanci V, et al. Comparison of two nutrition assessment techniques in hospitalized patients. Nutrition 2004;20:428–32.
[30] Baker J, Detsky AS, Wesson DE, et al. Nutritional assessment: a comparison of clinical judgment and objective measurements. N Engl J Med 1982;306:969–72.
[31] Detsky AS, Baker JP, O'Rourke K, et al. What is subjective global assessment of nutritional status. JPEN J Parenter Enteral Nutr 1987;11:8–13.
[32] Fiaccadori E, Lombardi M, Leonardi S, et al. Prevalence and clinical outcome associated with preexisting malnutrition in acute renal failure: a prospective cohort study. J Am Soc Nephrol 1999;10:581–93.
[33] Kyle UG, Kossovsky VL, Pichard C. Comparison of tools for nutritional assessment and screening at hospital admission: a population study. Clin Nutr 2006;25:409–17.
[34] Hasse J, Strong S, Gorman MA. Subjective global assessment: alternative nutrition-assessment technique for liver transplant candidates. Nutrition 1993;9:339–43.
[35] Guigoz Y, Vellas B, Garry PJ. Mini nutritional assessment, a practical assessment tool for grading the nutritional status of elderly patients. Facts Res Gerontol 1994;4(Suppl 2): 15–9.
[36] Katz S, Ford AB, Moskowitz RW, et al. Studies of illness in the aged. The index of ADL: a standardized measure of biological and psychosocial function. JAMA 1963;185: 914–21.
[37] Alves de Rezende CH, Marquez Cunha T, Alvarenga Junior V, et al. Dependence of mininutritional assessment scores with age and some hematological variables in elderly institutionalized patients. Gerontology 2005;5:316–21.
[38] Reilly HM. Screening for nutritional risk. Proc Nutr Soc 1996;55:841–53.
[39] Reilly HM, Martineau JK, Moran A, et al. Nutritional screening: evaluation and implementation of a simple risk score. Clinical Nutrition 1995;14:269–73.
[40] Sizer T, Russell CA, Wood S. Standards and guidelines for nutritional support of patients in a hospital. A report of the BAPEN working group 1996, monograph.
[41] Veterans Affairs Total Parenteral Nutrition Cooperative Study Group. Perioperative total parenteral nutrition in surgical patients. N Engl J Med 1992;325:525–32.
[42] Heslin MJ, Lutkary L, Leung D, et al. A prospective, randomized trial of early enteral feeding after resection of upper gastrointestinal tract malignancies. Ann Surg 1997;226: 567–80.
[43] Pablo AM, Izaga MA, Alday LA. Assessment of nutritional status on hospital admission: nutritional scores. Eur J Clin Nutr 2003;57:824–31.
[44] Boulillanne O, Morineau G, Dupont C, et al. Geriatric nutritional index: a new index for evaluating at-risk elderly medical patients. Am J Clin Nutr 2005;82:777–83.
[45] Stratton JS, Hackston A, Longmore D, et al. Malnutrition in hospital outpatients and inpatients: prevalence, concurrent validity, and ease of use of the Malnutrition Universal Screening Tool (MUST) for adults. Br J Nutr 2004;92:799–808.
[46] Guigoz Y, Vellas B, Garry P. Assessing the nutritional status of the elderly: the mini nutritional assessment as part of the geriatric evaluation. Nutr Rev 1996;54:59–65.
[47] Seltzer MH, Bastidas A, Cooper DM, et al. Instant nutritional assessment. JPEN J Parenter Enteral Nutr 1979;3:157–9.
[48] De Luis DA, Izaola O, Cuellar L, et al. Nutritional assessment: predictive variables at hospital admission related with length of stay. Ann Nutr Metab 2006;50:394–8.
[49] Churnla WC, Baumgartner RM. Status of anthropometry and body composition in elderly adults. Clin Nutr 1989;50:1158–65.
[50] Frishano AR. New norms of upper limb fat and muscle areas for assessment of nutritional status. J Physiol 1981;34:2540–7.
[51] Khaled MP, McCutcheon MJ, Reddy S. Electrical impedence is assessing human body composition by the BIA method. Am J Clin Nutr 1988;47:789–92.

[52] Kerr PG, Strauss BJ, Atkins RC. Assessment of nutritional status of dialysis patients. Blood Purif 1996;14:382–7.

[53] Borowitz D, Conboy K. Are bioelectrical impedence measurements valid in patients with cystic fibrosis. J Pediatr Gastroenterol Nutr 1997;18:453–6.

[54] Brodie D, Moscrip V, Hutcheon R. Body composition measurement: a review of hydrodensitometry, anthropometry, and impedance methods. Nutrition 1998;14:296–310.

[55] Heyward VH, Stolarczyk LM. Applied body composition assessment. Champaign (IL): Human Kinetics; 1996.

[56] Ward A, Pollock ML, Jackson AS, et al. A composition of body fat determined by underwater weighing and volume displacement. Am J Physiol 1978;234:E94–6.

[57] Jeejeebhouy KN. Nutritional assessment. Nutrition 2000;16:585–90.

[58] King S, Wilson J, Kotsimbos T, et al. Body composition in adults with cystic fibrosis: comparison of dual-energy x-ray absorptiometry with skinfolds and bioelectrical impedence analysis. Nutrition 2005;21:1087–94.

[59] Norris KH. Instrumental techniques for measuring quality of agricultural crops. In: Lieberman M, editor. Post-harvest physiology and crop preservation. New York: Plenum Publishing Corp; 1983. p. 84–93.

[60] Conway JM, Norris KH, Bodwell CE. A new approach for the estimation of body composition: infrared interactance. Am J Clin Nutr 1984;40:1123–30.

[61] Fornetti WC, Pivarnik JM, Foley JM, et al. Reliability and validity of body composition measures in female athletes. J Appl Physiol 1999;87:1114–22.

[62] Wagner DR, Heyward VH. Techniques of body composition assessment: a review of laboratory and field methods. Res Q Exerc Sport 1999;70:135–49.

[63] Ferrannini E. The theoretical bases of indirect calorimetry: a review. Metabolism 1988;37:287–301.

[64] Feurer ID, Crosby LO, Mullen JL. Measured and predicted energy expenditure in clinically stable patients. Clin Nutr 1984;3:27–34.

[65] Owen OE. Resting metabolic requirements of men and women. Mayo Clin Proc 1988;63:503–10.

[66] McClave SA, Snider HL. Use of indirect calorimetry in nutrition. Nutr Clin Pract 1992;7:207–22.

[67] Branson RD. The measurement of energy expenditure: instrumentation, practical considerations, and clinical application. Respir Care 1990;35:640–59.

[68] McClave SA, Lowen CC, Kebler MJ, et al. Is the respiratory quotient a useful indicator of over or underfeeding? [abstract]. JPEN J Parenter Enteral Nutr 1997;21:S11.

[69] McClave SA, McClain CJ, Snider HL. Should indirect calorimetry be used as part of nutritional assessment? J Clin Gastroenterol 2001;33:14–9.

[70] McClave SA, Spain DA, Skolnick JL, et al. Is achievement of steady state required when performing indirect calorimetry? JPEN J Parenter Enteral Nutr 1999;23:S8–14.

[71] Kalman HE. Monitoring energy metabolism with indirect calorimetry: instruments, interpretation, and clinical application. Nutr Clin Pract 2004;19:447–54.

[72] Sun M, Reed GW, Hill JO. Modification of a whole room indirect calorimeter for measurement of rapid changes in energy expenditure. J Appl Physiol 1994;76:2686–91.

[73] Harris JA, Benedict FG. Standard basal monitoring constants for physiologists and clinicians: a biometric study of basal metabolism in man. Philadelphia: JB Lippincott; 1919.

[74] Kruizenga HM, Van Tulder MW, Siedell JC, et al. Effectiveness and cost-effectiveness of early screening and treatment of malnourished patients. Am J Clin Nutr 2005;82:1082–9.

[75] Brugler L, Stankovic AK, Schlefer M, et al. A simplified nutrition screen for hospitalized patients using readily available laboratory and patient information. Nutrition 2005;21:650–8.

[76] Wu GH, Liu ZH, Zheng LW, et al. Prevalence of malnutrition in general surgical patients: evaluation of nutritional status and prognosis. Chinese Journal of Surgery 2005;43:693–6.

Gastroenterol Clin N Am 36 (2007) 23–46

GASTROENTEROLOGY CLINICS
OF NORTH AMERICA

Complications of Parenteral Nutrition

Andrew Ukleja, MD[a,*], Michelle M. Romano, RD, LD, CNSD[b]

[a]Department of Gastroenterology, Cleveland Clinic Florida, 2950 Cleveland Clinic Boulevard, Weston, FL 33331, USA
[b]Mayo Clinic College of Medicine, 4500 San Pablo Road, Jacksonville, FL 32224, USA

Parenteral nutrition (PN) has been lifesaving therapy for patients with intestinal failure and one of the greatest discoveries of the twenty-first century. The first patient who received PN was discharged home in 1968 [1]. PN allows delivery of essential nutrients and prolongation of life in patients with nonfunctioning intestinal tract. Patients with permanent dysfunction of intestinal tract, such as short-bowel syndrome, severe Crohn's disease, radiation enteritis, or chronic pseudo-obstruction, may require PN for life. Other patients may require PN temporarily for such conditions as malignancy, severe acute pancreatitis, bone marrow transplantation, perioperative period, and enteric fistulas. It is estimated that approximately 40,000 patients receive PN every year [2]. Several complications of PN have been recognized and some of them can be life threatening. Deficiencies of biotin, selenium, and essential fatty acid were discovered early in PN and eliminated. The complications of PN are divided into mechanical, infectious, and metabolic. Mechanical complications are related to insertion and care of the central venous catheter (CVC). Septic complications are the result of catheter-associated infections. Metabolic complications refer to high or low serum levels of any components of PN solution, liver disease, and metabolic bone disease. PN complications are associated with increased mortality and affect the quality of life of PN patients [3].

MECHANICAL AND SEPTIC COMPLICATIONS

Separate from the PN solution, complications can occur centered around the vascular access catheter. These catheters cannulate the subclavian, internal jugular, or antecubital fossa vein. They can be used for short-term (nontunneled) or long-term (tunneled, implanted) vascular access. Maintaining a central line is the key to providing PN. Obtaining central access, site care, and maintaining flow of nutrients through the catheter can provide its own set of complications. Early complications include injury to surrounding structures, such as vascular perforation, hemothorax, pneumothorax, and air embolism. Complications that develop over time include mechanical malfunction, occlusion, or infection.

*Corresponding author. E-mail address: uklejaa@ccf.org (A. Ukleja).

0889-8553/07/$ – see front matter
doi:10.1016/j.gtc.2007.01.009

Central Vascular Access Complications

Complications that occur when placing the vascular access catheter or device can develop immediately, early postprocedure, or delayed postprocedure. Placement methods include percutaneous, cut-down, and tunneled. The complication rate is approximately 7% when image guidance is used [4]. Published rates for individual types of complications are highly dependent of patient selection. Complications that occur early or at the time of procedure are related to injury of surrounding vital structures or malpositioning of the catheter tip. Pneumothorax, arterial puncture, and line malposition occur in 1% to 4% of central line placements. Between approaches to access, some differences were reported. Ruesch and colleagues [5] conducted a review of the internal jugular versus the subclavian approach. The jugular approach was significantly associated with arterial puncture than the subclavian approach (3% versus 0.5%; relative risk [RR] 4.70 [95% confidence interval (CI), 2.05–10.77]). Catheter malposition by the jugular approach, however, was significantly less reported. There was no difference in the incidence of hemothorax or pneumothorax (1.3% versus 1.5%; RR 0.76 [0.43–1.33]). A lower incidence of pneumothorax, but higher incidence of line malposition, has been reported with peripherally inserted central catheter (PICC) lines [6,7]. Femoral catheterization was shown to have similar risk for mechanical complication when compared with the subclavian site in critically ill patients [8]. In patients considered for home PN, the use of image-guided technology (ultrasound, fluoroscopy) should be strongly considered in placing Hickman catheters or ports [9].

Mechanical Complications

Inability to infuse nutrients or fluids or draw blood from a catheter is considered a mechanical malfunction. Causes include catheter dislodgement or fracture and catheter or venous thrombosis (the latter is discussed in the next section). Catheter breakage from the external segment can be repaired with proprietary repair kits. Catheters must be removed or replaced if unable to be repaired. Catheter "pinch-off" syndrome has been reported. Pinch-off syndrome occurs when the catheter is compressed between the first rib and the clavicle, causing an intermittent mechanical occlusion for both infusion and withdrawal, related to postural changes. Fracture of the catheter can occur. Findings should be confirmed radiographically. A more lateral replacement in the subclavian vein or using an alternative route avoids a recurrent complication [10,11].

Catheter-Related Infections

The Centers for Disease Control and Prevention guidelines for the Prevention of Intravascular Catheter-Related Infections estimate that 250,000 cases of CVC-associated bloodstream infections (BSI) occur in the United States annually [12]. This translated to nearly 5 cases per 1000 catheter-days. Mortality is estimated to be 12% to 25% for each infection. CVC infections can occur at the exit site, tunnel, or pocket, and be infusate-related and catheter-related BSI. The most prevalent organisms cultured include coagulase-negative staphylococci, *Staphylococcus aureus*, and *Klebsiella pneumoniae*. Patients receiving PN may also suffer from significant underlying diseases that may increase their risk of infection. The location of the catheter site, patient setting, and type of infusion also influence infection risk [13]. Patient location in the ICU, where CVC may be needed for a length of time and are frequently accessed, poses an increased risk of infection [14]. Maki and colleagues [15] recently reviewed 200 published prospective studies of infection associated with the various types of vascular devices to determine the RR of BSI. Included were catheters commonly used for PN support (PICC lines inpatient and outpatient, short-term noncuffed and long-term tunneled CVC, central venous ports, medicated and nonmedicated CVC). Based on their analysis, PICC rates of BSI for inpatients were 2.1 per 1000 catheter-days, and for outpatients 1 per 1000 catheter-days. For short-term nonmedicated, nontunneled CVC, rates of infection were 2.7 per 1000 catheter-days, and for short-term nonmedicated tunneled CVC, the rate was 1.7 per 1000 catheter-days. Of the various medicated CVC, the lowest rate was with the minocycline-rifampin–impregnated catheter at 1.2 per 1000 catheter-days, and the highest rate was with the silver-impregnated catheter at 4.7 per 1000 catheter-days. Cuffed and tunneled CVC had a rate of 1.6 per 1000 catheter-days, and central venous ports had a rate of 0.1 per 1000 catheter-days. Although the rate for PICC was lower than compared with short-term CVC, another study showed the infection rate of inpatient PICC lines to be 3.5 per 1000 catheter-days [16]. Many studies looked at infection risk with CVC used for multiple purposes (hemodialysis, blood sampling, and hemodynamic monitoring). One study collected prospective data on CVCs in 260 patients in the ICU [17]. In 61 of these patients, a single-lumen catheter was inserted by the subclavian route, through which only total parenteral nutrition (TPN) infused. The catheters were in place a mean of 4.3 days. Forty-nine percent of the total catheters were sent for culture, and from those 21% were colonized. Only one of the TPN catheters became colonized during the 1-year study period. For home PN patients with suspected line sepsis, a set of blood cultures should always be drawn before initiating antibiotic therapy, one from each lumen of the central catheter, and one from a peripheral vein. If the peripheral venous blood is not obtainable, two samples should be obtained from each lumen of the device. The device should be removed when the patient presents with severe sepsis and no other obvious source of infection is identified. Strong consideration should be given to removing any device if *S aureus* or a fungus is the source of infection [9].

Prevention of catheter-related BSI should include multiple fronts [18]. Box 1 includes selected guidelines from the Centers for Disease Control and Prevention [12]. Use of chlorhexidine gluconate for site care compared with povidone-iodine solution in patients with CVC was studied in a meta-analysis by Chaiyakunapruk and colleagues [19]. Eight studies with a total of 4143 catheters (in place from 1–10 days) in hospitalized patients met inclusion criteria. Chlorhexidine gluconate was found to reduce the risk for catheter-related BSI by approximately 50% in this population. Prevention of gram-positive

Box 1: Selected guidelines for the prevention of intravascular catheter-related infections

- For CVC, including PICC, replace gauze dressings every 2 days and transparent dressings every 7 days on short-term catheters.
- Replace dressing when the catheter is replaced; when the dressing becomes damp, loosened, or soiled; or when inspection of the site is necessary.
- Complete infusions of lipid-containing fluids within 24 hours of hanging the fluid.
- Complete the infusion of lipid emulsions alone within 12 hours of hanging the emulsion.
- Replace tube used to administer lipid-containing fluids every 24 hours. For dextrose and amino acid solution, the administration set does not need to be replaced more frequently than every 72 hours.
- Use either sterile gauze, transparent, or semi-permeable dressing to cover the catheter site.
- Select the catheter, insertion technique, and insertion site with the lowest risk of complications for the anticipated type and duration of therapy.
- Designate trained personnel for the insertion and maintenance of intravascular catheters.
- Do not administer transnasal or systemic antimicrobial prophylaxis routinely before insertion or during use of an intravascular catheter to prevent catheter colonization or bloodstream infection.
- Use totally implantable access devices for patients who require long-term, intermittent vascular access.
- Use an antimicrobial- or antiseptic-impregnated CVC in adults whose catheter is expected to remain in place more than 5 days if, after implementing a comprehensive strategy to reduce rates of BSI, the BSI rate remains above the goal set by the institution.
- In adults, use an upper-extremity instead of a lower-extremity site for catheter insertion.
- Do not routinely replace CVCs to prevent catheter-related infection.
- Do not remove CVC on the basis of fever alone.

catheter-related infections in oncology patients was reviewed [20]. This Cochran database review included randomized, controlled trials giving prophylactic antibiotics before insertion of the tunneled CVC, and trials using the combination of an antibiotic and heparin to flush the tunneled CVC in oncology patients. Eight trials were included with 527 patients. Four reported on vancomycin-teicoplanin before insertion, four reported on antibiotic flushing combined with heparin. The overall effect of an antibiotic before catheter insertion decreases the number for gram-positive tunneled CVC infection (odds ratio [OR] = 0.55; 95% CI, 0.29–1.04). Flushing with antibiotics and heparin proved to be beneficial (OR = 0.35; 95% CI, 0.16 –to 0.77). For intraluminal colonization the baseline infection rate was 15%, which leads to a number needed to treat of 13 (95% CI, 5–23). The authors concluded both interventions lead to a positive overall effect but should be considered with care because of the small number of studies.

Some studies have indicated that the type of dressing used for CVCs may affect the risk of infection. Gauze and tape, transparent polyurethane film dressings, or highly moisture-permeable transparent polyurethane film dressings are the most common types of dressing used. A recent Cochran database review looked at all randomized controlled trials evaluating the effects of dressing type [21]. Six studies were included, each one comparing one common type of dressing with another. All study data were limited because of small patient samples. There was no difference in the incidence of infectious complications between any of the dressing types compared. The study results suggest that the choice of dressing could be based on patient preference or cost.

Routine replacement of administration sets has been advocated to reduce intravenous infusion contamination. A Cochran database review was conducted to identify the optimal interval for the routine replacement of IV administration sets when infusate of PN (lipid and nonlipid) solutions are administered to hospitalized patients [22]. Randomized or quasirandomized controlled trials were reviewed and 15 were included, which contained 4783 participants. They concluded that administration sets that do not contain lipids, blood, or blood products may be left in place for intervals of up to 96 hours without increasing the incidence of infection. There was no evidence to suggest a change in the current recommendation that lipid-containing sets should be changed every 24 hours.

Catheter Occlusion and Thrombosis

The true incidence of catheter-related venous thrombus is not known because it can be asymptomatic. Risk factors for thrombus include underlying disease, such as patients with cancer, and type and location of the catheter. In a study of 50,470 home parenteral patients, the rate of thrombic catheter dysfunction was 0.23 per 1000 catheter-days [23]. This resulted in therapy interruption, catheter replacement, unscheduled emergency room visits, or hospitalization. Two deaths were attributed to venous thrombus in a study of home PN patients by Scolapio and colleagues [24]. In a study of 102 hospitalized patients receiving PN either through a PICC or subclavian or internal jugular placed catheters, PICC lines were associated with higher rate of clinically evident thrombophlebitis ($P < .01$) [6]. Thrombosis prophylaxis was reported in a systematic review by Klerk and colleagues [25] in patients with CVC for PN therapy. In five level 1 studies included in the analysis with a total of 204 patients, no bleeding events occurred. Prophylaxis with heparin added to PN was associated with a nonsignificant reduction in the incidence of catheter-related thrombosis. Per the consensus statement by the Home Parenteral and Enteral Working Group, when device occlusion or dysfunction occurs, mechanical causes should be ruled out and a history of recent infusions noted to rule out lipid, medication, or mineral precipitates as the cause of the dysfunction [9]. Tissue plasminogen activator is a useful modality for treating catheter obstruction or dysfunction related to thrombus. Seventy percent ethanol may be of value for occlusion related to lipid infusion, whereas 0.1-N sodium hydroxide may be of value when the occlusion is caused by mineral or drug precipitate. Heparin and saline are equally effective as a flushing agent. Central vein thrombosis should be treated with anticoagulation therapy in the absence of contraindication. Prophylactic anticoagulation therapy should be considered for those patients who are hypercoagulable or at high risk for catheter-related venous thrombosis.

METABOLIC COMPLICATIONS
Hyperglycemia

The most common cause of hyperglycemia is excess of dextrose infusion (Box 2). After the start of PN, a transient elevation of serum glucose can be observed followed by normalization of serum glucose after secretion of endogenous insulin is adjusted to the rate of dextrose infusion. Tolerance to dextrose depends on PN infusion rate and underlying medical condition. Patients at risk include the critically ill and those with sepsis, diabetes, acute pancreatitis, and corticosteroids use. Uncontrolled hyperglycemia from dextrose overfeeding can lead to immune system dysfunction and increased susceptibility to infection [26]. Suboptimal glucose control has been associated with higher rates of nosocomial and wound infections in critically ill and surgical patients [27]. A 50% reduction in mortality and 46% reduction in septicemia among patients in surgical ICU have been reported with intensive insulin therapy to maintain blood glucose levels between 80 and 110 mg/dL [28]. Dextrose infusion at rate 4 to 5 mg/kg/min seems to be optimal in stressed patients to avoid hyperglycemia and related complications [29]. Hyperglycemia should be corrected with insulin intravenous drip rather than with sliding scale in the critical care setting.

Box 2: Metabolic complications of PN

Hyperglycemia

Hyperlipidemia

Hypercapnia

Acid-base disturbance

Electrolyte abnormalities

Refeeding syndrome

Manganese toxicity

Hepatobiliary disorders

Bone disease

Hypoglycemia

Dextrose load in PN should be increased slowly to meet caloric goal, whereas insulin dosage adjustments are made in PN. Excess of caloric load stimulates glucose conversion to fat leading to hypertriglyceridemia and hepatic steatosis.

Sudden interruption of PN or excess of insulin in PN solution can result in hypoglycemia. Reactive hypoglycemia occurs 15 to 60 minutes after PN cessation as a result of prolonged elevated level of endogenous insulin in response to caloric load of PN [30]. Patients at risk are those with renal and liver disease, severe malnutrition, sepsis, starvation, hyperthyroidism, and infants. Infusion of 10% dextrose immediately after discontinuation of PN or gradual tapering of PN over 1 to 2 hours before complete discontinuation can prevent hypoglycemia if oral intake is not resumed [31]. A few studies, however, have shown no clinically significant hypoglycemia after tapered or abrupt cessation of PN [32,33]. Insulin dose in PN should be adjusted accordingly when underlying hyperglycemia is resolving. Monitoring of serum glucose levels is essential after discontinuation of PN [34].

Hyperlipidemia

Excess of lipids or dextrose in the PN solution, or impaired lipid clearance, is responsible for PN-induced hyperlipidemia. Obesity, diabetes, sepsis, pancreatitis, and liver disease predispose to hypertriglyceridemia because of decreased lipids clearance.

Composition of lipids (phospholipid/triglyceride ratio) in PN affects the rate of lipid clearance [35]. Hypertriglyceridemia from PN can precipitate acute pancreatitis, especially when serum triglyceride levels are above 1000 mg/dL [36]. In any case of hypertriglyceridemia in PN patients, dextrose overfeeding has to be considered. Dextrose load should be reduced first, followed by lipids reduction if hyperlipidemia is not corrected. Lipid infusion should not exceed 0.12 g/kg/h in critically ill patients or those with impaired lipid clearance [37]. Continuous infusion of lipids over 24 hours compared with cyclic lipid infusion has been associated with improved lipid oxidation and serum fatty acid profile, and less deleterious effects on reticuloendothelial system function [38]. Caution has to be used when a PN patient is also receiving propofol, a source of extra lipid calories [39]. Propofol, a lipid-based drug, provides 1.1 kcal/mL of infusion. Lipid amount has to be adjusted in PN to avoid lipid overload when a patient is given propofol infusion. Serum triglyceride levels should be monitored during PN therapy. Baseline serum triglyceride levels should be measured before initiation of PN and after lipid caloric goal is achieved. Daily lipid infusion should be discontinued when serum triglyceride concentration exceeds 400 mg/dL. Lipid emulsion two to three times weekly should be continued, however, to prevent essential fatty acid deficiency [40].

Hypercapnia

Overfeeding of total calories and dextrose can result in excess of carbon dioxide production during carbohydrates metabolism. This may occur within hours of overfeeding, particularly in severely malnourished patients. Increased carbon dioxide production stimulates minute ventilation and increases respiratory work load resulting in difficulty weaning off from mechanical ventilation [41]. Reduction of caloric load helps correct hypercapnia.

Refeeding Syndrome

Rapid nutritional repletion in severely malnourished individuals can result in severe fluid and electrolyte disturbances including hypernatremia, hypophosphatemia, hypokalemia, and hypomagnesemia [42]. Infusion of dextrose stimulates insulin secretion, which is responsible for shifting of phosphorus and potassium intracellularly. Severe hypophosphatemia can cause weakness, convulsions, respiratory failure, and cardiac decompensation leading to death [43]. In patients at risk, PN should be advanced gradually to achieve caloric goal over 3 to 5 days. The most important steps are to identify patients at risk for developing refeeding syndrome, provide nutrition support cautiously, and correct and supplement electrolyte and vitamin deficiencies to avoid refeeding syndrome.

Selenium Deficiency

Selenium deficiency has been reported in patients receiving long-term PN [44]. The recommended dietary allowance for selenium is 0.87 µg/kg, of which 80% is absorbed. In a study of adult long-term TPN patients who received 40 to 60 µg of selenium daily in their PN solution, 75% of patients had low serum selenium levels [45]. The findings were suggestive of impaired renal homeostasis of selenium conservation. Serum selenium levels should be monitored periodically in patients receiving long-term PN.

Renal Complications

Renal disorders associated with PN include hyperoxaluria, hypercalciuria, and tubular renal defects. Increased creatinine clearance resulting from glomerular hyperfiltration has been reported with short-term TPN infusion. TPN-associated nephropathy characterized by decline in creatinine clearance and impaired tubular function has been reported in adults and children receiving long-term PN [46]. Progression to chronic renal failure has not been documented in long-term PN patients. The renal dysfunction is multifactorial and related to amino acid load, use of nephrotoxic drugs, and possibly previous BSI [47]. The amount of parenteral amino acids and heavy metal contaminants has not been associated with decline in renal function except for chromium contaminant of PN in children [48]. Hypercalciuria, most likely related to vitamin C content, amino acid load, and cyclic PN, has been reported in adults on PN [49].

Gastrointestinal Complications

Intestinal atrophy

Numerous animal studies have demonstrated intestinal villous atrophy when PN is provided and enteral nutrition is withheld [50]. Intestinal morphologic and functional changes occur to a lesser degree in humans for whom PN is the only nutritional source [51]. Factors contributing to intestinal atrophy include lack of stimulation from luminal nutrients; lack of fuel source (glutamine); and impaired hormonal response. The loss of mucosal structure may be sufficient to increase intestinal permeability and bacterial translocation, the clinical significance of which remains to be determined. The use of concomitant oral feeding or enteral nutrition is important in restoring and prevention of intestinal changes associated with PN. Glutamine and arginine supplementation may be beneficial in this setting [52].

Gastroparesis
Abnormal gastric motility has been reported in patients with PN therapy [53]. Delayed gastric emptying has been documented in normal individuals receiving long-chain triglyceride-based lipid emulsion [54]. Hyperglycemia from dextrose load in PN can also induce gastroparesis. The rate of gastric emptying correlated with the increase in blood glucose induced by the parenteral nutrient load [55]. Early satiety and the intolerance to oral intake, displayed by some individuals receiving oral and high-caloric PN, can be explained by the previously mentioned mechanisms.

HEPATOBILIARY DISEASE
Numerous hepatobiliary complications have been associated with PN use in adults and pediatric patients (Box 3). The first case of PN-associated liver disease was reported in 1971 in an infant who presented with severe cholestasis [56]. Cholestasis has been reported more frequently in infants than in adults. Contrary, hepatic steatosis is predominantly seen in adults receiving PN. It is clinically characterized by elevated serum aminotransferases and hepatomegaly. Ultrasound or CT scan can confirm steatosis.

   Liver function test abnormalities have been reported in 20% to 90% of PN patients [57]. Asymptomatic increase in serum aminotransferases (>1.5 times normal) is commonly observed within the first 2 to 3 weeks from initiation of PN therapy [58]. Aminotransferases elevation is typically followed by increase in alkaline phosphatase and bilirubin. These mild biochemical abnormalities resolve with discontinuation of TPN therapy. The elevation of serum bilirubin is more often seen in children, particularly in preterm infants [59]. Immature bile acid transport and metabolism early in life may be partially responsible for an increased susceptibility to liver injury. The liver function

---

Box 3: PN-associated liver disorders

Steatosis

Steatohepatitis

Fibrosis

Cirrhosis

Gallstones or biliary sludge

Cholestasis

Cholecystitis

test abnormalities poorly correlate with histologic findings on the liver biopsy. Macrovesicular and microvesicular steatosis is the most common finding observed on biopsy specimen. The other histopathologic changes include steato-hepatitis, intrahepatic cholestasis, and phospholipidosis. More advanced changes can be found including steatonecrosis, fibrosis, and deposits of lipofuscin within Kupffer's cells. The progression of liver disease from mild steatosis to fibrosis and micronodular cirrhosis over a 5-year period in the patient with Crohn's disease and short-bowel syndrome receiving PN, documented by sequential liver biopsies, has been reported by Craig and colleagues [60]. Hepatic steatosis and steatohepatitis can be reversed by PN caloric manipulations [61]. End-stage liver disease has been reported in 15% of adults receiving PN and more often in neonates [62]. Pathogenesis of PN-associated liver disease is multifactorial.

Excess of Total Calories and Dextrose

Overfeeding is associated with increased lipogenesis in the liver and impaired fat mobilization and use leading to hepatic steatosis. Caloric overload and an imbalanced source of energy in PN play a pivotal role in steatosis. Increased insulin/glucagon ratio in portal circulation and resultant hyperinsulinemia from excess glucose in PN are responsible for glucose conversion to fat in the liver [63]. Replacement of dextrose by fat as a calorie source resulted in reduced severity of liver function test elevation. In a prospective study, Meguid and colleagues [64] showed the difference in liver function test elevation with glucose-based PN versus one third of calories from glucose replaced by lipids. Reduction in hepatic steatosis has been reported in 53% of patients who received only dextrose infusion, compared with 17% of those who received mixed dextrose and lipid emulsions (70:30 ratio of nonprotein calories) [65]. A balanced PN regimen should be used to provide 50% to 60% of total calories from dextrose and 25% to 30% of calories from lipids. Reducing the carbohydrate load in PN should be considered if elevated liver function tests are found to prevent steatosis.

Lipid Emulsions

Liver dysfunction has been reported with high dosages of lipid emulsions and essential fatty acid deficiency. Lipid emulsions may have a protective effect on the liver by allowing reduction of nonprotein calories in PN and providing essential fatty acids important for the production of hepatic phospholipids (protective from steatosis). Hepatic steatosis has been reported in patients with lipid-free PN, containing a mixture of dextrose and amino acids only, and resolution of steatosis was observed after lipid supplementation [66,67]. It was suggested, however, that essential fatty acid deficiency could be responsible for steatosis in those studies. It is recommended to provide a minimum 2% to 4% of calories as linoleic fatty acid to avoid essential fatty acid deficiency. The role of essential fatty acid deficiency in the development of steatosis, however, remains unclear. Excess of lipid infusion should be avoided. Fat overload syndrome has been reported with excess of lipid infusion at dosages greater than 4 g/kg/d [68]. The association between lipid emulsions and cholestasis has been reported in both adults and children [69,70]. Cholestasis is characterized by ballooning of hepatocytes, Kupffer cell hyperplasia, and bile duct plugging on liver biopsy. Lipid emulsions induce dose-dependent inhibition of cholesterol uptake by hepatocytes and reduce cholesterol availability for bile formation leading to decreased bile volume and reduced bile flow [71]. In the United States, lipid emulsions are made of long-chain triglycerides derived from soybean or soybean-safflower oil. Medium-chain triglycerides in comparison with long-chain triglycerides undergo faster oxidation and the medium-chain–long-chain triglyceride mixture may be better tolerated and may be less likely to cause hepatic dysfunction [72]. Such a mixture is not available, however, in the United States.

Amino Acids Excess
The development of PN-associated cholestasis (PNAC) in children has been linked to excess amounts of amino acids and their toxicity. The amino acids may have a direct effect on the canalicular membrane, with a tendency to reduce bile flow and bile salt secretion. The alteration in canalicular flow and membrane permeability leads to accumulation of hepatotoxic bile acids and impaired bile acid transport [73]. It seems prudent not to exceed limits of amino acids in PN to avoid hepatotoxicity. A definite relationship between plasma amino acid concentrations and liver dysfunction has not been established.

Methionine Toxicity
Methionine is an essential sulfur-containing amino acid that was found to be a contributing factor to development of cholestasis and steatosis [74]. Higher blood methionine levels were reported in infants receiving PN. In premature infants, a low cystathionase activity was found limiting conversion of methionine to taurine and glutathione [75]. Because taurine plays a role in bile acid conjugation, a deficiency may predispose these infants to cholestasis [76]. No good human data, however, have correlated cholestasis to methionine in PN. Lowering methionine concentrations in crystalline amino acid solution and providing alternative substrates should be considered to minimize possible hepatotoxic effects of methionine.

Carnitine Deficiency
Acquired carnitine deficiency has been linked to pathogenesis of hepatic steatosis [77]. Carnitine is involved in the transport of long-chain triglycerides across the mitochondrial membrane for lipid oxidation [59]. Carnitine deficiency has been described in premature neonates because of limited stores and reduced synthesis [78]. Carnitine deficiency is very rare in adults because carnitine is abundant in the diet. Carnitine supplementation in PN is controversial.

Choline Deficiency
Choline is required for synthesis of very low-density lipoproteins involved in triglyceride transport from the liver. Lower choline levels correlating with

aspartate transaminase–alanine transaminase concentrations and hepatic steatosis have been found in PN patients [79]. Choline supplementation in a form of lecithin in PN patients has been associated with amelioration or improvement in hepatic steatosis [80,81]. Choline may be an essential nutrient for PN-dependent patients.

Phytosterolemia

Phytosterols are contaminants in lipid emulsions. They impair the hepatocyte canalicular secretory activity by binding to membrane proteins and affecting membrane transporters, reduce bile synthesis and flow, and precipitate in the bile causing formation of biliary sludge and stones [81]. Phytosterolemia associated with cholestasis had been reported in children only after a high dose of lipid infusion (>1.4 g/kg/d) [82]. Higher plasma concentrations of phytosterols were seen in five children with severe PNAC than in those with less severe PNAC. Reduction or discontinuation of lipid emulsions in five patients resulted in decreased plasma phytosterol concentrations and improvement in liver function tests only in three patients. In the recent study, higher levels of phytosterols in short-bowel patients and long-term PN have been reported from excess of phytosterols in PN [83]. No convincing data are available to show a definite correlation between phytosterolemia and PNAC.

Therapy for Parenteral Nutrition–Associated Cholestasis

The pathophysiology of PNAC is multifactorial. Risk factors include prematurity, long duration of PN, sepsis, lack of bowel motility, and short-bowel syndrome [84,85]. Several measures can be undertaken to prevent PNAC, such as avoiding overfeeding, providing a balanced source of energy, cyclic PN infusion, and avoiding sepsis [86]. Initiation of enteral feeding and weaning off PN are the best method to prevent PNAC. Pharmacotherapy has been used for PNAC. Ursodeoxycholic acid at the dose 10 to 45 mg/kg/d has been shown to have a beneficial effect on cholestasis in preterm infants and children [87–89]. Improvement in cholestasis was also found in adults treated with ursodeoxycholic acid at a dose 6 to 15 mg/kg/d [90,91]. Initial studies with cholecystokinin (CCK) injections revealed a beneficial effect on bilirubin levels in neonates [92,93]. In a larger study by the same author, CCK failed to reduce significantly the incidence of PNAC and the levels of bilirubin [94]. CCK should not be recommended for the prevention of PNAC. Patients with short residual small bowel are at a higher risk of progressing to end-stage liver disease irrespective of duration of TPN [62,69]. Those patients with progressive chronic liver disease have a higher mortality rate, and they need to be referred early for combined liver and small bowel transplantation.

BILIARY COMPLICATIONS

Long-term PN has been associated with higher risk of acalculous and calculous cholecystitis [95]. Acalculous cholecystitis has been reported in approximately 4% of patients receiving PN for more than 3 months [96]. Lack of oral intake or enteral feeding decreases release of CCK and reduces gallbladder contractility.

Other contributing factors include bile stasis, increased bile lithogenicity, and opioid therapy [97]. To prevent development of cholecystitis, patients should be encouraged to maintain oral intake even if they are PN dependant. Formation of biliary sludge is very common in PN patients. Sludge was reported in 50% of the patients after 4 to 6 weeks of PN infusion and in almost 100% of patients after 6 weeks of PN therapy [98]. Reintroduction of enteral feeding was associated with sludge disappearance in all PN patients after a few weeks. Gallbladder stasis is responsible for sludge and gallstone formation. PN patients develop typically pigment stones composed of calcium bilirubinate [99]. The cause of pigment stones is unclear, but chronic bacterial infections of biliary tract are involved in their formation [100]. The best prevention of sludge formation is oral feeding. Potential therapy to prevent sludge formation includes CCK injections daily to induce gallbladder contractility and to reduce biliary stasis [101,102]. Nausea, flushing, and cholecystitis, however, limit CCK use. CCK has been found to be of no benefit in pediatric patients [103]. Ursodeoxycholic acid alters composition of the bile and has been shown to reduce gallstone formation, but has not been studied in PN patients [104]. Other preventive measures include rapid infusion of amino acids or lipids. Parenteral rapid high dose of amino acid infusion stimulates gallbladder contractions [105–107]. Similar results were found with rapid infusion of 10% lipid emulsion at 100 mL/h over 3 hours [108]. Contrary to their effects in adults, bolus infusions of amino acids or fat have not been associated with induction of gallbladder contractions in neonates on PN [109].

MANGANESE TOXICITY

Manganese is one of the trace elements routinely administered to PN patients as part of a multiple-trace-element additive. High blood levels of manganese have been associated with cholestasis, suggestive of a link between manganese and hepatic toxicity in patients receiving long-term PN [110]. Manganese is primarily eliminated in the bile, and it may accumulate to potentially toxic levels in patients with cholestasis and biliary obstruction [111]. The recommended dose of manganese supplementation is 100 to 800 μg/day. Manganese accumulation leads to neurotoxicity. Neurologic manifestations include Parkinson-type symptoms, tremor, muscle rigidity, mask-like face, abnormal gait, confusion, weakness, somnolence, and headaches [112]. Those neurologic symptoms can be reversed by manganese removal from PN solution [113]. Manganese deposition in basal ganglia can be detected by MRI. A significant correlation between blood manganese levels, plasma aspartate transaminase, and bilirubin concentrations was found in children with cholestasis [114]. Manganese and bilirubin levels declined after manganese supplementation was reduced or withdrawn in PN. Another study in infants showed no increase in cholestasis with large amounts of manganese supplement in PN [115]. It is uncertain whether hypermanganesemia causes the cholestasis, or vice versa. Periodic monitoring of manganese levels is important because patients can be asymptomatic [116]. Manganese should be eliminated from the solution if the manganese level is elevated and not be supplemented if the patient has liver disease with an elevated bilirubin.

BONE DISEASE

Bone disease is a common disorder in patients receiving prolonged PN, and some degree of bone demineralization was reported in between 40% and 100% of patients. In a cross-sectional study, osteopenia was observed in 84% and osteoporosis in 41% of patients on long-term PN [117]. Bone pain occurred in 35% and bone fracture in 10% of those patients. It is recognized that metabolic bone disease in PN patients is partially related to the underlying disease for which the PN was initiated [118,119]. PN-associated bone disease was first reported in 1980 [120,121]. Klein and colleagues [121] described insidious onset of severe bone pain and hypercalciuria in adults receiving PN for more than 3 months. Symptoms resolved within 1 to 2 months after discontinuation of the PN infusion despite nutritional deterioration. Many patients with PN-associated bone disease are asymptomatic. Other patients may suffer from mild to moderate bone or back pain or incidental fracture. Bone biopsy may be useful to establish the diagnosis. Histomorphometry of the bone shows patchy osteomalacia with reduced osteoid in adults, and osteopenia in children. Abnormalities in bone metabolism suggest a decrease in bone matrix-formation rather than a mineralization defect as the underlying mechanism [122]. PN-associated bone disease can be diagnosed by measurement of bone mineral density by dual energy x-ray absorptiometry revealing T score less than -1. Serum levels of calcium, phosphorus, and 25-hydroxyvitamin D may be normal [121]. Serum levels of immunoreactive parathyroid hormone (PTH) can be normal or low, consistent with physiologic hypoparathyroidism, even though Klein and colleagues [121] reported normal or elevated levels of PTH. Low serum levels of 1,25(OH)2-vitamin D have been demonstrated, but the significance of these reduced levels in the pathogenesis of the bone disease is not well defined [123]. The physiopathology of bone disease associated with long-term PN is multifactorial and poorly understood. Factors implicated as possible causes of bone disease include excess infusion of vitamin D, calcium, protein, or glucose; aluminum toxicity; cyclic TPN administration; and the patient's nutritional status. The underlying disorders and previous therapies may play an important role in the development of bone disease before PN initiation. Bone disease is a result of impaired calcium and phosphorus homeostasis. Abnormal calcium metabolism characterized by excessive urine calcium loss in PN patients has been observed. Hypercalciuria may be a result of cyclic TPN infusion, excess of amino acids infusion, vitamin A toxicity, hyperinsulinemia, or increased bone reabsorption [124,125]. Chronic acidosis has also been associated with hypercalciuria, and it can be corrected by acetate replacement for chloride [126]. Hypercalciuria can be corrected by increasing the amount of phosphorus in PN, but with a risk of precipitation with calcium in PN solution [127,128].

Aluminum Toxicity

Aluminum toxicity has been implicated in development of bone disease associated with PN. Large quantities of aluminum have been detected in the plasma, urine, and bone of patients treated with PN [129]. Infants are at a higher risk of aluminum toxicity because of reduced renal function. Significant aluminum contamination was found in the casein-based amino acids in the early 1980s, which were later substituted by crystalline free amino acid–based formulas [130]. Decreased serum 1,25(OH)2-vitamin D, reduced bone formation, and osteomalacia are typical features of aluminum toxicity. At present, components of TPN containing substantial amounts of aluminum include sodium phosphate, calcium gluconate, and multivitamins [131]. Contamination of PN solution by aluminum has to be suspected when serum aluminum level is over 100 μg/L or urine aluminum/creatinine ratio is greater than 0.3. Because PN patients continue to develop bone disease despite significant exposure to aluminum, the link between aluminum accumulation and bone disease in PN patients is uncertain.

Vitamin D Toxicity

The observation was made that vitamin D may have toxic effect on bones because the removal of vitamin D from PN solution was associated with improvement in bone formation [120,132]. The role of vitamin D in pathogenesis of bone disease is not well understood. Excess of vitamin D may suppress PTH secretion and may stimulate bone resorption. A long-term (mean, 4.5 years) vitamin D withdrawal in adult PN patients has been associated with normalization of PTH and 1,25(OH)-vitamin D levels and improved lumbar bone mineral density [133]. Vitamin D withdrawal for 2 years from PN in children resulted in markedly reduced levels of serum 25(OH)2-vitamin D and normal serum levels of 1,25(OH)2-vitamin D, calcium, and phosphorus, with no clinical sequelae [134]. The vitamin D requirement for PN patients does not differ from requirements for healthy individuals (200 IU daily for adults and children). Vitamin D in PN may be the only source of vitamin D in patients who avoid sun exposure. Normal vitamin D status should be maintained in PN patients to preserve maximal intestinal absorption of calcium and phosphorus. It is not recommended to discontinue completely vitamin D supplementation from PN formula. The data on vitamin D supplementation in PN patients remain controversial.

CALCIUM DEFICIENCY

Negative calcium balance is the most important factor contributing to PN-associated bone disease. Poor oral intake (dairy products), lactose maldigestion, and malabsorption in PN patients lead to reduced calcium absorption and resultant calcium deficiency. Adequate provision of calcium and phosphorus is critical in prevention of bone disease. Incompatibility of high concentration of calcium and phosphorus in the PN solution may result in precipitation of calcium and phosphorus. This has been observed more often in neonates because they have higher requirement for both calcium and phosphorus, while restricting fluid volume. The solubility can also be improved by acidification of PN solution by increasing concentration of amino acids [135]. The high protein load in PN solution may lead, however, to hypercalciuria and negative calcium balance [125]. Acidosis can negatively affect bone cell metabolism and bone mineralization. Other factors related to PN affecting urinary calcium loss include excessive fluid infusion, and increased load of magnesium, calcium, phosphorus, and sodium. It has been shown that patients on cyclic PN have greater urinary calcium excretion during the time of PN infusion [124,136]. This is a result of suppressed PTH secretion by calcium in PN infusion leading to hypoparathyroidism and reduced calcium renal reabsorption.

OTHER POTENTIAL CAUSES OF BONE DISEASE IN TOTAL PARENTERAL NUTRITION PATIENTS

Vitamin K regulates vitamin K–dependant osteocalcin involved in bone formation. Fat malabsorption and alteration in gut microflora from antibiotic use can result in vitamin K deficiency. Vitamin K is not provided routinely in PN solution and it should be added, 1 mg daily, to reduce hypercalciuria. The role of copper in bone disease in PN patients is unclear. At least one study showed that use of copper-free TPN was associated with bone disease in infants [137].

Underlying disease can be a major factor in development of bone disease including secondary hypoparathyroidism from magnesium deficiency, malabsorption, Crohn's disease, chronic inflammatory status, and drug use. Corticosteroids are a major culprit in development of metabolic bone disease by inhibition of bone formation and collagen synthesis. Long-term anticoagulation with warfarin has been shown to reduce bone mineral density.

TREATMENT OF PARENTERAL NUTRITION–ASSOCIATED BONE DISEASE

All patients at risk for metabolic bone disease should receive calcium supplements of 500 to 1000 mg/day, with total daily intake of at least 1500 mg. Intravenous calcium supplementation in PN solution is often limited by solubility with phosphorus. Vitamin D supplementation is questionable. Vitamin D should be given to correct deficiency, not for prevention, and serum levels of vitamin D 25-OH should be monitored. Estrogen replacement should be considered in postmenopausal women. Bisphosphonates have been used in PN patients with bone disease. In a double-blind, randomized, placebo-controlled trial, the effect of clodronate, 1500 mg, given intravenously every 3 months for 1 year, was studied on bone mineral density and markers of bone turnover in 20 home PN patients [138]. Clodronate was associated with significant improvement in biochemical markers of bone turnover and nonsignificant increase in spinal BMD. Calcitonin, given parenterally for 10 days, has been shown to be effective in relieving bone pain in PN patients and bone disease [139]. Long-term therapy with calcitonin has not been studied, however, in PN patients.

> **Box 4: Monitoring and management of PN-associated metabolic bone disease in long-term PN patients**
>
> *Monitoring*
>
> Symptoms: bone and back pain, atraumatic fractures
>
> Physical examination: loss of height
>
> Laboratory tests: serum calcium, phosphorus, magnesium, and acetate
>
> Obtain 24-hour urine collection for calcium and magnesium
>
> Obtain baseline dual energy x-ray absorptiometry scan, repeat every 1 to 2 years if abnormal scan
>
> *Management*
>
> Provide adequate amount of minerals in PN
>
>   Calcium >15 mEq/d
>
>   Phosphorus >15 mmol/d
>
>   Magnesium (adjust to maintain normal serum level)
>
>   Acetate (adequate amount to buffer excess acid and to avoid calcium absorption from bone)
>
> Decrease protein amount to 1 g/kg/d if stable nutrition status
>
> Suggest exercise program
>
> Avoidance of smoking
>
> Limit steroid use
>
> Treat metabolic bone disease if detected with bisphosphonates

Human PTH (teriparatide) has recently become available for treatment of osteoporosis [140]. PTH therapy has not been studied, however, in PN patients. A new promising treatment is glucagon-like peptide-2 for patients with short-bowel syndrome. In a 5-week study, glucagon-like peptide-2 (400 µg subcutaneously) given twice daily significantly increased spinal bone mass density in eight short-bowel patients with no colon (only four patients on PN) [141]. The mechanism by which glucagon-like peptide-2 affects bone metabolism is unclear, but may be related to improved intestinal calcium absorption. Regular exercise should be encouraged. Floor-based exercises are preferred at least twice a week. This has not been formally studied, however, in TPN patients. Recommended monitoring and management of PN-associated bone disease are shown in Box 4.

SUMMARY

PN is a highly complex therapy requiring close monitoring. The outcome of PN patients can be significantly affected by potentially serious PN-related complications. The knowledge about PN-related complications is helpful to intervene early and improve patient outcome. Infectious complications are the most common and are often related to suboptimal catheter care and inadequate patient education. Metabolic complications can be avoided if appropriate monitoring is implemented and if they are recognized early. PN-associated liver disease and bone disease can be quite debilitating, and both can be challenging to manage. Effective therapies are available for PN-associated bone disease. For long-term PN patients with severe and progressive liver disease, liver transplantation or combined liver and intestinal transplantation may be the only remaining treatment option.

References

[1] Shils ME, Wright WL, Turnbull A, et al. Long-term parenteral nutrition through an external arteriovenous shunt. N Engl J Med 1970;283:341–4.

[2] Howard L, Ament M, Fleming CR, et al. Current use and clinical outcome of home parenteral and enteral nutrition therapies in the United States. Gastroenterology 1995;109:355–65.

[3] Moreno JM, Planas M, de Cos AI, et al. The year 2003 national registry of home-based parenteral nutrition. Nutr Hosp 2006;21:127–31.

[4] Lewis CA, Allen TE, Burke DR, et al. Quality improvement guidelines for central access. J Vasc Interv Radiol 1997;8:475–9.

[5] Ruesch S, Walder B, Tramer MR. Complications of central venous catheters: internal jugular versus subclavian access-a systematic review. Crit Care Med 2002;30(2):454–60.

[6] Cowl CT, Weinstock JV, Al-Jurf A, et al. Complications and cost associated with parenteral nutrition delivered to hospitalized patients through either subclavian or peripherally-inserted central catheters. Clin Nutr 2000;19:237–43.

[7] Tran HS, Burrows BJ, Zang WA, et al. Brachial arteriovenous fistula as a complication of placement of a peripherally inserted central venous catheter: a case report and review of the literature. Am Surg 2006;72(9):833–6.

[8] Merrer J, DeJonghe B, Golliot F, et al. Complications of femoral and subclavian venous catheterization in critically ill patients, a randomized controlled trial. JAMA 2001;286:700–7.

[9] Steiger E, HPEN Working Group. Consensus statements regarding optimal management of home parenteral nutrition (HPN) access. JPEN J Parenter Enteral Nutr 2006;30(1):S94–5.

[10] Andris DA, Krzywda EA, Schulte W, et al. Pinch-off syndrome: a rare etiology for central venous catheter occlusion. JPEN J Parenter Enteral Nutr 1994;18:531–3.

[11] Mizra B, Vanek V, Kupensky DT. Pinch-off syndrome: care report and collective review of the literature. Am Surg 2004;70(7):635–44.

[12] O'Grady NP, Alexander M, Dellinger EP, et al. Guidelines for the prevention of intravascular catheter-related infections. Centers for Disease Control and Prevention. MMWR Morb Mortal Wkly Rep 2002;51:1–29.

[13] Moretti EW, Ofstead CL, Kristy RM, et al. Impact of central venous catheter type and methods on catheter-related colonization and bacteremia. J Hosp Infect 2006;61:139–45.

[14] NNIS System. National nosocomial infections surveillance (NNIS) system reports, data summary from January 1992 through June 2003, issued August 2003. Am J Infect Control 2003;31:481–98.

[15] Maki DG, Kluger DM, Crnich CJ. The risk of bloodstream infection in adults with different intravascular devices: a systematic review of 200 published prospective studies. Mayo Clin Proc 2006;81(9):1159–71.

[16] Safdar N, Make DG. Risk of catheter-related bloodstream infection with peripherally inserted central venous catheters used in hospitalized patients. Chest 2005;128:489–95.

[17] Dimick JB, Swaboda S, Talamini MA, et al. Risk of colonization of central venous catheters: catheters for total parenteral nutrition vs. other catheters. Am J Crit Care 2003;12:328–35.

[18] Ryder M. Evidence-based practice in the management of vascular access devices for home parenteral nutrition therapy. JPEN J Parenter Enteral Nutr 2006;30:S82–93.

[19] Chaiyakunapuruk N, Veenstra D, Lipsky BA, et al. Chlorhexidine compared with povidone-iodines solution for vascular catheter-site care: a meta-analysis. Ann Intern Med 2002;136:792–801.

[20] van de Wetering MD, van Woensel JBM. Prophylactic antibiotics for preventing early enteral venous catheter gram positive infections in oncology patients. Cochrane Database of Systematic Reviews 2006;4.

[21] Gilles D, O'Riordan L, Carr D, et al. Gauze and tape and transparent polyurethane dressings for central venous catheters. Cochrane Database of Systematic Reviews 2006;4.

[22] Gilles D, O'Riordan L, Wallen M, et al. Optimal timing for intravenous administration set replacement. Cochrane Database of Systematic Reviews 2006;4.

[23] Moureau N, Poole S, Murdock, et al. Central venous catheters in home infusion care: outcomes analysis in 50,470 patients. J Vasc Interv Radiol 2002;13:1009–16.

[24] Scolapio JS, Fleming CR, Kelly D, et al. Survival of home parenteral nutrition-treated patients: 20 years of experience at the Mayo Clinic. Mayo Clin Proc 1999;74:217–22.

[25] Klerk CPW, Smorenburg SM, Buller HR. Thrombosis prophylaxis in patient populations with a central venous catheter. Arch Intern Med 2003;163:1913–21.

[26] Kjersem H, Hilsted J, Madsbad S, et al. Polymorphonuclear leucocyte dysfunction during short term metabolic changes from normo- to hyperglycemia in type 1 (insulin dependent) diabetic patients. Infection 1988;16:215–21.

[27] Pomposelli JJ, Baxter JK 3rd, Babineau TJ, et al. Early postoperative glucose control predicts nosocomial infection rate in diabetic patients. JPEN J Parenter Enteral Nutr 1998; 22:77–81.

[28] Van den Berghe G, Wouters PJ, Bouillon R, et al. Outcome benefit of intensive insulin therapy in the critically ill: insulin dose versus glycemic control. Crit Care Med 2003;31: 359–66.

[29] Driscoll DF. Clinical issues regarding the use of total nutrient admixtures. DICP 1990;24: 296–303.

[30] Scribner BH. Hypoglycemia and home parenteral nutrition. Mayo Clin Proc 1986;61: 226.

[31] Fischer KF, Lees JA, Newman JH. Hypoglycemia in hospitalized patients: causes and outcomes. N Engl J Med 1986;315:1245–50.

[32] Krzywda EA, Andris DA, Whipple JK, et al. Glucose response to abrupt initiation and discontinuation of total parenteral nutrition. JPEN J Parenter Enteral Nutr 1993;17: 64–7.

[33] Nirula R, Yamada K, Waxman K. The effect of abrupt cessation of total parenteral nutrition on serum glucose: a randomized trial. Am Surg 2000;66:866–9.

[34] Bendorf K, Friesen CA, Roberts CC. Glucose response to discontinuation of parenteral nutrition in patients less than 3 years of age. JPEN J Parenter Enteral Nutr 1996;20:120–2.

[35] Jeejeebhoy KN, Anderson GH, Nakhooda AF, et al. Metabolic studies in total parenteral nutrition with lipid in man: comparison with glucose. J Clin Invest 1976;57:125–36.

[36] Cameron JL, Capuzzi DM, Zuidema GD, et al. Acute pancreatitis with hyperlipemia: the incidence of lipid abnormalities in acute pancreatitis. Ann Surg 1973;177:483–9.

[37] Iriyama K, Tsuchibashi T, Urata H, et al. Elimination of fat emulsion particles from plasma during glucose infusion. Br J Surg 1996;83:946–8.

[38] Jensen GL, Mascioli EA, Seidner DL, et al. Parenteral infusion of long- and medium-chain triglycerides and reticuloendothelial system function in man. JPEN J Parenter Enteral Nutr 1990;14:467–71.

[39] Mateu-de Antonio J, Barrachina F. Propofol infusion and nutritional support. Am J Health Syst Pharm 1997;54:2515–6.

[40] Hamilton C, Austin T, Seidner DL. Essential fatty acid deficiency in human adults during parenteral nutrition. Nutr Clin Pract 2006;21:387–94.

[41] Liposky JM, Nelson LD. Ventilatory response to high caloric loads in critically ill patients. Crit Care Med 1994;22:796–802.

[42] Kraft MD, Btaiche IF, Sacks GS. Review of the refeeding syndrome. Nutr Clin Pract 2005;20:625–33.

[43] Weinsier RL, Krumdieck CL. Death resulting from overzealous total parenteral nutrition: the refeeding syndrome revisited. Am J Clin Nutr 1981;34:393–9.

[44] van Rij AM, McKenzie JM, Robinson MF, et al. Selenium and total parenteral nutrition. JPEN J Parenter Enteral Nutr 1979;3:235–9.

[45] Buchman AL, Moukarzel A, Ament ME. Selenium renal homeostasis is impaired in patients receiving long-term total parenteral nutrition. JPEN J Parenter Enteral Nutr 1994;18:231–3.

[46] Buchman AL, Moukarzel A, Ament ME, et al. Serious renal impairment is associated with long-term parenteral nutrition. JPEN J Parenter Enteral Nutr 1993;17:438–44.

[47] Moukarzel AA, Ament ME, Buchman AL, et al. Renal function of children receiving long-term parenteral nutrition. J Pediatr 1991;119:864–8.

[48] Moukarzel AA, Song MK, Buchman AL, et al. Excessive chromium intake in children receiving total parenteral nutrition. Lancet 1992;339:385–8.

[49] Buchman AL, Moukarzel AA, Ament ME. Excessive urinary oxalate excretion occurs in long-term TPN patients both with and without ileostomies. Am Coll Nutr 1995;14:24–8.

[50] Illig KA, Ryan CK, Hardy DJ, et al. Total parenteral nutrition-induced changes in gut mucosal function: atrophy alone is not the issue. Surgery 1992;112:631–7.

[51] Buchman AL, Moukarzel AA, Bhuta S, et al. Parenteral nutrition is associated with intestinal morphologic and functional changes in humans. JPEN J Parenter Enteral Nutr 1995;19:453–60.

[52] Li J, Langkamp-Henken B, Suzuki K, et al. Glutamine prevents parenteral nutrition-induced increases in intestinal permeability. JPEN J Parenter Enteral Nutr 1994;18:303–7.

[53] Casaubon PR, Dahlstrom KA, Vargas J, et al. Intravenous fat emulsion (intralipid) delays gastric emptying, but does not cause gastroesophageal reflux in healthy volunteers. JPEN J Parenter Enteral Nutr 1989;13:246–8.

[54] MacGregor IL, Wiley ZD, Lavigne ME, et al. Slowed rate of gastric emptying of solid food in man by high caloric parenteral nutrition. Am J Surg 1979;138:652–4.

[55] Bursztein-De Myttenaere S, Gil KM, Heymsfield SB, et al. Gastric emptying in humans: influence of different regimens of parenteral nutrition. Am J Clin Nutr 1994;60:244–8.

[56] Peden VH, Witzleben CL, Skelton MA. Total parenteral nutrition. J Pediatr 1971;78:180–1.

[57] Kelly DA. Liver complications of pediatric parenteral nutrition: epidemiology. Nutrition 1998;14:153–7.

[58] Leaseburge LA, Winn NJ, Schloerb PR. Liver test alterations with total parenteral nutrition and nutritional status. JPEN J Parenter Enteral Nutr 1992;16:348–52.

[59] Btaiche IF, Khalidi N. Parenteral nutrition-associated liver complications in children. Pharmacotherapy 2002;22:188–211.

[60] Craig RM, Neumann T, Jeejeebhoy KN, et al. Severe hepatocellular reaction resembling alcoholic hepatitis with cirrhosis after massive small bowel resection and prolonged total parenteral nutrition. Gastroenterology 1980;79:131–7.

[61] Buzby GP, Mullen JL, Stein TP, et al. Manipulation of TPN caloric substrate and fatty infiltration of liver. J Surg Res 1981;31:46–54.

[62] Chan S, McCowen KC, Bistrian BR, et al. Incidence, prognosis, and etiology of end-stage liver disease in patients receiving home total parenteral nutrition. Surgery 1999;126:28–34.

[63] Lowry SF, Brennan MF. Abnormal liver function during parenteral nutrition: relation to infusion excess. J Surg Res 1979;26:300–7.

[64] Meguid MM, Akahoshi MP, Jeffers S, et al. Amelioration of metabolic complications of conventional total parenteral nutrition: a prospective randomized study. Arch Surg 1984;119:1294–8.

[65] Zagara G, Locati L. Role of total parenteral nutrition in determining liver insufficiency in patients with cranial injuries: glucose vs glucose + lipids. Minerva Anesthesiol 1989;55: 509–12.

[66] Tulikoura I, Huikuri K. Morphological fatty changes and function of the liver, serum free fatty acids, and triglycerides during parenteral nutrition. Scand J Gastroenterol 1982;17: 177–85.

[67] Reif S, Tano M, Oliverio R, et al. Total parenteral nutrition-induced steatosis: reversal by parenteral lipid infusion. JPEN J Parenter Enteral Nutr 1991;15:102–4.

[68] Heyman MB, Storch S, Ament ME. The fat overload syndrome: report of a case and literature review. Am J Dis Child 1981;135:628–30.

[69] Cavicchi M, Beau P, Crenn P, et al. Prevalence of liver disease and contributing factors in patients receiving home parenteral nutrition for permanent intestinal failure. Ann Intern Med 2000;132:525–32.

[70] Jobert A, Colomb B, Goulet O, et al. Cholestasis associated with parenteral nutrition in children: role of lipid emulsions [abstract]. Clin Nutr 1997;16:S51.

[71] Krawinkel MB. Parenteral nutrition-associated cholestasis: what do we know, what can we do? Eur J Pediatr Surg 2004;14:230–4.

[72] Ng VL, Balistreri WF. Treatment options for chronic cholestasis in infancy and childhood. Curr Treat Options Gastroenterol 2005;8:419–30.

[73] Schwenk RA, Bauer K, Versmold H. Parenteral nutrition associated cholestasis in the newborn. Klin Padiatr 1998;210:381–9.

[74] Lieber CS. S-adenosyl-L-methionine: its role in the treatment of liver disorders. Am J Clin Nutr 2002;76:1183S–7S.

[75] Moss RL, Haynes AL, Pastuszyn A, et al. Methionine infusion reproduces liver injury of parenteral nutrition cholestasis. Pediatr Res 1999;45:664–8.

[76] Cooper A, Betts JM, Pereira GR, et al. Taurine deficiency in the severe hepatic dysfunction complicating total parenteral nutrition. J Pediatr Surg 1984;19:462–6.

[77] Bowyer BA, Miles JM, Haymond MW, et al. L-Carnitine therapy in home parenteral nutrition patients with abnormal liver tests and low plasma carnitine concentrations. Gastroenterology 1988;94:434–8.

[78] Moukarzel AA, Dahlstrom KA, Buchman AL, et al. Carnitine status of children receiving long-term total parenteral nutrition: a longitudinal prospective study. J Pediatr 1992; 120:759–62.

[79] Bowyer BA, Fleming CR, Ilstrup D, et al. Plasma carnitine levels in patients receiving home parenteral nutrition. Am J Clin Nutr 1986;43:85–91.

[80] Buchman AL, Dubin MD, Moukarzel AA, et al. Choline deficiency: a cause of hepatic steatosis during parenteral nutrition that can be reversed with intravenous choline supplementation. Hepatology 1995;22:1399–403.

[81] Clayton PT, Whitfield P, Iyer K. The role of phytosterols in the pathogenesis of liver complications of pediatric parenteral nutrition. Nutrition 1998;14:158–64.

[82] Clayton PT, Bowron A, Mills KA, et al. Phytosterolemia in children with parenteral nutrition-associated cholestatic liver disease. Gastroenterology 1993;105:1806–13.

[83] Ellegard L, Sunesson A, Bosaeus I. High serum phytosterol levels in short bowel patients on parenteral nutrition support. Clin Nutr 2005;24:415–20.

[84] Luman W, Shaffer JL. Prevalence, outcome and associated factors of deranged liver function tests in patients on home parenteral nutrition. Clin Nutr 2002;21:337–43.

[85] Kumpf VJ. Parenteral nutrition-associated liver disease in adult and pediatric patients. Nutr Clin Pract 2006;21:279–90.

[86] Beath SV, Davies P, Papadopoulou A, et al. Parenteral nutrition-related cholestasis in postsurgical neonates: multivariate analysis of risk factors. J Pediatr Surg 1996;31:604–6.

[87] Spagnuolo MI, Iorio R, Vegnente A, et al. Ursodeoxycholic acid for treatment of cholestasis in children on long-term total parenteral nutrition: a pilot study. Gastroenterology 1996;111:716–9.

[88] Levine A, Maayan A, Shamir R, et al. Parenteral nutrition-associated cholestasis in preterm neonates: evaluation of ursodeoxycholic acid treatment. J Pediatr Endocrinol Metab 1999;12:549–53.

[89] Chen CY, Tsao PN, Chen HL, et al. Ursodeoxycholic acid (UDCA) therapy in very-low-birth-weight infants with parenteral nutrition-associated cholestasis. J Pediatr 2004;145: 317–21.

[90] Lindor KD, Burnes J. Ursodeoxycholic acid for the treatment of home parenteral nutrition-associated cholestasis: a case report. Gastroenterology 1991;101:250–3.

[91] Beau P, Labat-Labourdette J, Ingrand P, et al. Is ursodeoxycholic acid an effective therapy for total parenteral nutrition-related liver disease? J Hepatol 1994;20:240–4.

[92] Teitelbaum DH, Han-Markey T, Schumacher RE. Treatment of parenteral nutrition-associated cholestasis with cholecystokinin-octapeptide. J Pediatr Surg 1995;30: 1082–5.

[93] Teitelbaum DH, Han-Markey T, Drongowski RA, et al. Use of cholecystokinin to prevent the development of parenteral nutrition-associated cholestasis. JPEN J Parenter Enteral Nutr 1997;21:100–3.

[94] Teitelbaum DH, Tracy TF Jr, Aouthmany MM, et al. Use of cholecystokinin-octapeptide for the prevention of parenteral nutrition-associated cholestasis. Pediatrics 2005;115: 1332–40.

[95] Manji N, Bistrian BR, Mascioli EA, et al. Gallstone disease in patients with severe short bowel syndrome dependent on parenteral nutrition. JPEN J Parenter Enteral Nutr 1989;13:461–4.

[96] Roslyn JJ, Pitt HA, Mann LL, et al. Gallbladder disease in patients on long-term parenteral nutrition. Gastroenterology 1983;84:148–54.

[97] Barie PS, Eachempati SR. Acute acalculous cholecystitis. Curr Gastroenterol Rep 2003;5: 302–9.

[98] Messing B, Bories C, Kunstlinger F, et al. Does total parenteral nutrition induce gallbladder sludge formation and lithiasis? Gastroenterology 1983;84:1012–9.

[99] Muller EL, Grace PA, Pitt HA. The effect of parenteral nutrition on biliary calcium and bilirubin. J Surg Res 1986;40:55–62.

[100] Kaufman HS, Magnuson TH, Lillemoe KD, et al. The role of bacteria in gallbladder and common duct stone formation. Ann Surg 1989;209:584–91.

[101] Sitzmann JV, Pitt HA, Steinborn PA, et al. Cholecystokinin prevents parenteral nutrition induced biliary sludge in humans. Surg Gynecol Obstet 1990;170:25–31.

[102] Doty JE, Pitt HA, Porter-Fink V, et al. Cholecystokinin prophylaxis of parenteral nutrition-induced gallbladder disease. Ann Surg 1985;201:76–80.

[103] Tsai S, Strouse PJ, Drongowski RA, et al. Failure of cholecystokinin-octapeptide to prevent TPN-associated gallstone disease. J Pediatr Surg 2005;40:263–7.

[104] Tomida S, Abei M, Yamaguchi T, et al. Long-term ursodeoxycholic acid therapy is associated with reduced risk of biliary pain and acute cholecystitis in patients with gallbladder stones: a cohort analysis. Hepatology 1999;30:6–13.

[105] Kalfarentzos F, Vagenas C, Michail A, et al. Gallbladder contraction after administration of intravenous amino acids and long-chain triacylglycerols in humans. Nutrition 1991;7: 347–9.

[106] Shirohara H, Tabaru A, Otsuki M. Effects of intravenous infusion of amino acids on cholecystokinin release and gallbladder contraction in humans. J Gastroenterol 1996;31: 572–7.

[107] Wu ZS, Yu L, Lin YJ, et al. Rapid intravenous administration of amino acids prevents biliary sludge induced by total parenteral nutrition in humans. J Hepatobiliary Pancreat Surg 2000;7(5):504–9.

[108] de Boer SY, Masclee AA, Jebbink MC, et al. Effect of intravenous fat on cholecystokinin secretion and gallbladder motility in man. JPEN J Parenter Enteral Nutr 1992; 16:16–9.

[109] Phelps S, Dykes E, Pierro A. Bolus intravenous infusion of amino acids or lipids does not stimulate gallbladder contraction in neonates on total parenteral nutrition. J Pediatr Surg 1998;33:817–20.

[110] Fell JM, Reynolds AP, Meadows N, et al. Manganese toxicity in children receiving long-term parenteral nutrition. Lancet 1996;347:1218–21.

[111] Dickerson RN. Manganese intoxication and parenteral nutrition. Nutrition 2001;17: 689–93.

[112] Alves G, Thiebot J, Tracqui A, et al. Neurologic disorders due to brain manganese deposition in a jaundiced patient receiving long-term parenteral nutrition. JPEN J Parenter Enteral Nutr 1997;21:41–5.

[113] Fitzgerald K, Mikalunas V, Rubin H, et al. Hypermanganesemia in patients receiving total parenteral nutrition. JPEN J Parenter Enteral Nutr 1999;23(6):333–6.

[114] Hambidge KM, Sokol RJ, Fidanza SJ, et al. Plasma manganese concentrations in infants and children receiving parenteral nutrition. JPEN J Parenter Enteral Nutr 1989;13: 168–71.

[115] Beath SV, Gopalan S, Booth IW. Manganese toxicity and parenteral nutrition. Lancet 1996;347:1773–4.

[116] Siepler JK, Nishikawa RA, Diamantidis T, et al. Asymptomatic hypermanganesemia in long-term home parenteral nutrition patients. Nutr Clin Pract 2003;18:370–3.

[117] Pironi L, Labate AM, Pertkiewicz M, et al. Espen-Home Artificial Nutrition Working Group. Prevalence of bone disease in patients on home parenteral nutrition. Clin Nutr 2002;21: 289–96.

[118] Cohen-Solal M, Baudoin C, Joly F, et al. Osteoporosis in patients on long-term home parenteral nutrition: a longitudinal study. J Bone Miner Res 2003;18:1989–94.

[119] Haderslev KV, Tjellesen L, Haderslev PH, et al. Assessment of the longitudinal changes in bone mineral density in patients receiving home parenteral nutrition. JPEN J Parenter Enteral Nutr 2004;28:289–94.

[120] Shike M, Harrison JE, Sturtridge WC, et al. Metabolic bone disease in patients receiving long-term total parenteral nutrition. Ann Intern Med 1980;92:343–50.

[121] Klein GL, Targoff CM, Ament ME, et al. Bone disease associated with total parenteral nutrition. Lancet 1980;2:1041–4.

[122] Shike M, Shils ME, Heller A, et al. Bone disease in prolonged parenteral nutrition: osteopenia without mineralization defect. Am J Clin Nutr 1986;44:89–98.

[123] Klein GL, Horst RL, Norman AW, et al. Reduced serum levels of 1 alpha,25-dihydroxyvitamin D during long-term total parenteral nutrition. Ann Intern Med 1981;94: 638–43.

[124] Wood RJ, Bengoa JM, Sitrin MD, et al. Calciuretic effect of cyclic versus continuous total parenteral nutrition. Am J Clin Nutr 1985;41:614–9.

[125] Bengoa JM, Sitrin MD, Wood RJ, et al. Amino acid-induced hypercalciuria in patients on total parenteral nutrition. Am J Clin Nutr 1983;38:264–9.

[126] Berkelhammer CH, Wood RJ, Sitrin MD. Acetate and hypercalciuria during total parenteral nutrition. Am J Clin Nutr 1988;48(6):1482–9.

[127] Wood RJ, Sitrin MD, Cusson GJ, et al. Reduction of total parenteral nutrition-induced urinary calcium loss by increasing the phosphorus in the total parenteral nutrition prescription. JPEN J Parenter Enteral Nutr 1986;10:188–90.

[128] Berkelhammer C, Wood RJ, Sitrin MD. Inorganic phosphorus reduces hypercalciuria during total parenteral nutrition by enhancing renal tubular calcium absorption. JPEN J Parenter Enteral Nutr 1998;22:142–6.

[129] Ott SM, Maloney NA, Klein GL, et al. Aluminum is associated with low bone formation in patients receiving chronic parenteral nutrition. Ann Intern Med 1983;98:910–4.

[130] Vargas JH, Klein GL, Ament ME, et al. Metabolic bone disease of total parenteral nutrition: course after changing from casein to amino acids in parenteral solutions with reduced aluminum content. Am J Clin Nutr 1988;48:1070–8.

[131] Rabinow BE, Ericson S, Shelborne T. Aluminum in parenteral products: analysis, reduction, and implications for pediatric TPN. J Parenter Sci Technol 1989;43:132–9.

[132] Shike M, Sturtridge WC, Tam CS, et al. A possible role of vitamin D in the genesis of parenteral-nutrition-induced metabolic bone disease. Ann Intern Med 1981;95:560–8.

[133] Verhage AH, Cheong WK, Allard JP, et al. Increase in lumbar spine bone mineral content in patients on long-term parenteral nutrition without vitamin D supplementation. JPEN J Parenter Enteral Nutr 1995;19:431–6.

[134] Larchet M, Garabedian M, Bourdeau A, et al. Calcium metabolism in children during long-term total parenteral nutrition: the influence of calcium, phosphorus, and vitamin D intakes. J Pediatr Gastroenterol Nutr 1991;13:367–75.

[135] Fitzgerald KA, MacKay MW. Calcium and phosphate solubility in neonatal parenteral nutrient solutions containing TrophAmine. Am J Hosp Pharm 1986;43:88–93.

[136] de Vernejoul MC, Messing B, Modrowski D, et al. Multifactorial low remodeling bone disease during cyclic total parenteral nutrition. J Clin Endocrinol Metab 1985;60:109–13.

[137] Heller RM, Kirchner SG, O'Neill JA Jr, et al. Skeletal changes of copper deficiency in infants receiving prolonged total parenteral nutrition. J Pediatr 1978;92:947–9.

[138] Haderslev KV, Tjellesen L, Sorensen HA, et al. Effect of cyclical intravenous clodronate therapy on bone mineral density and markers of bone turnover in patients receiving home parenteral nutrition. Am J Clin Nutr 2002;76:482–8.

[139] Wasmuth HH, Verhage CC. Calcitonin treatment of metabolic bone disease induced by parenteral nutrition. Tidsskr Nor Laegeforen 1993;113:1987–9.

[140] Tashjian AH Jr, Gagel RF. Teriparatide [human PTH(1-34)]: 2.5 years of experience on the use and safety of the drug for the treatment of osteoporosis. J Bone Miner Res 2006;21: 354–65.

[141] Haderslev KV, Jeppesen PB, Hartmann B, et al. Short-term administration of glucagon-like peptide-2; effects on bone mineral density and markers of bone turnover in short-bowel patients with no colon. Scand J Gastroenterol 2002;37:392–8.

Gastroenterol Clin N Am 36 (2007) 47–63

GASTROENTEROLOGY CLINICS
OF NORTH AMERICA

ELSEVIER
SAUNDERS

Prebiotics, Probiotics, and Dietary Fiber in Gastrointestinal Disease

Jacqueline Park, MD, Martin H. Floch, MD, MACG, AGAF*

Digestive Disease Section, Yale University School of Medicine, 333 Cedar Street, 1080 LMP, PO Box 208019, New Haven, CT 06520, USA

Microecology of the gastrointestinal tract is the physiologic basis for the effect of dietary fiber, prebiotics and probiotics on the host [1–3]. The ecology consists of the gastrointestinal tract, primarily the intestines, the foods that are fed into the tract, and the flora living within [4]. Within this ecology, normal flora and probiotics ferment dietary fiber and prebiotics to produce short-chain fatty acids (SCFA) and substances that are absorbed and effect the host at the intestinal level and systemically [4,5]. In this review, we discuss the effects of prebiotics, probiotics, and dietary fiber in gastrointestinal disorders and diseases.

DEFINITIONS

Prebiotics are nondigested food ingredients that artificially affect the host by selectively stimulating the growth or activity of one or a number of bacteria in the colon that can improve the host's health [6]. Significant animal and human research have evolved on the subject so that the concept, which was first introduced in 1995, is now accepted [7]. Prebiotic substances are used around the world in varying degrees in different countries. Examples of this are the use of oligosaccharides in Asia and lactulose in the United States [8].

It is clear that prebiotics have little effect on mineral and lipid metabolism in the small bowel and experiments also reveal that they do not affect calcium metabolism. Their affect is primarily in the large intestines [9,10].

It is also clear that oligosaccharides and fructooligosaccharides (FOS) and inulin stimulate *Bifidobacterium* metabolism and growth. Nevertheless, they have not been used extensively in clinical trials but their use will be described below.

Probiotics as defined by Fuller in 1989 [11] are "supplements that benefit the host animal by improving its intestinal microbial balance." They are microbial organisms obtained from humans and used in supplements. Metchnikoff [12] first promulgated the theory of the importance of the intestinal microbial balance in maintaining health in his thesis where he felt that putrefying bacteria were harmful and saccharolytic organisms were beneficial. In 1926, Kipeloff

*Corresponding author. *E-mail address:* martin.floch@yale.edu (M.H. Floch).

0889-8553/07/$ – see front matter
doi:10.1016/j.gtc.2007.03.001

[13] began to introduce the importance of *Lactobacillus acidophilus* and then Rettger and colleagues [14] suggested its therapeutic use. A tremendous amount of research in humans and publications about humans have come forth in the second half of the twentieth century so that now we can finally make recommendations for the clinical use of probiotics [15].

A search of the recent literature reveals that there are approximately 20 organisms that are used as probiotics. These are used in a variety of gastrointestinal disorders and will be described [16]. The literature is now extensive, and at times there are controversies but there is no question that they are being used and that they can be important [16].

Dietary fiber is the nonstarch component of plant foods, but there has been controversy in clearly defining dietary fiber [4]. This is largely due to the chemical analysis of food to isolate specific fibers. There is no question of its importance in health. The theories of Cleave [17], Burkitt and Trowell [18], and Burkitt and colleagues [19] have been confirmed.

Because of its complexity, dietary fiber is difficult to analyze but, nevertheless, chemical analysis enables us to define the fibers as soluble or insoluble [20]. The soluble component is almost completely fermented by the bacterial flora to produce volatile fatty acids, whereas the insoluble component is only slightly fermented and excreted in stool [20]. Dietary fiber tends to have an inhibitory affect on pancreatic enzyme activity, slow the rate of absorbency, and increase stool bulk. Soluble fibers appear to slow transit and stimulate growth of the flora and by the affect on short-chain fatty acid production affect cholesterol metabolism [21].

The recommendation by health organizations is that humans consume anywhere from 25 to 30 g of dietary fiber per day in a mixture of soluble and insoluble fibers. Most studies to date feel that westernized and industrialized societies do not meet this goal, but yet this goal is reached by humans in underdeveloped countries. There is now a tremendous amount of literature on the subject and select references are included [8].

It is important to note that animal foods and diary foods contain no dietary fiber, whereas dietary fiber is contained in plant foods. There are numerous lists of examples of the varying content in plant foods [8].

COLON NEOPLASIA

In 1969, Burkitt [22] reported that common colorectal conditions in the western world, such as diverticulosis and colorectal cancer, were virtually nonexistent in East Africa. This furthered the hypothesis that increased dietary fiber may reduce the risk of colorectal cancer and diverticular disease. Since the early 1990s, with the first publications of prospective cohort studies exploring the relationship between dietary fiber intake and colorectal cancer risk, results have not been consistent; some have found an inverse association between high dietary fiber intake and colorectal neoplasms while others have found no relationship [23–27].

A recent pooled analysis of 13 prospective cohort studies compiled published data on 725,628 subjects followed for 6 to 20 years [28]. A comparison of the highest quintile to the lowest quintile of subjects grouped by dietary fiber intake found an inverse relationship between dietary fiber and colorectal cancer risk. This result was no longer significant when adjustments were made for other dietary risk factors.

Randomized controlled trials exploring the role of dietary fiber for the secondary prevention of colon neoplasia have come to similar conclusions [29–32]. These were large trials in different industrialized populations including Australia, Toronto, and the United States. They found no reduction in colorectal adenoma recurrence with dietary fiber supplementation with or without dietary fat reduction. A Cochrane Review of five randomized controlled trials with 4349 total subjects exploring the effect of dietary fiber on either adenoma recurrence or development of colorectal cancer in patients with a history of adenomatous polyps concluded that there is no evidence that dietary fiber reduces the incidence or recurrence of adenomatous polyps within a 2- to 4-year period [33].

The Women's Health Initiative published findings from a primary prevention trial to look at the effect of dietary modification, including reducing fat and increasing fiber intake on the incidence of colorectal cancer in postmenopausal women [34]. In this trial, 48,835 women over 50 years old were randomized to either a behavioral modification program that effectively decreased dietary fat and increased fiber intake among subjects in this group, or a comparison group. After a mean follow-up of 8 years, there was no evidence of reduced risk of invasive colorectal cancer with dietary intervention. Limitations in this study include failure to achieve their goals for the disparity in fiber intake between the groups. Also, the follow-up period may have been too brief to detect a change in their end point; in fact, the self-reported incidence of polyps or adenomas was lower in the intervention group.

Indeed, these limitations may also apply to other studies that have shown no relationship between dietary fiber and colorectal neoplasia; fiber intake may not have been sufficiently high, or the dietary intervention too late in life to be clinically significant. Also, the specific type or sources of dietary fiber that may ultimately be important in colon neoplasia have not yet been explored. The body of published work does not offer cohesive evidence for the protective role of dietary fiber in colon neoplasia. However, given the other beneficial effects of fiber, particularly in stroke and cardiovascular health, and the possibility that a benefit in colorectal neoplasia exists, it seems prudent to endorse a high-fiber diet to patients.

Although a role in colon neoplasia has been eluded to in some animal experiments employing prebiotics and probiotics, there has been no significant report of any study that demonstrates a clinical role for them in polyps or cancers in humans.

DIVERTICULAR DISEASE

Epidemiologic studies following Burkitt's observations described in colon neoplasia also revealed that diverticulosis is primarily a disease of industrialized and westernized populations [17–19,35–37]. A postmortem survey estimates its prevalence to be 50% of patients over age 70 in industrialized populations [38]. In addition to geographic patterns, epidemiologic studies have also confirmed an association between diverticulosis and low dietary fiber intake [39–42]. Physiologically, this is supported by our understanding of the Law of Laplace. Dietary fiber leads to bulkier stools, an increase in colonic diameter, and decreased intramural pressures [43]. A landmark study in rats reported that a fiber deficiency diet can cause diverticula. Experimentally, rats were divided into nine diet groups and their fiber intake, fecal output, transit time, and the development of acquired diverticula recorded [44]. Although this is an animal study it clearly demonstrates the formation of diverticula with fiber deficiency [44].

There is no evidence that dietary fiber can cause existing diverticula to regress, and no evidence for their use in acute diverticulitis; however, there were uncontrolled studies that did support its use in symptomatic diverticular disease. Patiner and associates [45] and Findlay and associates [46] report studies using unprocessed bran and a significant decrease in symptoms. Similarly, Taylor and Duthie [47] used bran tablets and showed significant relief, as did Brodribb [48] using a high-fiber diet. These four studies stimulated the medical community to prescribe high-fiber diets once diverticula had been identified. However, during acute diverticulitis the recommendation is to be off a high-fiber food diet until symptoms regress [8].

Two open label studies have explored the use of probiotic agents in the prevention of relapse of symptomatic diverticular disease. The first study, conducted in the Czech Republic, enrolled 15 patients with a history of symptomatic uncomplicated diverticular disease characterized by abdominal pain, irregular defecation, bloating, or excessive flatulence [49]. Each patient was treated with an antimicrobial and charcoal for their first episode of symptomatic diverticular disease after enrollment; the second episode was treated with the same therapy followed by *Escherichia coli Nissle 1917* for 6 weeks. The symptom-free period after treatment with the probiotic was significantly longer (mean 14 months) when compared with standard treatment (mean 2.4 months). Another trial similarly demonstrated that patients with a history of symptomatic uncomplicated diverticulosis had a higher likelihood of remaining asymptomatic after 1 year when treated with *Lactobacillus casei* and mesalamine compared with either therapy alone [50]. These studies are preliminary, small, and subject to bias given their open-label design and also limited by the subjective nature of their end points. The results should be followed by larger double-blinded randomized controlled trials to draw any conclusions about the utility of probiotics in diverticular disease.

We are unaware of any significant study of the use of prebiotics in diverticular disease.

IRRITABLE BOWEL SYNDROME

There are two excellent controlled studies using prebiotics. One was a multicenter, prospective, randomized, double-blind, placebo-controlled trial using FOS

[51]. The results were equivocal and did not show any definite benefit. The second study, a double crossover trial, used oligofructose in the clinical parameters of irritable bowel syndrome (IBS) with similar results [52]. Consequently, at the present time, we consider there is no evidence that prebiotics alone are of benefit in IBS [51,52].

Several controlled trials have explored the efficacy of probiotics in ameliorating IBS symptoms. They are quite varied in their use of probiotic strain, dose, and study design. Four results are encouraging to support further investigation, but data as a whole are presently not robust enough to support routine clinical use.

The most promising results may come from studies with *Bifidobacterium infantis*. A preliminary study randomized 77 IBS patients to take a malted drink with *B infantis, Lactobacillus salivarius,* or placebo for 8 weeks [53]. It demonstrated improvement in all IBS symptoms other than stool frequency or consistency in the *B infantis*–treated group, as well as coincident normalization of an abnormal interleukin (IL)-10/IL-12 ratio, suggesting an immune-modulating role of the probiotic. This study was followed by a large multicenter controlled trial [54] that randomized 362 women with IBS of any bowel habit subtype to placebo or one of three doses of *B infantis* for 4 weeks. An intermediate dose of the probiotic was superior to placebo for IBS symptom relief. The authors remark that a problem in the formulation of the highest-dose capsule uncovered in a post hoc experiment explained the lack of a dose-response relationship.

Other trials have been significantly smaller. Two used *Lactobacillus plantarum* [55,56] alone and one a mixture of *L plantarum* with either *Bifidobacterium breve* or *L acidophilus* [57]. These short-term trials resulted in modest improvement in a limited number of IBS symptoms.

Controlled studies with VSL #3 and *Lactobacillus rhamnosis GG (LGG)* did not seem to demonstrate significant improvement in IBS symptoms [58,59].

Regarding a possible role of dietary fiber for the treatment of IBS, a systematic review of 13 randomized controlled trials concluded that bulking agents were not more effective than placebo for global IBS symptoms [60]. These were graded as low to intermediate quality studies with small sample sizes, and used wheat bran, corn fiber, ispaghula husk, or psyllium.

Although that review comes to the conclusion that dietary fiber is not helpful in IBS [60], it must be kept in mind that IBS is a complex of symptoms and can be broken down into subtypes. There is IBS with pain and altered bowel pattern, IBS-D with primary diarrhea, and IBS-C with primary constipation. It is well accepted that dietary fiber can be helpful with constipation. Constipation is not IBS. Therefore, although it has been shown helpful with constipation, it does not clear the complex of defined IBS symptoms [61].

CONSTIPATION

Constipation is a symptom that depends on the patient's description and objective feelings. Most textbooks will accept the definition of less than three bowel movements per week of hard stools [62].

Prebiotics have been shown to be helpful in constipation. When constipated patients were fed inulin, there was change in the microflora that was associated with a high production of short-chain fatty acids. Stools became soft and more frequent with only mild discomfort during defecation [63]. However, except for this one study, there have been no significant reports of benefit with prebiotics or probiotics in the literature.

It is accepted that dietary fiber, by virtue of its water-holding capacity and flora nurturing produces an increase of the colonic microflora. The affect of a type of dietary fiber will affect the type of the stool. For example, high-soluble fibers increase the fermentation and increase the bacteria flora, whereas high-insoluble foods retain more fluid with a bulkier stool [36,64]. This has been demonstrated in clinical areas [21,36,63,64]. It has been shown that a combination of fiber substances such as wheat bran and resistant starch can have a more beneficial affect than simple wheat bran [65]. It is important that nutritionists keep this in mind when they prescribe and vary dietary fiber substances in accordance with the patient's response. It is important to remember facts like wheat bran is 90% insoluble, whereas oat bran is 50% soluble and insoluble, and psyllium seed is 90% soluble. Substances such as guar that are added to help decrease constipation are 100% soluble [8].

INFLAMMATORY BOWEL DISEASE (IBD)
Crohn's Disease

There are no significant uncontrolled studies in the use of prebiotics in Crohn's disease.

Several studies have explored the use of probiotic organisms in the treatment of Crohn's disease with varied results. As a whole, published studies are not consistent in their use or dose of particular probiotic strains, further confusing the evidence for specific therapies. An early double-blind randomized pilot study investigating the use of the nonpathogenic *E coli* strain, *Nissle 1917*, in maintaining remission in patients with Crohn's colitis found a trend toward reduced risk of relapse in the probiotic group compared with those receiving placebo (33% and 64% respectively); but statistical significance was not reached [66].

Subsequently, a number of studies using other probiotic strains have explored their efficacy in maintenance of medically induced remission of Crohn's disease. In a study with 32 patients, Guslandi and colleagues [67] demonstrated a significantly lower risk of clinical relapse over 6 months of follow-up in patients taking mesalamine and *Saccharomyces boulardii* (6%) compared with those take mesalamine alone (38%). Plein and Hotz [68] had first reported effectiveness in a small pilot study with *S boulardii*. A larger study in pediatric patients with Crohn's disease randomized to *LGG* or placebo in addition to standard medical therapy failed to show an improvement in incidence or time to relapse in patients taking the *LGG* [69].

Studies exploring the use of probiotics in the maintenance of postoperative Crohn's remission are similarly limited and inconsistent in their results.

A double-blind randomized controlled trial published only as an abstract [70] looked at VSL #3 in maintaining surgically induced remission of Crohn's disease. Forty patients were randomized in a blinded fashion to receive rifaximin followed by VSL #3 or mesalamine for 1 year following surgery. The probiotic group had a significantly higher rate of endoscopic remission (80%) compared with standard therapy (60%); the interpretation of these results is hampered by the additional variable of rifaximin in the probiotic group.

A subsequent study using *LGG* [71] failed to show efficacy in maintaining postoperative recurrence. Thirty-seven patients were randomized to receive *LGG* or placebo for 1 year following intestinal resection for Crohn's disease. There was no statistically significant difference between the groups in symptomatic or endoscopic recurrence. A larger, recent double-blind randomized controlled study with 98 patients failed to demonstrated the efficacy of *Lactobacillus johnsonii* in preventing postoperative endoscopic or clinical recurrence of Crohn's disease over 6 months of follow-up [72].

There have been two small open-label trials that demonstrate efficacy of probiotic therapy for the treatment of active Crohn's disease. Gupta and colleagues [73] reported a preliminary open-label pilot study using *LGG* in four children with mildly to moderately active Crohn's disease for 6 months. There was significant improvement in clinical activity beginning at 1 week following initiation of therapy that was sustained throughout the study period, and coincident improvement in intestinal permeability but there has been no published follow-up to these results [73].

Significant improvement in the Crohn's Disease Activity Index score was reported in an abstract [74] in another open-label study in 25 adult patients with mild to moderately active Crohn's disease treated with *Lactobacillus salivarius.*

In summary, there are varied results in the studies using varied probiotic strains in the maintenance of medically or surgically induced remission, as well as the treatment of active inflammation in patients with Crohn's disease. The particular strain of probiotic organism, and possibly the dose, may explain the variation in results. It is also possible that clinical efficacy may have not have been detected because of inadequate sample sizes or duration of follow-up. To date, however, there is insufficient evidence to support or discourage the use of probiotic therapy in patients with Crohn's except with the *S boulardii* results [67].

There have been no significant controlled studies on the use of dietary fiber in Crohn's disease patients.

Ulcerative Colitis

There have only been two reports on the use of prebiotics in ulcerative colitis (UC). Both of those employ germinated barley food [75,76]. In reality, it contains a large amount of FOS. In one study, they found a significant decrease in clinical activity index [75]. Unfortunately, this was a small number of patients. Another study open-label protocol for 24 weeks, the investigators also showed an improvement in clinical activity of UC [75]. These are only two small studies [75,76] and there is nothing else in the literature to substantiate the use of prebiotics.

Most studies investigating the use of probiotics for UC explore their efficacy in the maintenance of remission as opposed to the treatment of active disease.

Five studies have been reported for use as maintenance with varied success. Three with *E coli Nissle*, one with VSL, and one with *LGG*. The Italian investigators performed an open-label study exploring the efficacy of probiotic therapy for the maintenance of remission [77]. VSL #3 was administered for 12 months to 20 patients with UC in remission and intolerant or allergic to 5-ASA compounds. Fifteen of 20 patients remained in clinical and endoscopic remission over the course of the study. Fecal analysis demonstrated gut colonization by the strains contained in VSL #3, supporting the role of these probiotic organisms in preventing relapse.

Controlled studies using *E coli Nissle* have demonstrated equivalence with low-dose mesalamine in maintaining remission [78]. Superiority studies were not performed due to the proven efficacy of 5-ASA compounds in maintenance of UC and the ethical implications of using placebo. In this earliest study, 103 patients with quiescent UC were randomized to take mesalazine or *E coli Nissle* for 12 weeks. There was no significant difference between the two groups in rate or duration of clinical relapse.

Another double-blind, double-dummy randomized controlled trial investigating the equivalence of *E coli Nissle* to mesalamine in achieving and maintaining remission in UC reached similar conclusions [79]. In this trial, 116 patients with active UC were randomized to take either mesalamine or *E coli Nissle* with standard medical therapy (topical or systemic corticosteroids) to induce remission, and were continued on mesalamine or *E coli Nissle* following remission. Gentamicin was given to all patients at the start of the study to suppress native *E coli* flora. The primary end points were rate and time to relapse; secondary end points included rate and time to remission. There was no significant difference in end points between the two groups; the authors concluded that *E coli Nissle* was as effective as mesalazine in maintaining remission of UC.

Kruis and colleagues' initial study [78] was criticized for its short duration of follow-up; the second study with *E coli Nissle* may have been limited by the heterogeneity of the patient population, a relatively low mesalamine dose, and the high rate of relapse that limited the statistical power of the study [80]. In response to this, Kruis and colleagues [81] performed a much larger study to confirm the equivalence of *E coli Nissle* to mesalazine for maintenance of remission. In this double-blind, double-dummy trial, 327 patients were randomized to either *E coli Nissle* or mesalamine for 1 year. Almost one third of patients discontinued the study prematurely for varied reasons. Per protocol analysis of the remaining 222 patients as well as intention-to-treat analysis confirmed equivalence of probiotic and mesalazine therapy in maintenance of remission.

A recent randomized open-label study exploring the use of *LGG* in 187 patients with quiescent UC demonstrated equivalence of the probiotic with mesalamine in maintaining remission over a 1-year period [82]. It also demonstrated a longer duration of remission with probiotic therapy.

Five studies have reported on active UC. In 2003, bacteriotherapy was reported to be used in six patients with active, difficult-to-treat UC on steroids. Resolution of symptoms 4 months after administration of donor fecal suspension enemas was recorded [83]. There are many anecdotal and case reports on fecal bacteriotherapy but no large studies.

A pilot study investigating the use of probiotics for active UC using *S boulardii* in steroid-intolerant patients showed promising results; 17 of 24 patients taking the probiotic for 4 weeks achieved clinical and endoscopic remission [84].

An unblinded Italian study randomized 90 patients with active mild-to-moderate, primarily left-sided, UC to low-dose balsalazide with VSL #3, medium dose balsalazide, or mesalazine for 8 weeks [85]. More patients receiving VSL #3 with balsalazide achieved remission, and more quickly, when compared with the other groups. The data between the groups demonstrated overlap in confidence intervals for both intention-to-treat and per protocol data. In another uncontrolled study on 32 patients with active, severe UC, VSL #3 administered for 6 weeks achieved a 56% clinical remission, a response in 25%, and no response in 9% with worsening in 9% [86].

A coincident Japanese study randomized 20 patients with mild to moderate active UC to *Bifidobacteria*-fermented milk or placebo for 12 weeks along with standard medical therapy without steroids. Treatment with *Bifidobacteria*-fermented milk was more effective than placebo in diminishing UC clinically, endoscopically and histologically [87].

These 10 studies using probiotics in acute and remission UC report positive results in varying degrees but seem to be more promising than the experience in Crohn's disease. *LGG* and VSL are available worldwide, but *E coli Nissle* is not. More studies are needed before any firm recommendations can be made.

Although dietary fiber substances have not been used in inflammatory bowel disease, it should be noted that attempts to treat UC with the final product of fermentation, SCFA, particular butyric acids, have demonstrated varying results. Initially, diversion colitis was successfully treated with SCFA [88] but then attempts to treat UC proved inconsistent. There is no question that butyric acid is the main fuel for the colonicyte and there is some evidence that the colitis mucosa is unable to metabolize the butyric acid [89,90]. However, carefully controlled studies in 103 patients from several institutions using topical SCFA twice daily revealed conflicting results [91]. The consensus opinion from the data was that SCFA cannot be recommended consistently [91].

Pouchitis

Proctocolectomy with formation of an ileal reservoir, or pouch, followed by anastomosis to the anus (IPPA) is often performed for patients with UC or familial adenomatous polyposis syndrome (FAP). Inflammation of the pouch, or pouchitis, is a common complication particularly in those whose indication was UC with extraintestinal manifestations [92]. The cumulative risk of developing pouchitis in patients who had UC may exceed 50% at 4 years following surgery [93].

Standard therapy for pouchitis includes antibiotic therapy, most commonly metronidazole or ciprofloxacin. Given bacterial stasis as a possible etiological factor in the development of pouchitis, the use of probiotics and their ability to alter intestinal and pouch flora has been investigated for treatment or prevention of pouchitis. Three notable double-blinded random controlled trials have demonstrated the efficacy of the probiotic mixture VSL #3 in the primary prevention or maintenance of remission of pouchitis. VSL #3 contains a high concentration of eight strains of lactic acid bacteria, including *B breve, Bifidobacterium longum, B infantis, L acidophilus, L plantarum, L casei, Lactobacillus bulgaricus,* and *Streptococcus thermophilus.*

In the first controlled trial for the use of probiotics in prevention of pouchitis [94], 40 patients with relapsing pouchitis in remission were randomized in a double-blind manner to receive either VSL #3 at a dose of 6 g daily or placebo. A 9-month follow-up period consisted of monthly clinical assessments and bimonthly endoscopic surveillance with biopsies. There was a statistically significant decrease in the recurrence of pouchitis in the probiotic group; 15% of patients taking VSL #3 and 100% of the control group experienced relapse. The organisms contained in VSL #3 were recovered in feces from the probiotic group. Continued use of the probiotic formulation may be necessary, as fecal flora returned to pretreatment levels 1 month after discontinuation of VSL #3, and all of these patients experienced recurrent pouchitis within 3 months of cessation.

These results were replicated in another double-blind randomized controlled trial [95] in 36 patients with more severe recurrent pouchitis over a longer follow-up period of 1 year. It demonstrated that a significantly higher number of the patients taking VSL #3 (85%) maintained remission compared with the placebo group (6%). Over the course of the year, quality of life as assessed by the IBD Questionnaire (IBDQ) score remained high in the VSL #3 group, but significantly decreased in the placebo group.

Gionchetti and colleagues [96] also investigated the efficacy of VSL #3 in the primary prophylaxis of pouchitis. Forty patients who had undergone IPAA for UC were followed for 1 year after randomization to VSL #3 or placebo in a double-blinded fashion. By clinical, endoscopic, and histologic investigation, those in the VSL #3 group had significantly fewer (10%) episodes of pouchitis than those receiving placebo (40%), and also had a significant improvement in quality of life, measured by the IBDQ score.

Taken together, these Italian studies support the theory that pouchitis may result from fecal microbial imbalance, and that altering pouch bacteria with probiotics, specifically VSL #3, may play an important part in restoring the balance and preventing pouchitis. However, these results have not been replicated.

Shen and colleagues [97] reported an uncontrolled study to determine the compliance and efficacy of VSL#3 use in the maintenance of remission in routine care in a US population. Thirty-one patients with pouchitis effectively treated with ciprofloxacin were given VSL #3 for 8 months and followed for a mean of 14 months. At the 8-month follow-up period, the majority of patients had discontinued therapy because of either recurrence of pouchitis or adverse symptoms that were not clearly a result of VSL #3 use. The six (19%) who remained on therapy remained in symptomatic remission, but had endoscopic Pouchitis Disease Activity Index scores at the end of treatment that were not statistically different from their baseline score preceding antibiotics. This study demonstrated that only a minority of patients on VSL #3 will remain on therapy and remain in endoscopic remission during therapy. One notable difference in this patient population is that they all had a more severe, *antibiotic-dependent* pouchitis, requiring frequent or continuous low-dose antibiotic therapy to remain in remission. It is unclear if the higher severity of underlying disease affected study results.

Most authorities accept the evidence that VSL #3 is effective in controlling pouchitis, but further studies should prove the efficacy in various situations.

There have been no studies reporting the use of dietary fiber substances in pouchitis.

DIARRHEA

The most common gastrointestinal disorder worldwide is diarrhea. There have been no significant studies employing prebiotics; however, it is not surprising that the most common studies employing probiotics have been with diarrhea [16]. There are several studies reported in the literature in adults with diarrhea using a variety of organisms. Because of the range of doses of organisms, it is difficult to do any analysis of these studies but all six of the articles report improvement in diarrhea by either shortening the course or decreasing the severity [16].

Another analysis of diarrhea in children who had standard rehydration therapy plus a probiotic clearly revealed that the diarrhea is shortened by at least 1 day when a probiotic is used. A wide range of probiotics, again, have been used and it is difficult to make any recommendation. Nevertheless, consensus opinion of experts clearly reveal that probiotics shorten the course of diarrhea and the recommendation is that they should be used at the onset in children [98].

There are no clinically significant studies to demonstrate that dietary fiber is effective in treating diarrhea. Nevertheless, there are many that use foods to decrease diarrhea such as the classic rice/banana diets.

ANTIBIOTIC-ASSOCIATED DIARRHEA

Antibiotic-associated diarrhea was first described in the 1950s and early clinical correlations believed *Staphylococcus aureus* infection caused the disease [99]. It wasn't until the 1970s that it was firmly established that *C difficile* was the most common cause of diarrhea post antibiotic use [99]. At first, clindomycin was considered the antibiotic cause, but at this time almost any of the antibiotics can alter the bacterial flora so that *C difficile* causes diarrhea as a result of its toxins or even a severe enterocolitis [99].

There has been increasing interest in the use of probiotics to treat C difficile–associated diarrhea (CDAD), given the increasing frequency of recurrent and severe cases in many centers. Successful treatment of recurrent CDAD with donor stool delivered via nasogastric tube [100] or colonoscope [101] have been published in case reports. This strategy is based on the presumption that repopulation of the colon with normal nonpathogenic fecal flora may inhibit the proliferation of C difficile.

Alteration of the gut flora with specific probiotic therapy has been investigated more formally with randomized controlled trials. The following two articles have attempted to synthesize the data [102,103]. All of the primary outcome studies used in this systematic review were included in a recent meta-analysis of six blinded randomized controlled trials, with a total of 354 patients, to assess the efficacy of probiotics for the treatment of C difficile– associated diarrhea [104]. Probiotic strains included S boulardii, LGG, L plantarum, and a mixture of Bifidobacterium bifidus and L acidophilus. The pooled relative risk for CDAD in the probiotic group was 0.59 (95% confidence interval [CI] 0.41, 0.85). Of the probiotic strains, only S boulardii led to a significant reduction in recurrence. Consensus opinion of specialists evaluating the clinical use of probiotics felt that both S boulardii on the basis of the seminal work by Surawicz and colleagues [102] and the several studies reported on LGG were significant and, hence, both of these probiotics could be given a high recommendation in the treatment of recurrent infection [102]. No adverse events such as bacteremia or fungemia were reported in the trials.

A conflicting systematic review of controlled trials exploring probiotic therapy for CDAD based on four studies concluded that there is insufficient evidence to support the use of probiotics for prevention or treatment of CDAD [103]. Of the four eligible studies with CDAD prevention or treatment as the primary outcome, two studies had methodologic flaws that limited interpretation. The other two studies demonstrated benefit of probiotic therapy in subgroups with severe CDAD. Four trials with CDAD prevention as a secondary outcome provided no evidence that probiotic prophylaxis was beneficial, although the strength of these conclusions was limited by the small number of CDAD cases [103].

A positive result was reported in the only published controlled trial exploring the efficacy of prebiotics for CDAD recurrence. Hospitalized patients with CDAD were randomized in a double-blind fashion to 30 days of oligofructose or placebo in addition to standard antibiotic treatment and followed for an additional 30 days for recurrence of diarrhea [105]. An increase in fecal Bifidobacterium in patients receiving oligofructose confirmed its prebiotic effect. There was a significantly lower incidence of recurrent diarrhea in the prebiotic group when compared with placebo (8% versus 34% respectively, $P < .001$).

HEPATIC ENCEPHALOPATHY

It is now well accepted that one of the main treatments of hepatic encephalopathy is the prebiotic lactulose [106]. The mechanism by which lactulose works is still not totally clear but it definitely results in decreasing clinical hepatic encephalopathy, a drop in stool pH, and increased excretion of nitrogen. Fecal studies did show a change in the intestinal microflora and it can be assumed that lactulose as a prebiotic does alter the intestinal microecology resulting in these beneficial effects [107].

There have been a few probiotic studies but none have resulted in clinical significance.

A high vegetable diet has been recommended to be beneficial but rather than on the basis of dietary fiber, the basis has been presumed to be a difference in vegetable protein versus animal protein [108].

References

[1] Luckey TD. Introduction to intestinal microecology. Am J Clin Nutr 1992;25:1292–4.
[2] Vonk RJ. Manipulation of colonic flora as ecosystem and metabolic organ: consequences for the organism. Scand J Gastroenterol 1997;32(222):1–114.
[3] Hart AL, Stagg AJ, Graffner H, et al. Gut ecology. London: Martin Dunitz Ltd; 2002.
[4] Floch MH, Moussa K. Probiotics and dietary fiber. The clinical coming of age of intestinal microecology. J Clin Gastroenterol 1998;27:99–100.
[5] Floch MH. Soluble dietary fiber and short-chain fatty acids: an advance in understanding the human bacterial flora. Am J Gastroenterol 1990;85:1074–6.
[6] Gibson GR, Roberfroid MB. Dietary modulation of the human colonic microbiotia: introducing the concept of prebiotics. J Nutr 1995;125:1401–12.
[7] Cummings JH, Macfarlane GT, Englyst HN. Prebiotic digestion and fermentation. Am J Clin Nutr 2001;73(Suppl):4155–205.
[8] Floch MH. Prebiotics, probiotics and dietary fiber. In: Buchman AL, editor. Clinical nutrition in gastrointestinal disease. Thorofare (NJ): Slack; 2006.
[9] Crittenden RG. Prebiotics. In: Tannock GW, editor. Probiotics: a critical review. Wymondham (UK): Horizon Scientific Press; 1999. p. 141–56.
[10] Rastall RA, Gibson GR. Prebiotic oligosaccharides: evaluation of biological activities and potential future developments. In: Tannock GW, editor. Probiotics and Prebiotics: where are we going? Norfolk (UK): Calister Academic Press; 2002. p. 107–48.
[11] Fuller R. Probiotics in man and animals. J Appl Bacteriol 1989;66:365–78.
[12] Metchnikoff E. The prolongation of life: optimistic studies. London: Butterworth-Heinemann; 1907.
[13] Kipeloff N. Lactobacillus acidophilus. Baltimore (MD): Williams & Wilkins; 1926.
[14] Rettger LF, Levy MN, Weinstein L, et al. Lactobacillus acidophilus and its therapeutic application. London: Yale University Press; 1935.
[15] Montrose D, Floch MH. Probiotics used in human studies. J Clin Gastroenterol 2005;39:469–80.
[16] Floch MH, Montrose DC. Use of probiotics in humans: an analysis of the literature. Gastroenterol Clin North Am 2005;34:547–70.
[17] Cleave TL. The saccharine disease. New Canaan (CT): Keats Publishing, Inc.; 1975.
[18] Burkitt DP, Trowell HC. Refined carbohydrate foods and disease: some implications of dietary fiber. London: Academic Press; 1975.
[19] Burkitt DP, Walker ARP, Painter NS. Dietary fiber and disease. JAMA 1974;229:1068–74.
[20] Asp N-GL. Classification and methodology of food carbohydrates is related to nutritional effects. Am J Clin Nutr 1995;61(Suppl):930S–7S.
[21] Cummings JH, Englyst HN. Gastrointestinal effects of food carbohydrate. Am J Clin Nutr 1995;61(Suppl):938S–45S.
[22] Burkitt DP. Related disease—related cause? Lancet 1969;2:1229–31.

[23] Larsson SC, Giovannucci E, Bergkvist L, et al. Whole grain consumption and risk of colorectal cancer: a population-based cohort of 60,000 women. Br J Cancer 2005;92(9):1803–7.

[24] Peters U, Sinha R, Chatterjee N, et al. Dietary fibre and colorectal adenoma in a colorectal cancer early detection programme. Lancet 2003;361(9368):1491–5.

[25] Bingham SA, Day NE, Luben R, et al. Dietary fibre in food and protection against colorectal cancer in the European Prospective Investigation into Cancer and Nutrition (EPIC): an observational study. Lancet 2003;361(9368):1496–501.

[26] Fuchs CS, Giovannucci EL, Colditz GA, et al. Dietary fiber and the risk of colorectal cancer and adenoma in women. N Engl J Med 1999;340(3):169–76.

[27] Thun MF, Calle EE, Namboodiri MM, et al. Risk factors for fatal colon cancer in a large prospective study. J Natl Cancer Inst 1992;84(19):1491–500.

[28] Park Y, Hunter DJ, Spiegelman D, et al. Dietary fiber intake and risk of colorectal cancer: a pooled analysis of prospective cohort studies. JAMA 2005;294(22):2849–57.

[29] MacLennan R, Macrae F, Bain C, et al. Randomized trial of intake of fat, fiber, and beta carotene to prevent colorectal adenomas: the Australian polyp prevention project. J Natl Cancer Inst 1995;87:1760–6.

[30] McKeown-Eyssen GE, Bright-See E, Bruce WR, et al. A randomized trial of a low fat high fibre diet in the recurrence of colorectal polyps: Toronto Polyp Prevention Group. J Clin Epidemiol 1994;47:525–36.

[31] Schatzkin A, Lanza E, Corle D, et al. Lack of effect of a low-fat, high-fiber diet on the recurrence of colorectal adenomas. Polyp Prevention Trial Study Group. N Engl J Med 2000;342:1149–55.

[32] Alberts DS, Martinez ME, Roe DJ, et al. Lack of effect of a high-fiber cereal supplement on the recurrence of colorectal adenomas. Phoenix Colon Cancer Prevention Physicians' Network. N Engl J Med 2000;342:1156–61.

[33] Asano T, McLeod RS. Dietary fibre for the prevention of colorectal adenomas and carcinomas. Cochrane Database Syst Rev 2002;2:CD003430.

[34] Beresford SA, Johnson KC, Ritenbaugh C, et al. Low-fat dietary pattern and risk of colorectal cancer: the women's health initiative randomized controlled dietary modification trial. JAMA 2006;295(6):643–54.

[35] Almy TP, Howell DA. Diverticular disease of the colon. N Engl J Med 1980;302:324–30.

[36] Trowell H, Burkitt DP, Heaton K. Dietary fibre, fibre-depleted foods and disease. London: Academic Press; 1985.

[37] Painter NS. The cause of diverticular disease of the colon, its symptoms and complications: review and hypothesis. J R Coll Surg Edinb 1985;30:118–26.

[38] Hughes LE. Postmortem survey of diverticular disease of the colon. Gut 1969;10:336–51.

[39] Painter NS, Trowell H, Burkitt DP, et al. Diverticular disease of the colon. In: Trowell H, Burkitt D, Heaton D, editors. Dietary fibre, fibre-depleted foods and disease. London: Academic Press; 1985. p. 145–60.

[40] Aldoori WH, Giovannucci EL, Rimm EB, et al. A prospective study of diet and the risk of symptomatic diverticular disease in men. Am J Clin Nutr 1994;60:757–63.

[41] Nair P, Mayberry JF. Vegetarianism, dietary fibre and gastrointestinal disease. Dig Dis 1994;12:177–82.

[42] Korzenik JR. Case closed? Diverticulitis: epidemiology and fiber. J Clin Gastroenterol 2006;40:S112–6.

[43] Painter NS, Burkitt DP. Diverticular disease of the colon, a 20th century problem. Clin Gastroenterol 1975;4:3–12.

[44] Fisher N, Berry CS, Fearn T, et al. Cereal dietary fiber consumption and diverticular disease: a lifespan study in rats. Am J Clin Nutr 1985;42:788–804.

[45] Patiner NS, Almeida AZ, Colebourn KW. Unprocessed bran in treatment of diverticular disease of colon. Br Med J 1972;2:137–40.

[46] Findlay JM, Smith AN, Mitchell WD, et al. Effects of unprocessed bran on colon function in normal subjects and in diverticular disease. Lancet 1974;1:146–9.

[47] Taylor I, Duthie HL. Bran tablets and diverticular disease. Br Med J 1976;1:988–90.

[48] Brodribb AJM. Treatment of symptomatic diverticular disease with high-fibre diet. Lancet 1997;2:664–6.

[49] Fric P, Zavoral M. The effect of non-pathogenic *Escherichia coli* in symptomatic uncomplicated diverticular disease of the colon. Eur J Gastroenterol Hepatol 2003;15: 313–5.

[50] Tursi A, Brandimarte G, Elisei W, et al. Mesalamine and/or *Lactobacillus casei* for maintaining remission of symptomatic uncomplicated diverticular disease of the colon: a prospective, randomized study. Dig Liver Dis 2005;37; S20–26.

[51] Olesen M, Gudmand-Hoyer E. Efficacy, safety, and tolerability of fructooligosaccharides in the treatment of irritable bowel syndrome. Am J Clin Nutr 2000;72(6):1570–5.

[52] Hunter JO, Tuffnell Q, Lee AJ. Controlled trial of oligofructose in the management of irritable bowel syndrome. J Nutr 1999;129(7 Suppl):1451S–3S.

[53] O'Mahony L, McCarthy J, Kelly P, et al. *Lactobacillus* and *Bifidobacterium* in irritable bowel syndrome: symptom responses and relationship to cytokine profiles. Gastroenterology 2005;128(3):541–51.

[54] Whorwell PJ, Altringer L, Morel J, et al. Efficacy of an encapsulated probiotic *Bifidobacterium infantis* 35624 in women with irritable bowel syndrome. Am J Gastroenterol 2006;101(7):1581–90.

[55] Nobaek S, Johansson ML, Molin G, et al. Alteration of intestinal microflora is associated with reduction in abdominal bloating and pain in patients with irritable bowel syndrome. Am J Gastroenterol 2000;95(5):1231–8.

[56] Niedzielin K, Kordecki H, Birkenfeld B. A controlled, double-blind, randomized study on the efficacy of *Lactobacillus plantarum* 299V in patients with irritable bowel syndrome. Eur J Gastroenterol Hepatol 2001;13(10):1143–7.

[57] Saggioro A. Probiotics in the treatment of irritable bowel syndrome. J Clin Gastroenterol 2004;38(6 Suppl):S104–6.

[58] Kim HJ, Camilleri M, McKinzie S, et al. A randomized controlled trial of a probiotic, VSL#3, on gut transit and symptoms in diarrhea-predominant irritable bowel syndrome. Aliment Pharmacol Ther 2003;17(7):895–904.

[59] O'Sullivan MA, O'Morain CA. Bacterial supplementation in the irritable bowel syndrome. A randomised double-blind placebo-controlled crossover study. Dig Liver Dis 2000;32(4): 294–301.

[60] Jailwala J, Imperiale TF, Kroenke K. Pharmacologic treatment of the irritable bowel syndrome: a systematic review. Ann Intern Med 2000;133(2):136–47.

[61] Floch MH, Narayan R. Diet in the irritable bowel syndrome. J Clin Gastroenterol 2002; 35(Suppl):S45–52.

[62] Floch MH. Netter's gastroenterology. Philadelphia: Elsevier; 2005.

[63] Cummings JH, Southgate DAT, Branch W, et al. Colonic response to dietary fibre from carrot, cabbage, apple, bran and guar gum. Lancet 1978;1:5–9.

[64] Spiller GA. Dietary fiber in human nutrition. 2nd edition. Boca Raton (FL): CRC Press, Inc.; 1993.

[65] Muir JG, Yeow EGS, Keogh J, et al. Combining wheat bran with resistant starch has more beneficial effects on fecal indexes than does wheat bran alone. Am J Clin Nutr 2004;79: 1020–8.

[66] Malchow HA. Crohn's disease and *Escherichia coli*. A new approach in therapy to maintain remission of colonic Crohn's disease? J Clin Gastroenterol 1997;25(4): 653–8.

[67] Guslandi M, Messi G, Sorghi M, et al. *Saccharomyces boulardii* in maintenance treatment of Crohn's disease. Dig Dis Sci 2000;45:1462–4.

[68] Plein K, Hotz J. Therapeutic effects of *Saccharomyces boulardii* on mild residual symptoms in a stable phase of Crohn's disease with special respect to chronic diarrhea—a pilot study. Z Gastroenterol 1993;31:129–34.

[69] Bousvaros A, Guandalini S, Baldassano R, et al. A randomized, double-blind trial of *Lactobacillus GG* versus placebo in addition to standard maintenance therapy for children with Crohn's disease. Inflamm Bowel Dis 2005;11(9):833–9.

[70] Campieri M, Rizzello F, Venturi A, et al. Combination of antibiotic and probiotic treatment is efficacious in prophylaxis of post-operative recurrence of Crohn's disease: a randomized controlled study versus mesalamine. Gastroenterology 2000;118:A781.

[71] Prantera C, Scribano ML, Falasco G, et al. Ineffectiveness of probiotics in preventing recurrence after curative resection for Crohn's disease. A randomized controlled trial with *Lactobacillus GG*. Gut 2002;51:405–9.

[72] Marteau P, Lemann M, Seksik P, et al. Ineffectiveness of *Lactobacillus johnsonii* LA1 for prophylaxis of postoperative recurrence in Crohn's disease: a randomised, double blind, placebo controlled GETAID trial. Gut 2006;55(6):842–7. Epub 2005 Dec 23.

[73] Gupta P, Andrew H, Kirschner BS, et al. Is *Lactobacillus GG* helpful in children with Crohn's disease? Results of a preliminary, open-label study. J Pediatr Gastroenterol Nutr 2000; 31(4):453–7.

[74] McCarthy J, O'Mahony L, Dunne C, et al. An open trial of a novel probiotic as an alternative to steroids in mild/moderately active Crohn's disease. Gut 2001;49(Suppl 3):A2447.

[75] Kanauchi O, Mitsuyama K, Araki Y, et al. Modification of intestinal flora in the treatment of inflammatory bowel disease. Curr Pharm Des 2003;9:333–46.

[76] Kanauchi O, Mitsuyama K, Homma T, et al. Treatment of ulcerative colitis patients by long-term administration of germinated barley foodstuff: multi-center open trial. Int J Mol Med 2003;12(5):701–4.

[77] Venturi A, Gionchetti P, Rizzello F, et al. Impact on the composition of the fecal flora by a new probiotic preparation: preliminary data on maintenance treatment of patients with ulcerative colitis. Aliment Pharmcol Ther 1999;13:1103–8.

[78] Kruis W, Schutz E, Fric P, et al. Double-blind comparison of an oral *Escherichia coli* preparation and mesalazine in maintaining remission of ulcerative colitis. Aliment Pharmcol Ther 1997;11:853–8.

[79] Rembacken BJ, Snelling AM, Hawkey PM, et al. Non-pathogenic *Escherichia coli* versus mesalazine for the treatment of ulcerative colitis: a randomized trial. Lancet 1999;354: 635–9.

[80] Faubion WA, Sandborn WJ. Probiotic therapy with *E. coli* for ulcerative colitis: take the good with the bad. Gastroenterology 2000;118:630–1.

[81] Kruis W, Fric P, Pokrotnieks J, et al. Maintaining remission of ulcerative colitis with the probiotic *Escherichia coli Nissle1917* is as effective as with standard mesalazine. Gut 2004;53(11):1617–23.

[82] Zocco MA, Dal Verme LZ, Cremonini F, et al. Efficacy of *Lactobacillus GG* in maintaining remission of ulcerative colitis. Aliment Pharmacol Ther 2006;23(11):1567–74.

[83] Borody TJ, Warren EF, Leis SL, et al. Treatment of ulcerative colitis using fecal bacteriotherapy. J Clin Gastroenterol 2003;37(1):42–7.

[84] Guslandi M, Patrizia G, Testoni PA. A pilot trial of *Saccharomyces boulardii* in ulcerative colitis. Eur J Gastroenterol Hepatol 2003;15:697–8.

[85] Tursi A, Brandimarte G, Giorgetti GM, et al. Low-dose balsalazide plus a high-potency probiotic preparation is more effective than balsalazide alone or mesalazine in the treatment of acute mild-to-moderate ulcerative colitis. Med Sci Monit 2004;10(11):PI126–31. Epub 2004 Oct 26.

[86] Bibiloni R, Fedorak RN, Tannock GW, et al. VSL #3 probiotic mixture induces remission in patients with active ulcerative colitis. Am J Gastroenterol 2005;100:1539–46.

[87] Kato K, Mizuno S, Umesaki Y, et al. Randomized placebo-controlled trial assessing the effect of *Bifidobacteria*-fermented milk on active ulcerative colitis. Aliment Pharmacol Ther 2004;20:1133–41.

[88] Harig JM, Soegel KH, Komorowski RA, et al. Treatment of diversion colitis with short-chain fatty acid irrigation. N Engl J Med 1989;320:23–7.

[89] Roediger WEW, Nance S. Metabolic induction of experimental ulcerative colitis by inhibition of fatty acid oxidation. Br J Exp Pathol 1986;67:773–82.

[90] Scheppach W, Sommer H, Kirchner T, et al. Effect of butyrate enemas on the colonic mucosa in distal ulcerative colitis. Gastroenterology 1992;103:51–6.

[91] Breuer RI, Soergel KH, Lashner BA, et al. Short chain fatty acid rectal irrigation for left-sided ulcerative colitis: a randomized, placebo controlled trial. Gut 1997;40:485–91.

[92] Lohmuller JL, Pemberton JH, Dozois RR, et al. Pouchitis and extraintestinal manifestations of inflammatory bowel disease after ileal pouch-anal anastomosis. Ann Surg 1990;211(5): 622–7.

[93] Stahlberg D, Gullberg K, Liljeqvist L, et al. Pouchitis following pelvic pouch operation for ulcerative colitis. Incidence, cumulative risk, and risk factors. Dis Colon Rectum 1996;39: 1012–8.

[94] Gionchetti P, Rizzello F, Venturi A, et al. Oral bacteriotherapy as maintenance treatment in patients with chronic pouchitis: a double-blind, placebo-controlled trial. Gastroenterology 2000;119(2):305–9.

[95] Mimura T, Rizzello F, Helwig U, et al. Once daily high dose probiotic therapy (VSL#3) for maintaining remission in recurrent or refractory pouchitis. Gut 2004;53(1):108–14.

[96] Gionchetti P, Rizzello F, Helwig U, et al. Prophylaxis of pouchitis onset with probiotic therapy: a double-blind, placebo-controlled trial. Gastroenterology 2003;124(5):1202–9.

[97] Shen B, Brzezinski A, Fazio VW, et al. Maintenance therapy with a probiotic in antibiotic-dependent pouchitis: experience in clinical practice. Aliment Pharmacol Ther 2005;22(8): 721–8.

[98] Floch MH, Madsen KK, Jenkins DJA, et al. Recommendations for probiotic use. J Clin Gastroenterol 2006;40:275–8.

[99] Kelly CP, Lamont JT. Antibiotic-associated diarrhea, pseudomembranous colitis and *Colostrium difficile*-associated diarrhea and colitis. In: Feldman M, Friedman LS, Brandt LJ, editors. Gastrointestinal and liver disease. 8th edition. Philadelphia: Saunders; 2006. p. 2398–412.

[100] Aas J, Gessert CE, Bakken JS. Recurrent *Clostridium difficile* colitis: case series involving 18 patients treated with donor stool administered via a nasogastric tub. Clinical Infectious Diseases 2003;36:580–5.

[101] Persky SE, Brandt LJ. Treatment of recurrent *Clostridium difficile*-associated diarrhea by administration of donated stool directly through a colonoscope. Am J Gastroenterol 2000; 96:3283–5.

[102] Surawicz CM, Elmer GW, Speelman P, et al. Prevention of antibiotic associated diarrhea by *Saccharomyces boulardii*: a prospective study. Gastroenterology 1989;96:981–8.

[103] Dendukuri N, Costa V, McGregor M, et al. Probiotic therapy for the prevention and treatment of *Clostridium difficile*-associated diarrhea: a systematic review. CMAJ 2005; 173(2):167–70.

[104] McFarland LV. Meta-analysis of probiotics for the prevention of antibiotic associated diarrhea and the treatment of *Clostridium difficile* disease. Am J Gastroenterol 2006;101: 812–22.

[105] Lewis S, Burmeister S, Brazier J. Effect of the prebiotic oligofructose on relapse of *Clostridium difficile*-associated diarrhea: a randomized controlled study. Clin Gastroenterol Hepatol 2005;3:442–8.

[106] Fitz G. Hepatic encephalopathy, hepatopulmonary syndromes, hepatorenal syndrome, and other complications of liver disease. In: Feldman M, Friedman LS, Brandt LJ, editors. Gastrointestinal and liver disease. 8th edition. Philadelphia: Saunders; 2006. p. 1965–91.

[107] Elkington SG, Floch MH, Conn HO. Lactulose in the treatment of chronic portal-systemic encephalopathy. N Engl J Med 1969;281:408–11.

[108] Ballongue J, Schumann C, Quignon P. Effects of lactulose and lactitol on colonic microflora and enzymatic activity. Scand J Gastroenterol 1997;32(222):41–4.

ELSEVIER
SAUNDERS

Gastroenterol Clin N Am 36 (2007) 65–74

GASTROENTEROLOGY CLINICS
OF NORTH AMERICA

Nutrition Support in Acute Pancreatitis

Stephen A. McClave, MD

Division of Gastroenterology/Hepatology, Department of Medicine, University of Louisville
School of Medicine, 550 South Jackson Street, Louisville, KY 40202, USA

More than any other disease process, severe acute pancreatitis highlights the role of the gut in critical illness and the differential clinical response to feeding versus starvation [1]. Multiple factors contribute to the systemic inflammatory response syndrome (SIRS) seen in pancreatitis, including the nidus of inflammation within the gland, stimulation of exocrine enzyme secretion as a result of feeding, and loss of gut integrity. Late complications, such as infection, organ failure, shock, or hemorrhage, may further contribute to SIRS. Although the basic strategies of management for severe pancreatitis have evolved to some degree, the care remains mostly supportive. Early on, aggressive fluid resuscitation is needed while providing sufficient analgesia. Antibiotic prophylaxis for sterile necrosis is controversial, with the consensus opinion now suggesting that antibiotics should be reserved for documented infection [2]. Where indicated, management involves removal of impacted stones from the common bile duct and rapid surgical intervention for complications of infection or hemorrhage within the gland. In the past, the role of nutrition therapy has also been relegated to supportive care. Parenteral nutrition (PN) had seemed ideal for eliminating stimulation of pancreatic exocrine secretion while preventing deterioration of nutritional status and progression to protein energy malnutrition. Clinical experience, however, over the past decade suggests that a true window of opportunity exists early in admission, during which initiation of enteral feeding favorably impacts clinical outcome [3]. The degree to which gut integrity is maintained impacts systemic immunity and alters the degree of oxidative stress. In this sense, nutrition therapy through the provision of early enteral nutrition (EN) becomes a primary proactive component of management.

FACTORS RESPONSIBLE FOR SYSTEMIC INFLAMMATORY RESPONSE SYNDROME IN SEVERE ACUTE PANCREATITIS

The primary nidus of inflammation within the gland arises from a localized process of autodigestion, a process that is responsible for initiating SIRS in pancreatitis [4,5]. Although the events that trigger the process are unknown, factors

E-mail address: samcclave@louisville.edu

0889-8553/07/$ – see front matter
doi:10.1016/j.gtc.2007.01.002

involved in precipitating the initial injury include obstruction to outflow of pancreatic secretions, retrograde flow of duodenal contents into the pancreatic duct, transient impaction of a common bile duct stone with bile reflux into the pancreatic duct, direct stimulation of intracellular protease activation, lipolysis and generation of cytotoxic fatty acids from hypertriglyceridemia, and direct toxicity from ethanol [5,6]. A colocalization phenomenon occurs from the combination of the erroneously activated zymogen digestive enzymes within the acinar cell and lysosomal hydrolase cathepsin-B, a process that activates trypsinogen to trypsin and initiates the initial cell injury [7]. SIRS develops as a result of amplification of this acinar cell injury through the release of cytokines, mediators of inflammation, and inflammatory cell recruitment [6,7].

Stimulation of pancreatic exocrine secretion by enteral feeding may further exacerbate SIRS. The cephalic, gastric, and intestinal phases of pancreatic enzyme secretion represent different levels of stimulation of the pancreas within the gastrointestinal tract [8,9]. At each level, multiple factors may be used. Vagal stimulation may occur at any of the three levels of infusion. Within the gastric phase, additional factors include mechanical (gastric distention); hormonal (gastrin); and chemical (osmolarity, pH) stimuli [8,9]. A higher level of feeding within the gastrointestinal tract may invoke a greater number of stimulatory factors. Content of the feeding also influences the degree to which SIRS may be exacerbated [9,10]. Probably the most potent stimulus of pancreatic enzyme secretion is fat (with long-chain fat having greater effect than medium-chain triglycerides), whereas carbohydrate seems to have the least stimulatory effect [10]. Protein is probably intermediate between the other two macronutrients in its degree of pancreatic stimulation. Small peptides may have less of a stimulatory effect than intact protein or individual amino acids [10].

Loss of gut integrity may have an even greater impact on the generation of SIRS and the degree to which exocrine enzyme synthesis and secretion is stimulated. Loss of gut integrity from failure to use the gastrointestinal tract results in increased permeability, a process that allows bacteria to engage the gut-associated lymphoid tissue and subsequently up-regulate systemic immunity [1,11]. A proinflammatory process results from both the direct activation of macrophages involved in the innate immune response and the stimulation and proliferation of Th1 CD_4 helper lymphocytes in the acquired immune response. Starvation leads to reduced proliferation of anti-inflammatory Th2 lymphocyte subset cell populations [1]. The mass of secretory IgA-producing immunocytes at the gut (and distant sites like the liver, lungs, and kidneys) is reduced. Prolonged starvation leads to decreased intestinal contractility and bacterial overgrowth [12]. To an increasing degree, commensal bacteria resident in the gut lumen become displaced by pathogenic bacteria [12]. Because of these processes, the gut begins to contribute its own component to SIRS [13].

These three processes, which contribute to SIRS in acute severe pancreatitis, have tremendous implications for clinical practice. Little can be done to change the inciting events that start the initial injury to the acinar cell (other than removal of a gallstone, control of hypertriglyceridemia, and abstinence from ethanol to prevent disease recurrence). In the past, excessive emphasis on pancreatic rest and removal of any stimulatory factors of pancreatic enzyme secretion led inadvertently to the exacerbation of SIRS through the process mediated by loss of gut integrity. To minimize the exacerbation of SIRS by these latter two processes (stimulation of enzyme secretion and loss of gut integrity), enteral feeding must be used but manipulated in such a manner that stimulation of pancreatic enzyme secretion may be reduced to a subclinical level. Patient symptoms may be used by the clinician throughout feedings to indicate that a subclinical level of stimulation has been achieved, enough to allow resolution of inflammation within the gland and a decrease in the overall SIRS.

EVIDENCE FOR EARLY WINDOW OF OPPORTUNITY

In other disease processes within critical care (trauma, burns, respiratory failure on mechanical ventilation, and so forth), a large body of literature supports the concept of an early window of opportunity shortly after admission during which initiation of enteral feeding may change clinical outcome. In 15 prospective randomized controlled trials (PRCTs) and two meta-analyses, early versus delayed feeding was evaluated in critically ill patients, with the cutoff being 36 hours [14,15]. In these studies, feeds started within 36 hours of admission were shown to reduce infection by 55% ($P = .0006$); to shorten hospital length of stay by 2.2 days ($P = .0004$); and possibly to reduce mortality by as much as 48% ($P = .08$) [14,15]. In a separate body of literature, five studies evaluated the cumulative caloric deficit that is generated when delays in initiation of EN occur [16–20]. The most impressive study in critically ill patients on mechanical ventilation showed that an increasing caloric deficit corresponded to statistically significant increases in duration of mechanical ventilation ($P = .0002$); prolonged hospital length of stay ($P = .0001$); increased infectious morbidity ($P = .004$); and a higher rate of overall complications ($P = .0003$) [16].

For patients with acute pancreatitis, there is some evidence that a similar window of opportunity exists. Of six PRCTs of EN versus PN in acute pancreatitis randomized within 48 hours [21–26], five showed significant impact on clinical outcome. In these five studies, EN was associated with decreased infectious morbidity [22,24,25], shorter hospital length of stay [26], less overall complications [22], reduced duration of the disease process and length of nutritional therapy [25,26], and faster resolution of SIRS [23]. Only our study from Louisville failed to show an impact of early EN on patient outcome, which may be explained by the fact that patients in this study tended to have milder severity of pancreatitis than patients in the other studies (a mean Ranson's criteria for all study patients of 1.1) [21]. In contrast, one PRCT randomized patients after 4 full days of hospitalization [27]. Although the patients were clearly severely ill with a high mean number of Ranson's criteria (4.7–5), no beneficial effect of EN compared with PN was seen on any outcome parameter [27].

Delays in initiating EN in severe acute pancreatitis lead to prolonged ileus and reduced chances for tolerance. In a prospective nonrandomized series of

102 patients with acute pancreatitis, aggressive attempts at early placement of a feeding tube and minimizing the duration of ileus to less than or equal to 2 days resulted in 92% of patients achieving tolerance of enteral feeds [28]. Delays with initiating EN resulting in duration of ileus of up to 5 days decreased the rate of tolerance to 50%, whereas duration of ileus greater than or equal to 6 days resulted in a near 0% chance for tolerating early enteral feeding [28]. Through two prospective studies, Eatock and coworkers [29,30] noted that early onset of enteral feeding within 48 hours of admission served to maintain gut function and improve tolerance. Fewer problems were encountered with ileus and gastric stasis with this aggressive approach to feeding [29,30].

INFLUENCE OF DISEASE SEVERITY ON GUT INTEGRITY AND LIKELIHOOD FOR ENTERAL NUTRITION TO CHANGE OUTCOME

As has been shown in animal models [31,32] and in clinical studies involving other disease processes (eg, trauma) [33], pancreatitis patients with greater disease severity have greater degrees of intestinal permeability and are more likely to sustain a favorable response to early EN. In a study of patients with acute pancreatitis using urinary excretion of polyethylene glycol as a marker of intestinal permeability, Ammori and coworkers [34] showed that patients with mild pancreatitis had a degree of permeability that was no greater than that seen in controls without pancreatitis. Patients with severe but uncomplicated pancreatitis had a fourfold increase in permeability as measured by urinary polyethylene glycol levels, whereas patients with severe pancreatitis complicated by multiple organ failure had a fourfold higher increase in permeability [34]. Clearly, greater degrees of disease severity are associated with greater degrees to which the channels between the intestinal epithelial cells open and gut integrity is lost. Over the first four PRCTs evaluating EN versus PN in acute pancreatitis, the percentage of patients with severe pancreatitis seemed to be a key factor in whether the EN significantly altered clinical outcome [21–23,25]. In our Louisville study, only 19% of the study patients had severe pancreatitis, and no differences in clinical outcome were seen between the two routes of nutrition support [21]. In the studies by Abou-Assi and coworkers [25] and Windsor and coworkers [23], 35% to 38% of patients had severe pancreatitis and results indicated that early use of EN hastened resolution of SIRS and decreased the time to resolution of the disease process compared with PN [23,25]. In a Greek study by Kalfarentzos and coworkers [22], where 100% of patients had severe pancreatitis with necrosis on CT scan, early EN was shown to reduce the number of patients with complications significantly from 75% to 44%, and percent of patients with septic morbidity from 50% to 28% compared with use of PN.

Patients with severe pancreatitis (designated by APACHE II score ≥10 and ≥3 Ranson's criteria) had a high rate of complications (38%) and mortality (19%), and close to 0% chance of advancing to oral diet within 7 days [35–38]. For these patients, EN may be expected to change clinical outcome.

Patients with lower scores have mild to moderate pancreatitis; have a low rate of complications (6%); negligible mortality; and a greater than 80% chance of advancing to an oral diet within the first week of hospitalization [35–38]. The former group of patients needs specialized nutrition support and are most likely to experience an improved outcome with early enteral feeding. The latter group, in contrast, does not need specialized nutrition support, is not expected to experience improved outcome by the enteral or parenteral route of feeding, and instead simply needs supportive care with intravenous analgesia and fluid resuscitation.

PERCEPTION OF TOLERANCE EMERGES AS KEY FACTOR IN MANAGEMENT

The past decade of experience with PRCTs evaluating EN versus PN (especially the studies evaluating gastric versus jejunal feeding over the past year) has reshaped the perception of tolerance, has clarified the risk and consequences of providing early EN, and has raised the level of aggression with which clinicians pursue placement of feeding tubes and initiate early enteral feeds in acute pancreatitis. Distinguishing tolerance from true intolerance is better determined by understanding the adverse consequences associated with providing early EN in acute pancreatitis. Three potentially adverse scenarios occur in response to EN, the first of which is an asymptomatic stimulation of exocrine enzyme secretion (which is probably seen in 100% of patients placed on EN early in the course of hospitalization) [39]. In a study by O'Keefe and coworkers [39], all patients with acute pancreatitis randomized to EN showed significantly greater increases in trypsin, amylase, and lipase output than those patients randomized to PN. None of these increases, however, were associated with symptoms or any adverse clinical effect [39]. The second scenario is that of an uncomplicated exacerbation of symptoms, and may be expected in up to 21% of patients with pancreatitis placed on early EN [40]. In our study from Louisville, three patients placed on jejunal feeds that initially were well tolerated showed an exacerbation of abdominal pain and increases of amylase and lipase in response to early advancement to clear liquid oral diet [21]. Placement back on jejunal feeds resulted in rapid resolution of the symptoms. The third and more worrisome scenario is that of an exacerbation of the disease process and SIRS, an effect that could be expected in up to 4% of patients placed on EN [40]. A patient in our study from Louisville demonstrated an exacerbation of SIRS, as evidenced by increased white blood cell count and fever, when the tip of the feeding tube inadvertently became displaced from the jejunum back into the stomach [21]. Repositioning the tube back into the jejunum resulted in immediate improvement with decreasing fever and white blood cell count over the subsequent 12 hours [21]. There seems to be no evidence from the literature that early use of the enteral route increases intra-abdominal infection and pancreatic abscess (as suggested by Ranson and Spencer [41] almost 30 years ago). Collective experience suggests just the opposite, that infectious morbidity is reduced by use of the enteral route [3].

Tolerance to early EN in pancreatitis may be influenced by multiple factors. As the discussion in the previous paragraph alludes, the level of feeding within the gastrointestinal tract is a key factor in tolerance. Content of the formula infused also may impact tolerance [9,10]. At any given level of infusion within the gastrointestinal tract, formulas with lower fat content or with fat in the form of medium-chain triglycerides may cause less stimulation of pancreatic enzyme secretion (and lead to better tolerance) than formulas with higher fat content or fat in the form of long-chain fatty acids. Similarly, formulas with protein in the form of small peptides may be tolerated better with less stimulation of the pancreas than formulas with intact protein or protein in the form of free amino acids. Osmolarity is a tradeoff in this situation, because the nearly fat-free formulas tend to have higher osmolarity, a factor that increases stimulation of the pancreas, and may jeopardize tolerance [9]. Increasing duration of ileus may result in greater degrees of intolerance [28]. Institutional experience and the expertise with which tubes are placed and feeds are monitored may also be a factor in perceived tolerance and overall success of providing EN. In two studies from Great Britain, widely disparate results were achieved with initiation of EN between the separate institutions [23,42]. In the Windsor and coworkers [23] study, some degree of ileus was experienced in 5 out of the 16 patients placed on EN. This minor degree of intolerance was managed by decreasing the rate of infusion for 2 to 4 days before resuming the full rate. In contrast, in the Schneider and coworkers [42] study, EN was successfully initiated in only 53% of the 69 critically ill patients in whom EN was intended. The remaining 47% received PN alone or no specialized nutritional support. Individual variation by a specific patient may result in intolerance to EN that is unexpected from the experience incurred with the remainder of patients in a given study. In our Louisville study, a single patient was intolerant of gastric feeds (when the tube flipped back from the jejunum) [21], and yet early EN was tolerated in 100% of the 42 total patients randomized to gastric feeds in the Eatock and coworkers [30] and Kumar and coworkers [43] studies. In a similar fashion, two specific patients (one from our group in Louisville and one from Richmond described by O'Keefe and coworkers [39]) showed clear intolerance of nasojejunal feeds with an exacerbation of pain and an elevation of amylase and lipase in response to feeds infused 10 to 40 cm below the ligament of Treitz.

Preconceived expectations of problems and misconceptions of tolerance are common with use of EN in acute pancreatitis. The almost unbelievable recent experience with gastric feeding in the Eatock and coworkers [30] and Kumar and coworkers [43] studies seem to defy what most clinicians expect. In the Eatock and coworkers [30] study, 70.4% of patients in the nasogastric group tolerated more than 75% of goal calories within the first 48 hours of admission (versus 77.2% in the nasojejunal group). After 60 hours, 77.8% of goal calories were infused in the nasogastric group (versus 76.1% in the nasojejunal group). Only 2 patients out of the 27 randomized to gastric feeds experienced pain [30]. No change in rate of the nasogastric infusion was needed because there was no change in C-reactive protein levels, APACHE scores, or need for intravenous analgesia [30]. In the Kumar and coworkers [43] study, one patient in each group (both nasogastric and nasojejunal) experienced pain in response to feeding, with no change in amylase levels. Partial PN was required in the first week for six of the patients randomized to nasogastric feeding (versus four patients in the nasojejunal group), and no supplemental PN was required during the second week of feeding [43].

The clinical experience from these studies indicates that clinicians should avoid misinterpreting "intolerance." Such misinterpretation may result from low set points for gastric residual volumes (which are a poor marker for gastric emptying [44,45] or for risk of aspiration) [46]; mild increases in pain; or asymptomatic increases in amylase and lipase. Excess caution may result in loss of opportunity to impact outcome. Delays in waiting to achieve jejunal placement, slow advances in the rate of infusion of EN, and frequent inappropriate cessation may result in an insufficient volume of EN infused.

Vigilant monitoring and quick changes in feeding strategy, however, may promote improved tolerance in those patients experiencing difficulty with initiation of EN. Diverting the level of infusion of EN lower in the gastrointestinal tract, while changing the content of formula to that which is less stimulating to the pancreas, has been shown quickly to ameliorate intolerance and allow continuation of EN [21]. Basic protocols for delivery of EN may further enhance tolerance. Measures should be used to provide strict glucose control; to reduce aspiration by elevating the head of the bed and providing scheduled chlorhexidine mouthwash; and to promote intestinal motility by reversing the effects of opioid narcotics at the level of the gut (by infusing naloxone through the nasoenteric tube).

APPROPRIATE USE OF PARENTERAL NUTRITION

Experience in the past with PN infused early in the course of acute pancreatitis showed that such practice results in adverse clinical outcome. In a study by Sax and coworkers [37], patients randomized to early PN initiated within the first 24 hours of admission had a longer hospital length of stay and a higher rate of central line catheter sepsis than controls who received no specialized nutrition support. Certainly, PN is not needed for pancreatic rest. Shortly after admission throughout the period corresponding to the early window of opportunity (during which the route of feeding may alter clinical outcome), PN may serve as a liability. Increases in serum glucose levels in response to PN and provision of immunosuppressive parenteral omega-6 fatty acids may adversely affect the risk/benefit ratio for this route of nutritional support. In a more recent study, delays in the initiation of PN because of time required for full fluid resuscitation and subsequent randomization altered the timing of PN in such a way as to reduce liability and significantly improve outcome in response to its provision [47].

In a Chinese study by Xian-Li and coworkers [47], patients had to undergo full fluid resuscitation, and then had 48 hours to be randomized to standard therapy (no specialized nutrition support), PN, or PN with parenteral gluta-mine. Although details were not provided in the manuscript, such practice may have resulted in PN being started between the third and fifth day of hos-pitalization, possibly past the peak of inflammation and SIRS. Possibly as a result of the altered timing, use of PN in this study significantly reduced mortality from 43.5% to 14.3%, overall complications from 21% to 11%, and hospital length of stay from 39.1 to 28.6 days (all differences, $P < .05$) compared with those patients randomized to standard therapy [47]. The addition of paren-teral glutamine significantly improved these clinical end points even further.

Although use of EN is always the first choice of nutrition support, use of PN should be considered in that patient with severe acute pancreatitis shown to be intolerant of EN. PN is generally not indicated in patients with mild to moder-ate pancreatitis, because standard therapy with no specialized nutrition support is appropriate for these patients. If use of PN is indicated in a particular patient, initiation of therapy should be delayed until after the first 5 days of hospitali-zation. When PN is started, strict control of glucose is mandatory, as is mon-itoring of serum calcium and triglyceride levels. Permissive underfeeding may improve insulin sensitivity, and patients should receive approximately 80% of caloric requirements by this route of nutrition therapy (K.N. Jeejeebhoy, per-sonal communication, 2003).

SUMMARY

The benefit of early EN for the disease process and for patient outcome in severe acute pancreatitis is dramatic. A narrow window of opportunity exists, possibly over the first 48 to 72 hours, during which there is potential for EN to decrease disease severity and reduce overall complications. Delays in initiating EN beyond this point may result in loss of the chance for EN to improve out-come. Most patients with severe pancreatitis tolerate enteral feeds. Minimizing the duration of ileus may improve tolerance. The consequences of inadvertent pancreatic stimulation are minimal, and with vigilant monitoring, there is little chance of doing net harm. Any signs of symptom exacerbation or increasing inflammation in response to EN may be ameliorated by subtle adjustments in the feeding strategy. In this manner, provision of EN represents primary therapy in the management of the patient with acute pancreatitis and is emerg-ing as the gold standard of therapy in nutrition support for this disease process.

References
[1] Jabbar A, Chang WK, Dryden GW, et al. Gut immunology and the differential response to feeding and starvation. Nutr Clin Pract 2003;18(6):461–82.
[2] Mazaki T, Ishii Y, Takayama T. Meta-analysis of prophylactic antibiotic use in acute necro-tizing pancreatitis. Br J Surg 2006;93(6):674–84.
[3] McClave SA, Chang WK, Dhaliwal R, et al. Nutrition support in acute pancreatitis: a system-atic review of the literature. JPEN J Parenter Enteral Nutr 2006;30(2):143–56.
[4] Bradley EL III. Acute pancreatitis: clinical classification and terminology. Pract Gastroenterol 1996;20:8–24.

[5] Soergel KH. Acute pancreatitis. In: Sleisenger MH, Fordtran JS, editors. Gastrointestinal disease. Philadelphia (PA): WB Saunders; 1989. p. 1814–42.

[6] McClave SA, Ritchie CS. Artificial nutrition in pancreatic disease: what lessons have we learned from the literature? Clin Nutr 2000;19(1):1–6.

[7] Saluja AK, Steer MLP. Pathophysiology of pancreatitis: role of cytokines and other mediators of inflammation. Digestion 1999;60(Suppl 1):27–33.

[8] Deng X, Whitcomb DC. Neurohumoral control of the exocrine pancreas. Curr Opin Gastroenterol 1998;14:362–8.

[9] Corcoy R, Ma Sanchez J, Domingo P, et al. Nutrition in the patient with severe acute pancreatitis. Nutrition 1998;4:269–75.

[10] Parekh D, Lawson HH, Segal I. The role of total enteral nutrition in pancreatic disease. S Afr J Surg 1993;31(2):57–61.

[11] DeWitt RC, Kudsk KA. The gut's role in metabolism, mucosal barrier function, and gut immunology. Infect Dis Clin North Am 1999;13(2):465–81.

[12] Alverdy JC, Laughlin RS, Wu L. Influence of the critically ill state on host-pathogen interactions within the intestine: gut-derived sepsis redefined. Crit Care Med 2003;31(2): 598–607.

[13] Moore EE, Moore FA. The role of the gut in provoking the systemic inflammatory response. Journal Critical Care Nutrition 1994;2:9–15.

[14] Heyland DK, Dhaliwal R, Drover JW, et al. Canadian Critical Care Clinical Practice Guidelines Committee. Canadian clinical practice guidelines for nutrition support in mechanically ventilated, critically ill adult patients. JPEN J Parenter Enteral Nutr 2003;27(5): 355–73.

[15] Marik PE, Zaloga GP. Early enteral nutrition in acutely ill patients: a systematic review. Crit Care Med 2001;29(12):2264–70.

[16] Villet S, Chiolero RL, Bollmann MD, et al. Negative impact of hypocaloric feeding and energy balance on clinical outcome in ICU patients. Clin Nutr 2005;24(4):502–9.

[17] Rubinson L, Diette GB, Song X, et al. Low caloric intake is associated with nosocomial bloodstream infections in patients in the medical intensive care unit. Crit Care Med 2004;32(2): 350–7.

[18] Mault J. Energy balance and outcome in critically ill patients: results of a multicenter prospective randomized trial by the ICU Nutrition Study Group. JPEN J Parenter Enteral Nutr 2000;24:S4.

[19] Bartlett RH, Dechert RE, Mault JR, et al. Measurement of metabolism in multiple organ failure. Surgery 1982;92(4):771–9.

[20] Kleber MJ, Lowen CC, McClave SA, et al. Is there a role for indirect calorimetry in maximizing patient outcome from nutritional alimentation in the long-term nursing care setting? Nutr Clin Pract 2000;15(5):1–7.

[21] McClave SA, Greene LM, Snider HL, et al. Comparison of the safety of early enteral vs parenteral nutrition in mild acute pancreatitis. JPEN J Parenter Enteral Nutr 1997;21(1):14–20.

[22] Kalfarentzos F, Kehagias J, Mead N, et al. Enteral nutrition is superior to parenteral nutrition in severe acute pancreatitis: results of a randomized prospective trial. Br J Surg 1997;84(12):1665–9.

[23] Windsor AC, Kanwar S, Li AG, et al. Compared with parenteral nutrition, enteral feeding attenuates the acute phase response and improves disease severity in acute pancreatitis. Gut 1998;42(3):431–5.

[24] Olah A, Pardavi G, Belagyi T, et al. Early nasojejunal feeding in acute pancreatitis is associated with a lower complication rate. Nutrition 2002;18(3):259–62.

[25] Abou-Assi S, Craig K, O'Keefe SJ. Hypocaloric jejunal feeding is better than total parenteral nutrition in acute pancreatitis: results of a randomized comparative study. Am J Gastroenterol 2002;97(9):2255–62.

[26] Gupta R, Patel K, Calder PC, et al. A randomised clinical trial to assess the effect of total enteral and total parenteral nutritional support on metabolic, inflammatory and oxidative

markers in patients with predicted severe acute pancreatitis (APACHE II > or = 6). Pancreatology 2003;3(5):406–13.

[27] Louie BE, Noseworthy T, Hailey D, et al. Enteral or parenteral nutrition for severe pancreatitis: a randomized controlled trial and health technology assessment. Can J Surg 2005;48(4):298–306.

[28] Cravo M, Camilo ME, Marques A, et al. Early tube feeding in acute pancreatitis: a prospective study. Clin Nutrit 1989;8(Suppl):14.

[29] Eatock FC, Brombacher GD, Steven A, et al. Nasogastric feeding in severe acute pancreatitis may be practical and safe. Int J Pancreatol 2000;28(1):23–9.

[30] Eatock FC, Chong P, Menezes N, et al. A randomized study of early nasogastric versus nasojejunal feeding in severe acute pancreatitis. Am J Gastroenterol 2005;100(2):432–9.

[31] Sax HC, Illig KA, Ryan CK, et al. Low-dose enteral feeding is beneficial during total parenteral nutrition. Am J Surg 1996;171(6):587–90.

[32] Nelson JL, Foley-Nelson TL, Gianotti L, et al. Caloric intake and bacterial translocation following burn trauma in guinea pigs. Nutrition, in press.

[33] Kudsk KA, Croce MA, Fabian TC, et al. Enteral versus parenteral feeding: effects on septic morbidity after blunt and penetrating abdominal trauma. Ann Surg 1992;215(5):503–11.

[34] Ammori BJ, Leeder PC, King RF, et al. Early increase in intestinal permeability in patients with severe acute pancreatitis: correlation with endotoxemia, organ failure, and mortality. J Gastrointest Surg 1999;3(3):252–62.

[35] Larvin M, McMahon MJ. APACHE-II score for assessment and monitoring of acute pancreatitis. Lancet 1989;2(8656):201–5.

[36] Corfield AP, Cooper MJ, Williamson RC, et al. Prediction of severity in acute pancreatitis: prospective comparison of three prognostic indices. Lancet 1985;2(8452):403–7.

[37] Sax HC, Warner BW, Talamini MA, et al. Early total parenteral nutrition in acute pancreatitis: lack of beneficial effects. Am J Surg 1987;153(1):117–24.

[38] Wilson C, Heath DI, Imrie CW. Prediction of outcome in acute pancreatitis: a comparative study of APACHE II, clinical assessment and multiple factor scoring systems. Br J Surg 1990;77(11):1260–4.

[39] O'Keefe SJ, Broderick T, Turner M, et al. Nutrition in the management of necrotizing pancreatitis. Clin Gastroenterol Hepatol 2003;1(4):315–21.

[40] Levy P, Heresbach D, Pariente EA, et al. Frequency and risk factors of recurrent pain during refeeding in patients with acute pancreatitis: a multivariate multicentre prospective study of 116 patients. Gut 1997;40(2):262–6.

[41] Ranson JH, Spencer FC. Prevention, diagnosis, and treatment of pancreatic abscess. Surgery 1977;82(1):99–106.

[42] Schneider H, Boyle N, McCluckie A, et al. Acute severe pancreatitis and multiple organ failure: total parenteral nutrition is still required in a proportion of patients. Br J Surg 2000;87(3):362–73.

[43] Kumar A, Singh N, Prakash S, et al. Early enteral nutrition in severe acute pancreatitis: a prospective randomized controlled trial comparing nasojejunal and nasogastric routes. J Clin Gastroenterol 2006;40(5):431–4.

[44] Tarling MM, Toner CC, Withington PS, et al. A model of gastric emptying using paracetamol absorption in intensive care patients. Intensive Care Med 1997;23(3):256–60.

[45] Cohen J, Aharon A, Singer P. The paracetamol absorption test: a useful addition to the enteral nutrition algorithm? Clin Nutr 2000;19(4):233–6.

[46] McClave SA, Lukan JK, Stefater JA, et al. Poor validity of residual volumes as a marker for risk of aspiration in critically ill patients. Crit Care Med 2005;33(2):324–30.

[47] Xian-Li H, Qing-Jiu M, Jian-Guo L, et al. Effect of total parenteral nutrition (TPN) with and without glutamine dipeptide supplementation on outcome in severe acute pancreatitis (SAP). Clinical Nutrition Supplements 2004;1:43–7.

Gastroenterol Clin N Am 36 (2007) 75–91

GASTROENTEROLOGY CLINICS
OF NORTH AMERICA

Food Allergies and Eosinophilic Gastrointestinal Illness

Nirmala Gonsalves, MD

Division of Gastroenterology, Northwestern University, The Feinberg School of Medicine, 676 North St. Claire Street, Suite 1400, Chicago, IL 60611, USA

Eosinophilic gastrointestinal disorders are characterized by eosinophilic infiltration and inflammation of the gastrointestinal tract in the absence of previously identified causes of eosinophilia, such as parasitic infections, malignancy, collagen vascular diseases, drug sensitivities, and inflammatory bowel disease. These disorders include eosinophilic esophagitis (EE), eosinophilic gastroenteritis (EG), eosinophilic enteritis, and eosinophilic colitis. This article focuses mainly on EE and EG.

In the body, eosinophils are normally present in the gastrointestinal tract, spleen, lymph nodes, and the thymus. Within the gastrointestinal tract, eosinophils are located in the lamina propria of the stomach, small intestine, cecum, and colon and are not usually found in the esophagus. They serve a protective role in defending the host against parasitic infections. Fig. 1 shows the normal eosinophil levels in the gastrointestinal tract [1]. When these levels are elevated, and other causes for tissue eosinophila are excluded, one must consider eosinophilic gastrointestinal disorders as a diagnosis.

EOSINOPHILIC ESOPHAGITIS

Over the last several years, EE has become the topic of an increasing number of articles in the adult and pediatric gastrointestinal and allergy literature. First reported in an adult patient by Landres and coworkers [2] in 1978, EE was further characterized by Attwood and coworkers [3] in a series of 12 adults in 1993. Since that time, the main clinical and research focus has been in the pediatric population. Over the last several years, however, EE has been recognized as one of the most common causes of dysphagia and food impaction in adults [4].

EPIDEMIOLOGY OF EOSINOPHILIC ESOPHAGITIS

EE may occur in isolation or in conjunction with EG [5]. Previously considered a rare condition, there has been a dramatic increase in reports of EE from North and South America, Europe, Asia, Australia, and the Middle East

E-mail address: n-gonsalves@northwestern.edu

0889-8553/07/$ – see front matter
doi:10.1016/j.gtc.2007.01.003
gastro.theclinics.com

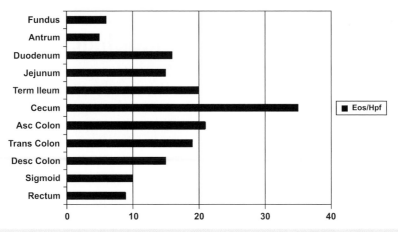

Fig. 1. Normal level of tissue eosinophilia in various sites in the gastrointestinal tract.

over the last several years [6–15]. The cause for this rise is likely a combination of an increasing incidence of EE and a growing awareness of the condition among gastroenterologists, allergists, and pathologists. Noel and colleagues [16] calculated an incidence of EE in a population of children in Ohio to be 1 in 10,000 per year and a prevalence of 4 in 10,000 in 2003. Straumann and Simon [17] estimated an incidence of 0.15 cases per 10,000 adult inhabitants with a prevalence of 2.9 per 10,000 inhabitants of their catchment area in Switzerland. These numbers are likely to underestimate the true incidence and prevalence, because these data are based on patients with symptoms sufficient to warrant endoscopy. A recent population-based study in Sweden randomly surveyed 3000 adult members of the population. A total of 1563 were invited to have endoscopy, and 1000 agreed and underwent esophageal biopsies. This group found that esophageal eosinophilia was present in nearly 5% of the population and histologic criteria for EE was met in 1% of the population [18]. These numbers suggest that EE is becoming as common as other immunologically influenced diseases, such as inflammatory bowel disease [19]. In addition, the many publications about EE in the last several years are contributing to increasing the awareness of this condition in both the gastroenterology and pathology community [13].

CLINICAL FEATURES OF EOSINOPHILIC ESOPHAGITIS
The clinical features of EE in both adults and children are described in Table 1. The most common presenting symptoms in adults include dysphagia, food impaction, heartburn, and chest pain, whereas those in children include vomiting, regurgitation, and abdominal pain [20,21]. Although younger children rarely present with dysphagia and food impaction, these presentations were more commonly seen in older children and adolescents [22]. A male predisposition has been seen in both adults and pediatric cases [20,21]. In adults, this diagnosis

Table 1
Clinical features of eosinophilic esophagitis in children and adults

Study	N	Age (range)	Male (%)	Allergy (%)	% Patients with Peripheral Eosinophilia	Endoscopic Findings
Pediatric						
Boston 2002	19	8 (1–16)	74	84	58	NA
Philadelphia 2002	26	7 (2–14)	85	81	NA	NA
Australia 2003	21	10 (2–16)	76	67	NA	Wrinkled or thickened mucosa 67%, mild redness 10%, NI 33%
Philadelphia 2003	51	8 (3–16)	65	51	NA	Furrows 41%
Philadelphia 2005	381	9 (NA)	66	53	NA	NI 32%, rings 12%, furrows 41%, plaques 15%
Adult						
United Kingdom 2003	12	40 (22–64)	58	50	NA	NI 17%, rings 17%, furrows 33%, rings and furrows 25%
Australia 2003	31	34 (14–77)	77	46	36	Furrows ± furrows 97%
Mayo 2003	21	40 (28–55)	81	29	5	Rings 71%, stricture 14%, NI 14%
Switzerland 2003	30	41 (16–71)	73	29	50	Minimal 57%, moderate 27%, severe 10%, NI 7%
Milwaukee 2004	29	35 (19–65)	72	48	NA	Rings 72%, stricture 90%, small caliber 17%, esophagitis 14%, NI 9%
Chicago 2005	74	38 (14–76)	76	70	9	Rings 81%, furrows 74%, strictures 31%, plaques 15%, small caliber 10%, edema 8%
Australia 2006	26	36 (17–65)	69	77	31	Furrows 77%, rings 62%, small caliber 27%, plaques 15%, stricture 12%

has often been overlooked and many patients have had endoscopies with alternate diagnoses, including Schatzki's rings or gastroesophageal reflux disease (GERD) before a diagnosis of EE [23,24]. In many cases, these patients had undergone repeated endoscopies, esophageal dilations, and a delay in the institution of appropriate medical therapy [23,24]. In previous years, the presence of eosinophils in esophageal mucosal biopsies was equated with GERD [25,26]. More recent series demonstrated the absence of erosive esophagitis and normal ambulatory esophageal pH studies in patients with esophageal mucosal eosinophilia [3]. Additional studies have demonstrated that the degree of tissue eosinophilia in the esophagus negatively correlates with response to conventional therapy for GERD, further supporting an association with EE [27–30]. Nevertheless, because of this potential overlap, gastroenterologists who suspect a diagnosis of EE should specifically request tissue eosinophil counts by the pathologist to help differentiate this diagnosis from GERD.

ENDOSCOPIC FINDINGS

The most common endoscopic features in adults with EE include linear furrows (80%); mucosal rings (64%); small-caliber esophagus (28%); white plaques or exudates (16%); and strictures (12%) (Fig. 2) [20]. In a large clinical series of 381 children, the most common endoscopic features were linear furrows (41%); normal appearance (32%); esophageal rings (12%); and white plaques (15%) [21]. It is important to note that the classic endoscopic features may be subtle and missed during endoscopy [11]. Therefore, it is suggested that biopsies be taken for the clinical indication of unexplained dysphagia, refractory heartburn, or chest pain despite normal endoscopic findings [23].

HISTOLOGIC FEATURES

Although certain endoscopic features are characteristic of EE, this condition is ultimately diagnosed by obtaining biopsy specimens that demonstrate histologic findings of increased intramucosal eosinophils in the esophagus without concomitant eosinophilic infiltration in the stomach or duodenum (Fig. 3) [11,13]. Other histologic features of this condition include superficial layering of the eosinophils; eosinophilic microabscesses (clusters of ≥ 4 eosinophils); intercellular edema; degranulation of eosinophils; and the presence of other inflammatory cells, such as lymphocytes. Another histologic finding in EE is epithelial hyperplasia, defined by papillary height elongation and basal zone proliferation [11–13,30]. Epithelial hyperplasia is also a cardinal feature of the histopathology of reflux esophagitis. Studies have also shown evidence of subepithelial fibrosis in biopsies of adults with EE [7].

Although a single diagnostic threshold of eosinophil density has not been determined, most centers use a value of greater than or equal to 15 to 20 eosinophils per high-power field to differentiate EE from GERD, with the latter generally demonstrating less than 5 eosinophils per high-power field [28]. It has also been demonstrated that the eosinophilic infiltration of the esophagus may not be evenly distributed. It is suggested that biopsies be obtained from both

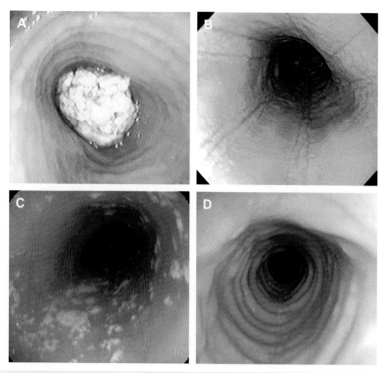

Fig. 2. Endoscopic photographs showing common features of eosinophilic esophagitis. (*A*) Concentric mucosal rings seen throughout the length of the esophagus in a patient presenting with a food impaction. (*B*) Linear furrows or creases in the esophageal mucosa. (*C*) White exudates and plaques seen in some patients, which correspond to areas of eosinophilic abscess eruption through the esophageal mucosa. (*D*) Endoscopic photo of a patient with concentric mucosal rings and small-caliber esophagus.

the proximal and distal esophagus to obtain a higher diagnostic yield and perhaps increase the specificity of the diagnosis. A retrospective review suggested that at least five biopsies maximizes the sensitivity based on a diagnostic threshold of greater than or equal to 15 eosinophils per high-power field [24]. Prospective studies need to be performed to validate this recommendation.

ADDITIONAL DIAGNOSTIC TESTING

Radiologic studies, such as barium esophagrams, may be used in the work-up of patients with EE but are often nondiagnostic [11]. A recent study that correlated endoscopic and radiologic features in EE demonstrated that both esophageal strictures and esophageal rings may be identified on barium studies of patients with EE [12]. Several studies have examined the manometric findings in these patients and the most common finding has been a nonspecific motility pattern [11]. Endoscopic ultrasound has also been used to demonstrate that eosinophilic infiltration may include deeper layers of the esophagus [31–33]. It is speculated that

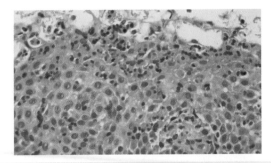

Fig. 3. Common histologic appearance in eosinophilic esophagitis. This image demonstrates superficial layering of eosinophils in the esophageal mucosa with presence of microabscesses seen in most patients with eosinophilic esophagitis (H&E, original magnification ×200).

this mucosal and submucosal fibrosis may lead to decreased compliance of the esophagus, contributing to the symptoms of dysphagia even in the absence of an identifiable stricture.

PATHOPHYSIOLOGY: THE ROLE OF FOOD ALLERGENS

Studies have shown that the infiltration of eosinophils in the esophagus may be related to an allergic response to either food or aeroallergens [34–42]. This section focuses on the data behind the implication of food allergens. One of the first links between food allergies and EE was demonstrated by Kelly and colleagues [27] in 1995. This group evaluated 10 pediatric patients with intractable symptoms attributed to GERD who also had histologic changes of epithelial hyperplasia and eosinophilic infiltration in the esophagus. The patients had all been treated with several courses of antireflux therapy without resolution of symptoms or histologic changes. Six of the children had undergone a Nissen fundoplication. These authors speculated that the symptoms and histologic changes were caused by a hypersensitivity reaction to intact dietary proteins rather than acid reflux. These children underwent a dietary trial consisting of the substitution of a protein-free, 1-crystalline amino acid–based formula for 6 weeks. After the dietary trial, endoscopic abnormalities normalized in six patients. There was a significant reduction in the degree of esophageal eosinophilia in all 10 patients, and complete resolution in five patients. Findings of epithelial hyperplasia also significantly decreased after the dietary trial. These results helped link dietary allergens to the development of esophageal eosinophilia unresponsive to antireflux therapy.

Further support to this association came when the patients underwent an open food challenge. Reintroduction of foods recreated the patients' symptoms in 9 of 10 patients a median of 1 hour (0.5–8 hours) after the introduction of specific foods. Specific food triggers were cow milk in seven patients, soy protein in four patients, wheat in two patients, peanut in two patients, and egg in one patient. The authors concluded that in patients with a diagnosis of GERD who have esophageal eosinophilia and fail conventional therapy, consideration of a food-related hypersensitivity response should be considered.

Another study that linked EE with food allergens was performed by Liacouras and colleagues [43] in 1998. In this study, 20 patients with EE with symptoms of refractory reflux were treated with methylprednisolone (1.5 mg/kg/d, divided into twice daily dosing) for 4 weeks. A total of 65% of patients became asymptomatic, whereas the remainder had significant improvement in symptoms within 4 weeks. The average time for clinical improvement was 8 ± 4 days. All patients in this group had histologic improvement demonstrated by decreased tissue eosinophilia in addition to decreased peripheral eosinophilia and IgE levels. They also demonstrated recurrence of symptoms on discontinuation of the steroids.

This association of food allergens to EE created challenges regarding identification of these agents given current limitations of allergy testing. Spergel and colleagues [44] demonstrated that the use of both skin prick and patch testing was helpful in identifying causative foods contributing to EE. In their study, 26 pediatric patients with EE underwent both skin prick and patch testing to identify potential food triggers. They found that milk and egg were the most common foods to be positive with skin prick testing, whereas wheat was the most common food identified by patch testing. The most common allergens implicated in this study were milk, egg, soy, peanut, and wheat. They found that dietary elimination of these agents resulted in resolution of symptoms in 18 patients and partial improvement in 6 patients. Two patients were lost to followup. They also demonstrated that esophageal eosinophil counts decreased from 55.8 to 8.4 eosinophls per high-power field on the diet. Their finding that patients with EE have both positive skin prick results and patch test results indicate both Th1-mediated and IgE-mediated reactions may be involved in the pathogenesis of this condition. This is further supported by the finding that the time frame for symptom resolution varied from minutes to days, also implicating both IgE and a delayed mechanism in the pathogenesis.

Another study showing the association of food allergens and EE was by Markowitz and colleagues [45] in 2003. This study focused on a series of pediatric patients with chronic symptoms of GERD who had persistent esophageal eosinophilia despite antireflux therapy for 3 months and who were ultimately diagnosed with EE. This group was subsequently placed on an elemental diet for 1 month followed by a repeat esophagogastroduodenoscopy. They found that all but two patients experienced symptomatic improvement on the elemental diet and that the average time to clinical improvement was 8.5 ± 3.8 days. They found that the number of eosinophils significantly decreased from prediet (33.7 ± 10.3) to postdiet (1 ± 0.6) levels $(P < .01)$. This study further supported the role of dietary allergens as a trigger for EE in children.

Although the previous studies have shown an association with food allergens and EE, the treatment of the condition with dietary alterations can be challenging. Elemental diets have been found to be unpalatable, requiring the use of nasogastric tube feedings or placement of gastostomy tubes. Elimination diet solely based on allergy testing may have limitations of sensitivity of the available allergy testing methods. Kagalwalla and colleagues [46] demonstrated another approach that can help identify causative food allergens using a standardized six-food (milk, soy, egg, wheat, nuts, and seafood) elimination diet in their pediatric group. During 2001 to 2003, 27 children underwent treatment with an elemental diet, and from 2003 to 2005, 39 children completed a six-food elimination diet. Their main outcome was histologic improvement after the 6-week diet, and there was a significant decrease of histologic eosinophilia with both treatments. They found that 74% of the patients in the food elimination group and 88% in the elemental diet group achieved significant improvement of esophageal inflammation defined as less than 10 eosinophls per high-power field. This group concluded that the six-food elimination diet is a reasonable and often more palatable option than the elemental diet in their cohort.

Although food allergens have been demonstrated to play a role in the cause of children with EE, this has not formally been tested in adults. In a recent study, 26 adult patients with EE underwent allergy testing for both food and environmental allergens by skin prick testing [47]. This group found that 72% of adults had food allergens and 96% had environmental allergens found on skin prick testing. The most common food allergens were milk (40%); tree nuts (40%); soy (38%); peanuts (33%); egg (21%); seafood (21%); and wheat (20%). The most common environmental allergens were grass (83%); ragweed (83%); tree (74%); dust mite (74%); cats (48%); and roach (48%). Patients who had undergone allergy testing were offered treatment with a six-food elimination diet for 6 weeks. Preliminary results suggest a significant improvement both in symptoms and histologic changes after a 6-week dietary trial in some patients (N. Gonsalves, unpublished data, 2007). This suggests that in a subset of adults, the etiology of EE may also be related to food allergies.

PATHOPHYSIOLOGY: THE ROLE OF ENVIRONMENTAL ALLERGENS

Although these studies have shown an association with food allergies and EE, environmental allergens and atopy have also been implicated in the pathophysiology of this condition. About half of both pediatric and adult patients with EE have also been shown to have evidence of other allergic conditions including asthma, allergic rhinitis or sinusitis, and eczema [11,20]. Peripheral eosinophilia can be seen in approximately 30% of adults and 60% of children, and increased IgE level in 55% of adults and 40% to 73% of children [20,21]. Mishra and colleagues [38] have induced EE in their mouse model by exposing mice to an aeroallergen, *Aspergillus fumigates*. This group further investigated the roles of cytokines in the pathogenesis of this inflammatory response using interleukin-5 and eotaxin knockout mice [36,37]. They demonstrated that in response to aeroallergen exposure, eotaxin knockout mice showed decreased esophageal eosinophilia, whereas interleukin-5 knockout mice did not demonstrate any esophageal eosinophilia. They concluded that both interleukin-5 and eotaxin have important roles in eosinophil recruitment in this murine model of EE and may be potential therapeutic targets.

The role of environmental allergens contributing to esophageal eosinophilia has also been suggested in humans. A case report of an adult with allergic rhinoconjunctivitis and asthma demonstrated an increase in symptoms and esophageal eosinophilia during pollen seasons [34]. Interestingly, biopsies obtained during nonpollen months were normal, suggesting that tissue eosinophilia was triggered by pollen exposure. Future studies regarding the pathogenesis of this illness are underway and are critical to developing appropriate treatments.

NATURAL HISTORY

Limited short-term studies addressing the natural history of EE are available. A study by Straumann and coworkers [7] followed a cohort of 30 adults with EE for a mean of 7 years. Although their main symptom of dysphagia persisted in almost every patient, eosinophil levels in the esophagus decreased in the absence of treatment. No patient had concomitant eosinophilic infiltration of the stomach or duodenum either on the index or follow-up endoscopy. Furthermore, none of the patients progressed to hypereosinophilic syndrome or developed a malignancy. An important question raised is whether children with EE outgrow the condition or progress to long-term sequelae, such as fibrosis and strictures. Additional long-term follow-up studies in both the pediatric and adult population are needed to address this concern.

TREATMENT

Treatment approaches for EE vary between children and adult patients (Table 2). In children, the most common approach is to embark on elimination or elemental diets. Preliminary data in adults suggest that elimination diet may also be an effective approach (N. Gonsalves, unpublished data, 2007). Systemic corticosteroids may also effectively treat the symptoms and histologic changes in children with EE. More recently, topical corticosteroids have demonstrated effectiveness [23,41,48,49]. A study by Teitelbaum and colleagues [41] showed that the use of swallowed fluticasone propionate (44 µg/puff for 2–4 years old, 110 µg/puff for 5–10 years old, 220 µg/puff for >11 years old), two puffs twice daily for 8 weeks, significantly reduced the number of eosinophils and lymphocytes in esophageal specimens of children with EE. This treatment has also been tested in adults [23,49]. A recent study by Remedios and colleagues [23] tested this approach in 19 adults. In this group, topical fluticasone (250 µg, two puffs swallowed twice daily for 4 weeks) resulted in significant reduction in symptom score and esophageal eosinophilia posttreatment. This therapy tends to be well tolerated and side effects of oral candidiasis are rare.

Attwood and colleagues [50] studied the use of montelukast in eight adult patients with EE. An initial dose of 10 mg daily was used and increased if needed to a total of 100 mg daily. Maintenance dosages for all patients were

Table 2
Current therapeutic options for patients with eosinophilic esophagitis

Study	N	Treatment	% Response	Mean time to Recurrence
Pediatric				
Liacouras 2000 [43]	20	Methylprednisolone	95	NA
Spergel 2002 [44]	24	Elimination diet x 6 wk	75	NA
Markowitz 2003 [45]	51	Elemental diet x 4 wk	96	NA
Teitelbaum 2002 [41]	11	Fluticasone propionate, 2 puffs twice daily x 8 wk	100	NA
Garrett 2003 [51]	1	Anti–interleukin-5	100	NA
Kagalwalla 2006 [46]	35	Six-food elimination diet	74	NA
Adult				
Arora 2003 [49]	21	Fluticasone propionate, twice daily for 6 wk	100	12–18 mo
Remedios 2006 [23]	19	Fluticasone propionate, twice daily for 4 wk	100	3 mo
Attwood 2003 [50]	8	Montelukast	88	3 wk
Attwood 1993 [3]	12	Esophageal dilation	100	3–6 mo
Straumann 2003 [7]	11	Esophageal dilation	90	8 mo
Potter 2003 [14]	13	Esophageal dilation	54	3 mo

between 20 and 40 mg per day for 4 months. Therapy resulted in resolution of dysphagia symptoms while continuing the medication; however, 75% of patients had recurrence within 3 weeks of cessation or reduction in the medication. Also, treatment with montelukast for 4 months did not reduce the density of eosinophils on repeat biopsy. Another agent that has shown to improve symptoms and histology of EE is anti–interleukin-5 (mepolizumab) [51]. In an open-label trial of anti–interleukin-5 in a patient with EE, this agent improved peripheral eosinophilia, tissue eosinophilia, clinical symptoms, and structural changes of the esophagus. This agent is currently being investigated in clinical trials both for EE and EG.

Esophageal dilation has also been used to treat patients with strictures. Attwood and colleagues [3] performed esophageal dilations in 12 adults with EE. Although dysphagia improved initially, symptoms recurred in all patients 3 to 6 months after dilation. In another adult cohort studied by Straumann and colleagues [7], 10 of 11 patients had symptom resolution after dilation; however, symptoms recurred an average of 8 months later. In another adult group studied by Potter and colleagues [14], transient improvement in symptoms was seen in 7 of 13 adults after dilation. Duration of improvement in this group was less than 3 months, with most patients requiring repeat dilation an average of twice per year. This group, like others, noticed extensive esophageal wall disruption postdilation in their cohort [14,52]. Although dilation may be helpful in the short term, repeated dilations may be required to maintain symptom resolution. Moreover, given the risk of wall disruption and potential for perforation, it is recommended that medical therapy be attempted before dilation.

NEW INSIGHTS IN 2006

In the past year, several important studies have been reported. One study by Liacouras and colleagues [21] described a single center, 10-year experience of a large cohort of children with EE. This retrospective review from January 1, 1994 to January 1, 2004 included 381 patients (66% male; age, 9.1 ± 3.1 years). A total of 312 patients presented with reflux symptoms, with the remainder presenting with dysphagia. Although most patients had abnormal findings at endoscopy, 32% had a normal-appearing esophagus. Endoscopic abnormalities consisted of esophageal furrowing (41%); white plaques (15%); and esophageal rings (12%). The average number of eosinophils in the proximal and distal esophagus was 23.3 ± 10.5 and 38.7 ± 13.3, respectively.

This group found that patients who underwent pharmacologic therapy with either oral methylprednisolone or swallowed fluticasone improved symptomatically and had histologic improvement, but that symptoms recurred on withdrawal of medication. None of 14 patients treated with cromolyn sodium experienced improvement in symptoms. Of the patients who had undergone a dietary restriction based on allergy testing, 57% had demonstrated significant improvement in symptoms and histology for a period of 9 months. Of the 172 patients who underwent complete dietary replacement with an elemental formula, including the 57 patients who failed the elimination diet, 98% experienced significant histologic and dietary improvement. These data suggest that dietary alteration may be a better long-term therapy than steroids for children with EE.

Another study tried to delineate better the prevalence of EE among 31 adult patients with food impaction presenting to a single center [4]. They found that 17 of 31 patients had EE based on more than 20 eosinophils per high-power field. The EE patients were younger and had other endoscopic and histologic findings, such as white exudates and eosinophilic microabscesses. Based on their finding that most food impactions were related to underlying EE, the authors recommended that biopsies be routinely obtained at the time of a food impaction. Making a diagnosis of EE at the time of a food impaction obviates the need for a repeat endoscopy with dilation.

Another important study examined the histopathologic variability in biopsy specimens in 74 adults with EE [24]. This group found that using diagnostic criteria of greater than or equal to 15 eosinophils per high-power field, five biopsies are needed to achieve a 100% sensitivity of diagnosing EE. Using a stricter diagnostic threshold (ie, 30 eosinophils per high-power field), additional biopsies are needed to achieve the same sensitivity. The authors also found that although there was no significant difference between eosinophilia in proximal and distal biopsy locations, taking biopsies from just one site may miss the diagnosis. The authors conclude that obtaining four-quadrant biopsies from both proximal and distal esophagus locations helps maximize sensitivity.

Additional investigations using a murine model of EE have also provided deeper insight into the pathophysiology of this condition, suggesting evidence that epicutaneous exposure to allergens can lead to eosinophil infiltration in the esophagus in mice [53]. Because epidemiologic studies have suggested that atopic dermatitis in childhood is a risk factor for persistence of allergic disease, these authors hypothesized that atopic dermatitis may precede the development of EE in their murine model. They found that epicutaneous antigen exposure to the allergens ova or *A fumigatus* creates an atopic dermatitis-like skin reaction but did not cause eosinophils to migrate to the esophagus. Only when they subsequently exposed these mice to intranasal allergen were they able to induce significant esophageal eosinophilia. They concluded that epicutaneous sensitization by allergens primes the esophagus for respiratory allergen-induced EE in their murine model.

Another pivotal study published by the same group analyzed esophageal tissue in patients with EE, non-EE chronic esophagitis, and controls using a genome-wide microarray expression analysis [54]. They found that patients with EE had a unique transcript signature involving 1% of the human genome. This transcriptome was conserved across sex, age, and allergic status. This group found that the gene encoding for eotaxin-3 (an eosinophil-specific chemoattractant) was the most highly induced gene in EE patients compared with controls, and that esophageal eotaxin-3 mRNA protein levels strongly correlated with tissue eosinophilia and mastocytosis. They also found that a single-nucleotide polymorphism in the human eotaxin-3 gene was associated with disease susceptibility and that eotaxin receptor knockout mice were protected from experimental EE. These results suggest eotaxin-3 is a critical effector molecule for EE and targeted blockers of eotaxin-3 or its receptor may be beneficial in the treatment of EE. These studies and many other investigative efforts in EE are ongoing and it is hoped they will shed more insight into the pathophysiology of this interesting illness.

EOSINOPHILIC GASTROENTERITIS

Although the incidence of EE seems to be rising over the years, EG remains a rare condition. First described by Kaijser [55] in 1937, EG is characterized by tissue eosinophilia that can involve any layer or layers of the gut wall. This diagnosis has further been defined to include demonstration of eosinophilic tissue infiltration of one or more areas of the gastrointestinal tract and the presence of gastrointestinal symptoms in the absence of parasitic infection. Because the disease is so infrequent, incidence is difficult to estimate. Although the disease may affect all ages, typical presentations are in the third through fifth decades. Unlike EE, which has a marked male preponderance, EG tends to have an equal gender distribution [56]. The etiology of EG is still unknown but several theories include an autoimmune, immunologic, or allergic condition. Clinical classification of this condition is based on the predominant layer of gut wall involved [57]. The most common form is characterized by mucosal and submucosal disease. Symptoms may include abdominal pain, nausea, vomiting, regurgitation, diarrhea, weight loss, and protein-losing enteropathy. In this group, 50% of patients may be atopic and 50% may have a history of food intolerance of allergy. Allergic history tends to be more common in children with this condition [58].

Patients with disease affecting predominantly the muscle layer typically present with obstructive symptoms secondary to pyloric or upper intestinal obstruction [59]. Food intolerance or allergic history is not usually present in this subtype. The rarest form is serosal disease, which usually affects all layers of the bowel wall. As a result, eosinophilic ascites may be present. An allergic history may be common in this group [60].

Peripheral eosinophilia is common in EG and is found in up to 80% of patients. The absolute eosinophil count averages 2000 cells/µL in patients with mucosal disease and 1000 cells/µL in patients with muscular involvement. Patients with serosal disease tend to have marked eosinophilia, with counts as high as 8000 cells/µL [56].

TREATMENT OF EOSINOPHILIC GASTROENTERITIS

Treatment of EG tends to be much more challenging than treatment of isolated EE. Because this entity is seen so infrequently, there are no large controlled treatment trials and current management of this condition is guided by supportive evidence from case reports and small clinical series. Once other etiologies of eosinophilic infiltration, such as parasitic infection or drug reaction, are ruled out, an initial approach is to try and identify any causative food allergens followed by a dietary elimination trial. Both elimination and elemental diet have been shown to have efficacy in some series [58,61]. Although some patients may achieve resolution of their symptoms, this may be temporary.

The use of sodium cromoglycate (cromolyn) has been shown to be helpful in some cases. This agent prevents the release of toxic mast cell mediators including histamine, platelet-activating factor, and leukotrienes and also acts to reduce absorption of antigens by the small intestine. The typical doses are usually 200 mg three or four times per day and tend to be well tolerated [62].

Patients who do not respond to dietary therapy or those with nonallergic EG may be tried on glucocorticoids. Approximately 90% of patients respond quickly to a daily dose of 20 to 40 mg per day after 1 to 2 weeks. At this time, a slow taper over several weeks may be attempted. If the patient relapses, a maintenance regimen may be needed [56,63]. Recent reports of the use of budesonide in the treatment of patients with right colon and ileum involvement is also promising [64]. Some suggest that if maintenance with high-dose steroids is needed, immunomodulating agents, such as azathioprine, may be added, but its efficacy is not well established.

Ketotifen, which is not available in the United States, is an H_1-antihistamine that has been shown to reduce symptoms and tissue eosinophilia in patients with EG. It is administered in a dose of 2 to 4 mg per day for 1 to 4 months [65,66]. There is also limited experience with the use of montelukast in EG [67,68]. This agent competitively antagonizes the leukotriene receptor cys-LT1 expressed on bronchial smooth muscle cells and eosinophils, subsequently blocking the action of LTD4, which is a potent and specific eosinophil chemoattractant.

There has also been limited experience with newer biologic agents for this condition. The results of an open-label uncontrolled study of patients with hypereosinophilic syndrome treated with a humanized monoclonal antibody against interleukin-5 have been encouraging [51]. A newer agent, omalizumab, a recombinant IgG1 antibody that binds IgE, has previously been used for the treatment of moderate to severe asthma [69]. There is currently a National Institutes of Health study investigating the use of this agent for patients with EG, and results are eagerly anticipated.

SUMMARY

Although the last several years have led to increased awareness of the prevalence and presentations of eosinophilic gastrointestinal disorders, research over the next several years will be critical to improving the understanding of the pathophysiology, treatment, and natural history of this condition. Further studies delineating the molecular mechanisms behind these conditions should lead to the development of targeted therapeutic agents. The results from these and other studies are eagerly awaited.

References

[1] Lowichik A, Weinberg AG. A quantitative evaluation of mucosal eosinophils in the pediatric gastrointestinal tract. Mod Pathol 1996;9(2):110–4.
[2] Landres RT, Kuster GG, Strum WB. Eosinophilic esophagitis in a patient with vigorous achalasia. Gastroenterology 1978;74:1298–301.
[3] Attwood S, Smyrk T, Demeester T, et al. Esophageal eosinophilia with dysphagia: a distinct clinicopathologic syndrome. Dig Dis Sci 1993;38:109–16.
[4] Desai TK, Stecevic V, Chang C, et al. Association of eosinophilic inflammation with esophageal food impaction in adults. Gastrointest Endosc 2005;61(7):795–801.
[5] Rothenberg M. Eosinophilic gastrointestinal disorders (EGID). J Allergy Clin Immunol 2004;113:11–28.
[6] Croese J, Fairley S, Masson J, et al. Clinical and endoscopic features of eosinophilic esophagitis in adults. Gastrointest Endosc 2003;58(4):516–22.
[7] Straumann A, Spichtin H, Grize L, et al. Natural history of primary eosinophilic esophagitis: a follow-up of 30 adult patients for up to 11.5 years. Gastroenterology 2003;125:1660–9.
[8] Lucendo A, Carrion G, Navarro M, et al. Eosinophilic esophagitis in adults: an emerging disease. Dig Dis Sci 2004;49(11):1884–8.
[9] Esposito S, Marinello D, Paracchini R, et al. Long-term follow-up of symptoms and peripheral eosinophil counts in seven children with eosinophilic esophagitis. J Pediatr Gastroenterol Nutr 2004;38:452–6.
[10] Khan S, Orenstein S, Di Lorenzo C, et al. Eosinophilic esophagitis: strictures, impactions, dysphagia. Dig Dis Sci 2003;48(1):22–9.
[11] Fox V, Nurko S, Furuta G. Eosinophilic esophagitis: it's not just kid's stuff. Gastrointest Endosc 2002;56(2):260–70.
[12] Zimmerman S, Levine M, Rubesin S, et al. Idiopathic eosinophilic esophagitis in adults: the ringed esophagus. Radiology 2005;236(1):159–65.
[13] Arora A, Yamazaki K. Eosinophilic esophagitis: asthma of the esophagus? Clin Gastroenterol Hepatol 2004;2:523–30.
[14] Potter J, Saeian K, Staff D, et al. Eosinophilic esophagitis in adults: an emerging problem with unique esophageal features. Gastrointest Endosc 2004;59(3):355–61.
[15] Cheung KM, Oliver MR, Cameron DJ, et al. Esophageal eosinophilia in children with dysphagia. J Pediatr Gastroenterol Nutr 2003;37(4):498–503.

[16] Noel R, Putnam P, Rothenberg M. Eosinophilic esophagitis. N Engl J Med 2004;351(9): 940–1.

[17] Straumann A, Simon H. Eosinophilic esophagitis: escalating epidemiology? J Allergy Clin Immunol 2005;115(2):418–9.

[18] Ronkainen J, Talley N, Aro P, et al. Prevalence of eosinophilia and eosinophilic esophagitis in adults: the population based Kalixanda study. Gut 2007, in press.

[19] Kugathasan S, Judd R, Hoffman R, et al. Epidemiologic and clinical characteristics of children with newly diagnosed inflammatory bowel disease in Wisconsin: a statewide population-based study. J Pediatr 2003;143:525–31.

[20] Sgouros S, Bergele C, Mantides A. Eosinophilic esophagitis in adults: a systematic review. Eur J Gastroenterol Hepatol 2006;18:211–7.

[21] Liacouras C, Spergel J, Ruchelli E, et al. Eosinophilic esophagitis: a 10-year experience in 381 children. Clin Gastroenterol Hepatol 2005;3(12):1198–206.

[22] Gonsalves N, Kagalwalla A, Kagalwalla A, et al. Distinct features in the clinical presentations of eosinophilic esophagitis in children and adults [abstract]. Gastroenterology 2005;128(4)S2:A7.

[23] Remedios M, Campbell C, Jones D, et al. Eosinophilic esophagitis in adults: clinical, endoscopic, histologic findings, and response to treatment with fluticasone propionate. Gastrointest Endosc 2006;63(1):3–12.

[24] Gonsalves N, Policarpio-Nicolas M, Zhang Q, et al. Histopathologic variability and endoscopic correlates in adults with eosinophilic esophagitis. Gastrointest Endosc 2006;64(3): 313–9.

[25] Morrow J, Vargo J, Goldblum J, et al. The ringed esophagus: histologic features of GERD. Am J Gastroenterol 2001;96(4):984–9.

[26] Winter HS, Madara JL, Stafford RJ, et al. Intraepithelial eosinophils: a new diagnostic criterion for reflux esophagitis. Gastroenterology 1982;83:818–23.

[27] Kelly K, Lazenby A, Rowe P, et al. Eosinophilic esophagitis attributed to gastroesophageal reflux: improvement with an amino-acid based formula. Gastroenterology 1995;109: 1503–12.

[28] Ruchelli E, Wenner W, Voytek T, et al. Severity of esophageal eosinophilia predicts response to conventional gastroesophageal reflux therapy. Pediatr Dev Pathol 1999;2: 15–8.

[29] Steiner S, Gupta S, Croffie J, et al. Correlation between number of eosinophils and reflux index on same day esophageal biopsy and 24 hour esophageal pH monitoring. Am J Gastroenterol 2004;59(7):801–5.

[30] Lee R. Marked eosinophilia in esophageal mucosal biopsies. Am J Surg Pathol 1985;7: 475–9.

[31] Stevoff C, Rao S, Parsons W, et al. EUS and histopathologic correlates in eosinophilic esophagitis. Gastrointest Endosc 2001;54:373–7.

[32] Lutsi B, Hirano I, Alasadi R. Manometric, endoscopic and histopathologic correlates of diffuse esophageal spasm secondary to eosinophilic esophagitis. Am J Gastroenterol 2006;101(9):S394.

[33] Fox V, Nurko S, Teitelbaum J, et al. High-resolution EUS in children with eosinophilic "allergic" esophagitis. Gastrointest Endosc 2003;57(1):30–6.

[34] Fogg M, Ruchelli E, Spergel J. Pollen and eosinophilic esophagitis. J Allergy Clin Immunol 2003;112(4):796–7.

[35] Fujiwara H, Morita A, Kobayashi H, et al. Infiltrating eosinophils and eotaxin: their association with idiopathic eosinophilic esophagitis. Ann Allergy Asthma Immunol 2002;89: 429–32.

[36] Mishra A, Rothenberg M. Intratracheal Il-13 induces eosinophilic esophagitis by an Il-5, eotaxin-1 and STAT6-dependent mechanism. Gastroenterology 2003;125:1419–27.

[37] Mishra A, Hogan S, Brandt E, et al. Il-5 promotes eosinophil trafficking to the esophagus. J Immunol 2002;168:2464–9.

[38] Mishra A, Hogan S, Brandt E, et al. An etiological role for aeroallergens and eosinophils in experimental esophagitis. J Clin Invest 2001;107:83–90.

[39] Rothenberg M, Mishra A, Collins M, et al. Pathogenesis and clinical features of eosinophilic esophagitis. J Allergy Clin Immunol 2001;108:891–4.

[40] Straumann A, Bauer M, Fischer B, et al. Idiopathic eosinophilic esophagitis is associated with a Th2-type allergic inflammatory response. J Allergy Clin Immunol 2001;108(6): 954–61.

[41] Teitelbaum J, Fox V, Twarong F, et al. Eosinophilic esophagitis in children: immunopathological analysis and response to fluticasone propionate. Gastroenterology 2002;122: 1216–25.

[42] Straumann A, Simon H. The physiological and pathophysiological roles of eosinophils in the gastrointestinal tract. Allergy 2004;59:15–25.

[43] Liacouras CA, Wenner WJ, Brown K, et al. Primary eosinophilic esophagitis in children: successful treatment with oral corticosteroids. J Pediatr Gastroenterol Nutr 1998;26(4):380–5.

[44] Spergel J, Beausoleil J, Mascarenhas M, et al. The use of skin prick tests and patch tests to identify causative foods in eosinophilic esophagitis. J Allergy Clin Immunol 2002;109: 363–8.

[45] Markowitz J, Spergel J, Ruchelli E, et al. Elemental diet is an effective treatment for eosinophilic esophagitis in children and adolescents. Am J Gastroenterol 2003;98(4):777–82.

[46] Kagalwalla A, Sentongo T, Ritz S, et al. Effect of six-food elimination diet on clinical and histologic outcomes in eosinophilic esophagitis. Clin Gastroenterol Hepatol 2006;4: 1097–102.

[47] Gonsalves N, Le Thuy, Zhang Q, et al. Distinct allergic predisposition of children and adults with eosinophilic esophagitis. [abstract]. Gastroenterology 2006;130(4):T1947.

[48] Noel R, Putnam P, Collins M, et al. Clinical and immunopathologic effects of swallowed fluticasone for eosinophilic esophagitis. Clin Gastroenterol Hepatol 2004;2:568–75.

[49] Arora A, Perrault J, Smyrk T. Topical corticosteroid treatment of dysphagia due to eosinophilic esophagitis in adults. Mayo Clin Proc 2003;78:830–5.

[50] Attwood S, Lewis C, Bronder C, et al. Eosinophilic esophagitis: a novel treatment using Montelukast. Gut 2003;52:181–5.

[51] Garrett J, Jameson S, Thomson B, et al. Anti-interleukin-5 (mepolizumab) therapy for hypereosinophilic syndromes. J Allergy Clin Immunol 2004;113:115–9.

[52] Kaplan M, Mutlu EA, Jakate S, et al. Endoscopy in eosinophilic esophagitis: "feline" esophagus and perforation risk. Clin Gastroenterol Hepatol 2003;1(6):433–7.

[53] Akei H, Mishra A, Blanchard C, et al. Epicutaneous antigen exposure primes for experimental eosinophilic esophagitis in mice. Gastroenterology 2005;129:985–94.

[54] Blanchard C, Wang N, Stringer K, et al. Eotaxin-3 and a uniquely conserved gene-expression profile in eosinophilic esophagitis. J Clin Invest 2006;116:536–47.

[55] Kaijser R. Allergic disease of the gut from the point of view of the surgeon. Langenbecks Arch Klin Chir Ver Dtsch Z Chir 1937;188:34–64.

[56] Talley NJ, Shorter RG, Phillips SF, et al. Eosinophilic gastroenteritis: a clinicopathological study of patients with disease of the mucosae, muscle layer, and subserosal tissues. Gut 1990;31:54–8.

[57] Klein NC, Hargrove RL, Sleisenger MH, et al. Eosinophilic gastroenteritis. Medicine 1970;49:299–319.

[58] Khan S. Eosinophilic gastroenteritis. Best Pract Res Clin Gastroenterol 2005;19(2): 177–98.

[59] Khan S, Orenstein SR. Eosinophilic gastroenteritis masquerading as pyloric stenosis. Clin Pediatr 2000;39:55–7.

[60] McNabb PC, Fleming CR, Higgins JA, et al. Transmural eosinophilic gastroenteritis with ascites. Mayo Clin Proc 1979;54:119–22.

[61] Chen MJ, Chu CH, Lin SC, et al. Eosinophilic gastroenteritis: 10 years experience. Am J Gastroenterol 2003;9:2813–6.

[62] Perez-Millan A, Martin-Lorente JL, Lopez-Morante A, et al. Subserosal eosinophilic gastroenteritis treated efficaciously with sodium cromoglycate. Dig Dis Sci 1997;42:342–4.

[63] Kalantar SJ, Marks R, Lambert JR, et al. Dyspepsia due to eosinophilic gastroenteritis. Dig Dis Sci 1997;42:2327–32.

[64] Tan AC, Kruimel JW, Naber TH. Eosinophilic gastroenteritis treated with non-enteric coated budesonide tablets. Eur J Gastroenterol Hepatol 2001;13:425–7.

[65] Suzuki J, Kawasaki Y, Nozawa R, et al. Oral disodium cromoglycate and ketotifen for a patient with eosinophilic gastroenteritis, food allergy and protein-losing enteropathy. Asian Pac J Allergy Immunol 2003;21:193–7.

[66] Melamed I, Feanny SJ, Sherman PM, et al. Benefit of ketotifen in patients with eosinophilic gastroenteritis. Am J Med 1991;90:310–4.

[67] Neustrom MR, Friesen C. Treatment of eosinophilic gastroenteritis with montelukast. J Allergy Clin Immunol 1999;104:506.

[68] Schwartz DA, Pardi DS, Murray AJ. Use of montelukast as steroid sparing agent for recurrent eosinophilic gastroenteritis. Dig Dis Sci 2001;46:1787–90.

[69] Nowak D. Management of asthma with anti-immunoglobulin E: a review of clinical trials of omalizumab. Respir Med 2006;100(11):1907–17.

Gastroenterol Clin N Am 36 (2007) 93–108

GASTROENTEROLOGY CLINICS
OF NORTH AMERICA

Nutritional Deficiencies in Celiac Disease

Susan H. Barton, MD, Darlene G. Kelly, MD, PhD*,
Joseph A. Murray, MD

Division of Gastroenterology and Hepatology, Mayo Clinic, 200 First Street SW,
Rochester, MN 55905, USA

C eliac disease is characterized by small bowel enteropathy, precipitated in genetically susceptible individuals by the ingestion of "gluten," a term used to encompass the storage proteins of wheat, rye, and barley. Although the intestine heals with removal of gluten from the diet, the intolerance is permanent and the damage recurs if gluten is reintroduced. The major site of damage is in the proximal small intestine. This damage causes a wide variety of consequences, including maldigestion and malabsorption. These derangements result in the characteristic, although not universal, features of malnutrition. This article examines recent advances in the understanding of the spectrum of celiac disease, illustrates the impact of celiac disease on nutrition, and describes approaches to the management of the disease.

EPIDEMIOLOGY

Celiac disease was previously thought to be quite rare in the United States, affecting 1 per 10,000 to 1 per 4800 based on two epidemiologic studies performed before 2000 [1,2]. A more recent study showed an increase in the incidence, particularly in adults [3]. A large multicenter study in 2003 determined the frequency of celiac disease in at-risk and not-at-risk groups and found the overall prevalence in the United States to be much higher, at 1 per 133 persons. In addition, they demonstrated the prevalence rates in first-degree relatives to be 1:22, in second-degree relatives to be 1:39, and in symptomatic patients to be 1:6 [4]. Prevalence in European countries ranges from 1 in 85 to 1 in 540, and additional reports from South America, Asia, and Africa indicate that celiac disease has a much higher occurrence than previously thought [5–28]. A frequency of 1 per 133 in the United States comprises approximately 2 million people who have active or more often silent celiac disease. The "celiac iceberg" is often used to illustrate the distribution of cases, with the smallest tip portion being composed of the active, clinically apparent

*Corresponding author. E-mail address: kelly.darlene@mayo.edu (D.G. Kelly).

0889-8553/07/$ – see front matter
doi:10.1016/j.gtc.2007.01.006

cases of malabsorption. Most cases are silent, with complete absence of gastrointestinal symptoms.

In European countries, Italy has one of the higher rates of undiagnosed celiac disease at 1 per 184 of the population [23]. A large multicenter trial assessing prevalence demonstrated regional variation within Italy, with the highest rates in the Lombardia and Piedmont regions and the lowest rates within Sardinia and Umbria [24]. A recent follow-up study in Carcare, a region of Italy previously thought to have an exceptionally low prevalence of celiac disease, screened patients using antitransglutaminase and antiendomysial antibody (AEA) titers and found a prevalence rate of 1 per 100, suggesting significant underdiagnosis of celiac disease [19]. Table 1 compares prevalence rates between the United States, additional European countries, and the Middle East.

One recent study characterized the prevalence of immigrants in Italy and found a disease occurrence of 1.9 per 100 immigrant children; the highest rates were among children of Eastern European and North African descent [25]. The highest European prevalence rate found was in 1 per 85 Hungarian children, detected only by AEA titer [18]. The highest rate found worldwide is reported from the Western Sahara, in which the prevalence was 5.6 per 100 from a group of 989 children [7].

True prevalence data are not known in India, although a retrospective analysis from a single medical center revealed an increased rate of incidence from 1995 to 2000 [5,6]. Among South and Central American countries, recent data from Argentina show a prevalence rate of 1 per 167 [14], lower prevalence in Brazil at 1 per 417 [12], and the highest prevalence in the Mexican mestizo population of Spanish European heritage with 2.6 per 100 [11].

Table 1
Prevalence rates within the United States, European and Middle Eastern countries

Country	Prevalence rate (undiagnosed celiac disease)
United Kingdom [22]	1 per 100
Finland [21]	1 per 130
Northern Ireland [28]	1 per 122
Northern Spain [26]	1 per 389
Dresden, Germany [17]	1 per 500 (pediatric population)
	1 per 540 (adult population)
Sweden [15]	1–2 per 100 (pediatric population)
Israel [16]	1 per 157
Turkey, Central Anatolia [10]	1 per 100
Iran [8]	1 per 104
United States [4]	1 per 133

PATHOGENESIS

The development of celiac disease is the result of an unchecked immune response to the ingestion of gluten. Both innate and adaptive immunologic responses are up-regulated at the level of the small intestinal mucosa in the setting of gluten exposure. The innate immune response is the initial activation step in the presence of foreign antigens (ie, food and microbial cell surface proteins) and is mediated primarily by $CD8^+$ T cells, enterocytes, macrophages, and dendritic cells. In genetically susceptible individuals, ingestion of gluten results in expansion of specific intraepithelial lymphocyte populations and dysregulated expression of the proinflammatory cytokine, interleukin-15, on the enterocytes [29]. This chronic inflammatory state contributes to increased permeability of the intestinal mucosa and presumably increases the risk of loss of immune tolerance given the heightened interaction with foreign antigens present in the gut milieu [30]. Current ongoing research suggests that the innate immune response of celiac disease patients is inherently dysfunctional and the consequences of this dysregulation in response to continual exposure to the food proteins and possibly microbial antigens in the gut are key factors in the initiation events preceding development of celiac disease [31,32]. Specific immunogenic peptides within wheat and the other grains protein have been found to produce a potent response of the adaptive immune system. The adaptive arm of the immune response has been well-characterized with $CD4^+$ T cells responding to gluten in a major histocompatibility complex class II–restricted manner and within the context of DQ2-DQ8 T-cell receptors [33]. This immune response, which is required for the development of celiac disease, results in an inflammatory cascade with the release of interferon-γ, further perpetuating the proinflammatory state within the mucosa [33]. This leads to recruitment of many other inflammatory mediators and eventual remodeling of the mucosa that ultimately causes the nutritional consequences of the disease.

There is also a substantial humoral response to gluten with both secreted and circulating antibodies directed against the dominant immunogenic protein, gliadin. In addition to this response to the exogenous antigen, antibodies are also produced against an autoantigen [33]. Initially, this was characterized as the endomysial antibody and subsequently determined to be tissue transglutaminase. The role of tissue transglutaminase and the humoral response to it, in initiation and perpetuation of celiac disease pathogenesis, remains unclear. Transglutaminases are ubiquitous enzymes with diverse functions within the human body, including catalysis of protein cross-linking and angiogenesis [34]. Transglutaminase class 2, which is the relevant enzyme form in celiac disease, functions to deamidate specific glutamine residues within the gluten peptide to glutamate, thereby increasing the gluten peptide's immunogenicity [33]. The prevailing hypothesis is that gluten ingestion stimulates the $CD4^+$ T cells in the lamina propria, which in turn stimulate proinflammatory cytokine production and also production of autoantibodies in the form of antitransglutaminase and AEA [35].

DIAGNOSIS

In the past, celiac disease was defined solely by the clinical picture of severe malabsorption. In the 1950s, however, the characteristic gluten-induced changes in the small intestinal mucosa were described. Currently, celiac disease is detected with serologic tests, specifically antitransglutaminase or anti-AEA antibodies, but requires confirmation by intestinal biopsy. AEA is highly specific (approaching 100%), although it has a variable sensitivity and may be less sensitive than antitransglutaminase [36,37]. One study noted that AEA levels were always positive in the setting of total villous atrophy, but were less sensitive in those cases of less severe damage, and concluded that several cases of celiac disease in that particular series would have been missed if the patients had not been recommended for biopsy [38]. In general use, most studies have reported a high sensitivity of transglutaminase antibody for untreated celiac disease [39].

The gold standard for diagnosis is traditionally small intestinal biopsy and subsequent response to a gluten-free diet. The biopsies can be assessed or staged according to the degree of injury that has occurred. This staging is based on characterizing the histologic evolution of the celiac intestinal lesion after challenging healed celiacs with gluten. Marsh 1 comprises increased intraepithelial lymphocytes (infiltrative type); Marsh 2 comprises Marsh 1 changes and crypt hyperplasia (hyperplastic type); and Marsh 3 consists of partial to total villous atrophy (atrophic type) [40]. It is the damage to villous architecture that has traditionally been thought to give rise to the clinical symptoms and nutritional deficiencies associated with celiac disease.

CLINICAL PRESENTATION

The clinical presentation of celiac disease has traditionally been one of diarrhea, weight loss, abdominal pain, refractory iron deficiency anemia, and malabsorption, although recent studies have increasingly characterized celiac disease patients as having symptoms less typical for classic malabsorption. Extraintestinal manifestations of celiac disease affecting multiple organ systems are becoming increasingly recognized. Additional features associated with celiac disease are low birth weight and intrauterine growth retardation among infants born to untreated celiac mothers, recurrent abortions, infertility, late menarche, early menopause, persistent transaminitis, short stature, premature osteopenia and osteoporosis, aphthous stomatitis, folate-zinc deficiency, macrocytosis, depression, and chronic fatigue [41]. Conditions associated with celiac disease include dermatitis herpetiformis, Sjögren's syndrome, type I diabetes mellitus, autoimmune thyroid disease, microscopic colitis, IgA nephropathy, and selective IgA deficiency [41,42].

Because of the high prevalence of celiac disease in both Europe and the United States, and the emerging prevalence being found in South America, Asia, and North Africa, much debate has focused on mass screening of the population for this chronic disease. Given the lack of evidence as to the natural history of silent celiac disease, mass screening is not wholly supported [37]. More aggressive screening for high-risk groups has been advocated based on the reports of increased prevalence within these select groups [4]. Several cases highlight the nutritional deficiencies relevant to both classic and silent forms of celiac disease.

Case 1

A 32-year-old man with type I diabetes mellitus and chronic anemia presented to his physician, complaining of chronic epigastric pain and fatigue. He reports adequate blood sugar control and no recent illnesses. He has two young children who are healthy. His family history is negative for known celiac disease. His mother has rheumatoid arthritis. His laboratory results reveal elevated transglutaminase and AEA levels and his small bowel biopsy shows partial villous atrophy consistent with celiac disease. In addition, ferritin and vitamin B_{12} levels are low. He asks if his children (ages 3 and 5) should undergo screening for celiac disease in the absence of gastrointestinal symptoms and normal growth and development.

Type I diabetics and first-degree relatives of celiac patients are considered high-risk groups for celiac disease, and testing for celiac disease should be considered in all patients, but especially in those with any gastrointestinal symptoms. Additional at-risk groups include those patients with Sjögren's syndrome, connective tissue diseases, autoimmune liver, thyroid disease, Downs and Williams syndromes, selective IgA deficiency, and relatives of celiac patients [4,41]. The association of celiac disease with autoimmune disease has been recognized, although a causal basis has not been clearly established. Ventura and colleagues [43] showed that length of exposure to gluten increased the risk of developing autoimmune disease, supporting a causal relationship between chronic gluten exposure and dysregulation of innate and adaptive immune mechanisms. Prevalence testing has used several methods for screening: AEA only, antigliadin IgA followed with AEA if antigliadin titers are positive, and antitransglutaminase antibody in conjunction with AEA. In the case of IgA deficiency, IgG class antitransglutaminase levels should be obtained.

Initial evaluation for newly diagnosed celiac disease includes testing for iron, folate, and vitamin B_{12} deficiencies. Because the proximal small intestine is the predominant site of inflammation and also the site of iron absorption, malabsorption of iron is markedly impaired and the association of celiac disease to refractory iron deficiency anemia is well established. The frequency of iron deficiency anemia in celiac disease varies from 12% to 69% [44] and is reportedly higher in patients with long-standing, untreated disease [45]. Malabsorption is likely the cause of iron deficiency anemia, but the frequency of occult gastrointestinal bleeding as a contributing factor in celiac disease is more controversial, with conflicting results from various studies [46–49]. In the absence of blood loss, iron deficiency anemia resolves with adherence to a gluten-free diet, although normalization of the iron stores may require months in tandem with healing of the small intestinal mucosa.

Incidence of vitamin B_{12} deficiency in untreated celiac patients ranges from 11% to 41% [50,51]; the more recent study controlled for underlying pernicious anemia. Given that site of vitamin B_{12} absorption is ileal and the relative sparing of villous atrophy in the ileum of celiac patients, the mechanisms inducing deficiency are unclear. A recent study of histologic changes in celiac disease by Dickey and Hughes [52] revealed an increase in the degree of ileal intraepithelial lymphocytosis, and that this finding correlated to duodenal villous atrophy. No data are available investigating the impairment of vitamin B_{12} absorption in the setting of increased ileal intraepithelial lymphocytosis. Although ileal inflammatory changes and functional impairment have not been extensively studied in the context of celiac disease, the basis for the observed vitamin B_{12} deficiency is considered most likely caused by underlying mucosal changes [51].

In patients presenting with the classic malabsorption of celiac disease, deficiencies in fat-soluble vitamins (vitamins A, D, E, and K) are commonly encountered. Serum retinol is used to measure vitamin A deficiency with clinical manifestations including night blindness, conjunctival dryness, and keratomalacia [53]. Vitamin D is ingested in a prohormone form, converted in the liver to 25-hydroxyvitamin D, and then later changed to the active form 1,25-hydroxyvitamin D at the level of the kidneys [53]. The recommended range of 25-hydroxyvitamin D is 30 to 50 ng/dL [54]. Vitamin D malabsorption may result in osteomalacia, which clinically manifests as muscle weakness and musculoskeletal pain; diagnosis is established with low serum 25-hydroxyvitamin D levels less than 20 [54]. Osteomalacia secondary to vitamin D deficiency has become increasingly recognized in relation to celiac disease in several recently published case reports [55,56]. In the event of vitamin D deficiency, repletion recommendations are 50,000 IU of oral vitamin D per week for 8 weeks [54]. Vitamin E is an antioxidant with deficiency states associated with hemolytic anemia, gait disturbance, and neuropathy. Low vitamin K levels are detected by prolonged prothrombin time, result in decreased synthesis of clotting factors II, VII, IX, and X, and predispose to hemorrhage [53].

Case 2

A 35-year-old woman with hypothyroidism and refractory iron deficiency anemia presented to a primary care clinic complaining of chronic fatigue of several months duration. She reports sleeping 10 hours per night, but continues to have chronic fatigue, which is negatively impacting her work and ability to care for her young son. Her hemoglobin has improved minimally on iron supplementation and thyroid-stimulating hormone is normal on levothyroxine replacement. She reports two spontaneous abortions before her son's birth 4 years ago. There were no complications during her pregnancy, except for mild intrauterine growth retardation of the fetus. Her parents are healthy and she reports her paternal grandmother had type I diabetes mellitus. Her transglutaminase and AEA antibody titers were found to be elevated and small bowel biopsy revealed total villous atrophy consistent with celiac disease.

Additional nutritional screening considered in the setting of newly diagnosed celiac disease includes copper, zinc, and folate deficiency. Folic acid is absorbed in the jejunum, the proximal segments of which can be inflamed and damaged in active celiac disease. Red blood cell macrocytosis is often present, although the presence of iron deficiency anemia may result in a mixed picture on the blood smear. In nonfasting states, decreased serum folate levels less than 2 ng/mL establish the diagnosis [57]. Howard and colleagues [58] noted that 4.7% of 258 patients with evidence of iron and folate deficiency had celiac disease, yet did not exhibit clinical signs of malabsorption. Moreover, Haapalahti and coworkers [59] in 2005 reported 31% of young celiac patients, detected by screening alone and without overt malabsorption, showed evidence of subnormal folate levels. Given these results, folate supplementation is recommended to ensure that the goal daily allowance is consumed until the damaged, functionally impaired villous architecture normalizes in the absence of gluten.

Early studies measuring serum zinc concentrations indicate significant deficiency in patients with active disease [60]. Zinc absorption occurs primarily in the jejunum; following digestion, zinc complexes with various ligands in the intestine and is transported through both active and passive processes into the circulation [61]. Zinc is used as a cofactor for multiple metalloenzymes and mild deficiency states cause impaired immune function, hypogonadism, oligospermia, alopecia, poor wound healing, and skin changes (eg, pustular and vesiculobullous lesions) [62]. Zinc pools are stored in the bone, plasma, and liver and fluctuate in response to stress and infection, casting doubt on the accuracy of serum zinc concentrations to measure deficiency states [63]. Plasma zinc concentrations have traditionally been used to this end, although plasma metallothionen levels are also considered a useful tool in terms of measuring hepatic stores of zinc [63].

The exact prevalence of copper deficiency in active celiac disease is unclear. This micronutrient is primarily absorbed in the small intestine, bound to albumin in the portal circulation, and subsequently transferred to copper-dependent ceruloplasmin [64]. Copper is used as a cofactor by multiple enzymes involved in redox reactions and is essential for ceruloplasmin ferroxidase function. Of the few, small studies on copper deficiency and celiac disease, there is an association between unexplained anemia or neutropenia and low copper levels [65,66]. Although copper deficiency is considered quite rare, groups at increased risk include patients on long-term parenteral nutrition, those with postgastrectomy malabsorption syndromes, and malnourished infants [67]. One study reported hematologic abnormalities among patients dependent on enteral feedings as caused by underlying copper deficiency. These abnormalities included anemia and neutropenia with preservation of normal platelet levels (bicytopenia), macrocytosis, and elevated serum ferritin and erythropoietin. Normalization of these changes occurred with copper repletion [67]. Copper deficiency states have also been associated with microcytic and normocytic anemia; the mechanism causing these hematologic changes is unknown [68]. Serum copper levels are used to screen for deficiency.

Several studies have implicated subclinical celiac disease in the cause of recurrent abortions, infertility, decreased age of menopause, low birth weight infants, and increased risk of intrauterine growth retardation [69–73]. Prevalence of undiagnosed celiac disease in mothers of small-for-gestational age infants is increased in one study at 1.60% from the baseline prevalence of celiac disease among Italian women, 0.9% to 1% [69]. Mechanisms to explain this association have included occult malnutrition of the mother and immunologically based pathogenic mechanisms [70]. Ludviggson and colleagues [74] performed a retrospective study of 2078 Swedish children born to mothers with celiac disease (varied time of diagnosis, before and after pregnancy). There was an increased rate in intrauterine growth retardation, low birth weight, preterm labor, and cesarean section; these risks were reportedly reduced when celiac disease had been diagnosed and presumably treated with gluten-free diet. Severe malabsorption has not been associated with decreased fetal growth per studies by Ciacci and coworkers [75] and Sher and Mayberry [71], increasing the likelihood of an immunologically based mechanism; investigators have implicated decreased placental angiogenesis secondary to elevated antitransglutaminase antibody in untreated celiac patients (which occurs in early disease phases before development of intestinal lesions and subsequent severe malnutrition) [76]. In the setting of pregnancy, the potential for folic acid deficiency is of particular importance, although the authors found no reports of increased incidence of neural tube defects.

Case 3

A 45-year-old obese woman with a history of depression presented to clinic complaining of chronic constipation and mild dyspepsia. She reports past episodes of atopic dermatitis secondary to nickel exposure in jewelry. Her family history is notable for a mother with gastroesophageal reflux disease and hypothyroidism. Laboratory studies revealed mild hypothyroidism. Following correction of the elevated thyroid-stimulating hormone, her symptoms persisted and screening transglutaminase and AEA antibody titers were elevated. Small bowel biopsy showed partial villous atrophy consistent with celiac disease. Bone densitometry revealed evidence of early osteoporosis.

A recent study from Northern Ireland found that only 5% of 371 celiac patients were underweight, 57% had normal body mass index, 39% were obese, and 13% were morbidly obese [77]. Moreover, these obese patients were less likely to present clinically with iron deficiency anemia or diarrhea. The authors suggest that variations in the body mass index of patients are related variable percentages of the small intestine affected by inflammation, consider the prediagnosis dietary modification by patients for gluten-free foods, and cite prior studies indicating that weight gain can occur following initiation of gluten-free diet. Weight gain has been attributed to replacement of high-fat foods for gluten-containing products [78]. In the study, no correlation between

AEA titers and body mass index was noted. They suggest that low clinical suspicion in the setting of normal or high body mass index may result in delay of diagnosis resulting in increased morbidity and mortality within the silent celiac population. These findings further underscore the celiac iceberg model of disease prevalence, with most patients existing beneath the surface without overt malabsorption and weight loss.

One notable alteration in lipid metabolism, following the initiation of a gluten-free diet, was reported in a recent study by Brar and colleagues [79] that found significant increases in total cholesterol and high-density lipoprotein levels and a decrease in the low-density/high-density lipoprotein ratio in both symptomatic and silent patients following dietary modification. Low total cholesterol and serum high-density lipoprotein in association with celiac disease have been reported in the literature [79–81]. The authors proposed two possible mechanisms for these changes: increased intestinal synthesis of both high-density lipoprotein and apolipoprotein A-I (the main high-density lipoprotein apoprotein), given the reported decreased intestinal production of apolipoprotein A-I during active celiac disease; and increased fat absorption from the diet with the high high-density lipoprotein levels reflecting a change of the type of fat consumed. Notably, the patients with the most significant fluctuations were noted to have the lowest total cholesterol levels before initiation of a gluten-free diet. High high-density lipoprotein conveys a cardioprotective effect, although no reduction in myocardial infarction was observed in a population-based study by West and colleagues [82].

Diminished bone density may be caused by osteomalacia or osteoporosis in the context of active celiac disease and is related, in part, to decreased calcium absorption in the proximal small intestine, subsequent elevation in parathyroid hormone levels, and resultant loss of cortical bone. Measurement of bone density, serum calcium, alkaline phosphatase, and parathyroid hormone levels is thereby recommended at the time of diagnosis [83]. Additional recommended measures include ensuring adequate calcium intake to maintain the 1500 mg per day, adhering to a strict gluten-free diet, exercise, abstaining from tobacco usage, minimizing alcohol intake, obtaining a baseline bone mineral density by dual energy x-ray absorptiometry scan, and screening for vitamin D deficiency. For men older than 55 years, postmenopausal women, and patients with a history of a prior "fragility fracture" (ie, resulting from a minimal fall or without obvious trauma), bisphosphonate and calcitonin therapy are potential treatment options [83]. Some propose the excessive bone loss seen in untreated celiac disease patients is multifactorial because of calcium malabsorption from mucosal lesions and secondary effects of proinflammatory cytokines (eg, interleukin-6, tumor necrosis factor-α, interleukin-1) [84,85]. Interleukin-6, specifically, has been shown to up-regulate osteoclast activity and be inversely proportional to bone mineral density [86]. Children with celiac disease demonstrate decreased bone mineral density, which has been shown to recover following initiation of gluten-free diet, yet complete recovery may require over 12 months [87]. The risk of fractures has been shown to be increased in celiac patients, although a recent study by West and colleagues [88] found only a moderately increased risk in hip, ulnar, and radial fractures in patients with an established diagnosis of celiac disease [89,90]. Some have recommended that bone mineral density measurements be repeated in 1 year following strict adherence to a gluten-free diet among patients with evidence of malabsorption at diagnosis [91], yet the study by West and colleagues [88] raises the overall question of the cost effectiveness in recommending universal screening for bone disease.

Dermatologic conditions associated with celiac disease are considered primarily immune-mediated and less caused by nutritional deficiency states. The classic skin condition linked with celiac disease is dermatitis herpetiformis, although additional associated skin disorders include urticaria, hereditary angioneurotic edema, cutaneous vasculitis, and erythema nodosum [92]. Moreover, prevalence of silent celiac disease in patients with atopic histories including asthma, rhinoconjunctivitis, atopic dermatitis, and angioedema was shown to be 1% in a study from Bologna, Italy [93].

Case 4

A 52-year-old man with known celiac disease diagnosed in his early 20s, with a long-standing history of noncompliance with a gluten-free diet, presented with acute onset of severe abdominal pain. CT imaging revealed evidence of small bowel perforation. On laparotomy, a perforated tumor of the jejunum was found and resected. Pathology from the resected bowel showed evidence of ulcerative jejunitis at the site of perforation and lesions consistent with T-cell lymphoma. Positron emission tomography revealed multiple, additional lesions in the jejunum suggestive of malignancy.

Corrao and colleagues [94] report an increase in overall mortality of patients with delayed diagnosis and those who are noncompliant with gluten-free diet [94]. Green and colleagues [95] estimated that in the United States, symptoms are present for a mean of 11 years before diagnosis and report marked improvement in quality of life following diagnosis, even in the age 60 and above group. One study from Sweden found an elevation in mortality from all causes in a group of 828 celiac patients and found risks elevated in multiple areas, notably non-Hodgkin's lymphoma, small intestinal cancer, rheumatoid arthritis, connective tissue disease, and diabetes [96]. A recently published study from the United Kingdom found that of 4732 celiac patients, there was a 30% overall increased risk of any malignancy [82]. Specifically, an increased risk in gastrointestinal cancers and lymphoproliferative cancer types was observed, in addition to a decreased risk of lung and breast cancer. The mechanisms to explain the decreased risk of breast cancer among celiac patients is unknown and is an area of ongoing research. These findings were consistent, albeit lower, than malignancy rates reported by Askling and colleagues [97], who found increased risks of malignant lymphomas, small-intestinal, oropharyngeal, esophageal, large intestinal, hepatobiliary, and pancreatic carcinomas [97].

TREATMENT

Adherence to gluten-free diet remains the mainstay of therapy for celiac disease. Although a gluten-free diet seems simple theoretically, its implementation is much more difficult. It requires dedicated well-motivated patients who are provided with adequate personalized instruction by an expert dietitian and family and community support. The diet should avoid foods and any other ingestants (eg, lipstick and communion wafers) that are made with wheat, barley, or rye. Oats has been controversial but probably are safe for most celiacs if pure oats are used. Detection and correction of nutritional deficiencies is also important. Emphasis on education for patients and their families, and consistent follow-up with a knowledgeable nutritionist, is essential [98].

Symptoms resolve in most cases following compliance with gluten-free diet. Follow-up is important to ensure compliance and to detect any complications that may have occurred. Surveillance transglutaminase antibody serology is sensitive for large amounts of gluten contamination, and when persistently positive should prompt a careful re-evaluation of the gluten-free diet [99]. Vahedi and colleagues [100] reports that transglutaminase and AEA antibody levels are not reliable markers of low-level contamination with gluten. Teenagers are especially likely to cheat, and the absence of symptoms with gluten ingestion may give a false sense of safety to some. Excess weight gain, elevation in cholesterol and lipids, excess food restriction, and social isolation may occur following the institution of a gluten-free diet and dietary consultation should be sought. On a societal level, a greater awareness of celiac disease and the need for gluten-free foods prompted changes in food labeling laws in the United States and elsewhere and has made life a little easier (Box 1).

REFRACTORY SPRUE

A few patients either relapse after an initial response to a gluten-free diet or have never responded to gluten withdrawal. Often older in age, these patients have persistent malabsorption and villous atrophy despite a strict gluten-free diet. These patients are very ill and malnourished, characterized by low

---

Box 1: Overview of management recommendations at time of diagnosis

Referral to dietitian with expertise in celiac disease

Obtain baseline bone mineral density (dual energy x-ray absorptiometry), screen for vitamin D deficiency

Basic hematologic indices to assess for anemia and depletion of iron stores, screen for vitamin B_{12}, folic acid, zinc, and copper deficiency

Referral to support group for education of both patients and their family members

Follow-up with clinician within 1 year to obtain surveillance transglutaminase serology and to assess clinical progression following initiation of gluten-free diet

albumin, anemia, severe metabolic bone disease, and multiple vitamin and micronutrient deficiencies. They require a careful evaluation for coexistent or evolving lymphoma. They also need intensive nutritional support often including parenteral nutrition. Some patients respond to steroids in these rare cases [98].

SUMMARY

Celiac disease is common and presents in a wide variety of ways. It can result in a wide spectrum of nutritional deficits. Once identified, it readily responds to a gluten-free diet that needs to be continued for life. Complications are rare once it is treated.

References

[1] Rossi TM, Albini CH, Kumar V. Incidence of celiac disease identified by the presence of serum endomysial antibodies in children with chronic diarrhea, short stature, or insulin-dependent diabetes mellitus. J Pediatr 1993;123(2):262–4.

[2] Talley NJ, Valdovinos M, Petterson TM, et al. Epidemiology of celiac sprue: a community-based study. Am J Gastroenterol 1994;89(6):843–6.

[3] Murray JA, Van Dyke C, Plevak MF, et al. Trends in the identification and clinical features of celiac disease in a North American community, 1950–2001. Clin Gastroenterol Hepatol 2003;1(1):19–27.

[4] Fasano A, Berti I, Gerarduzzi T, et al. Prevalence of celiac disease in at-risk and not-at-risk groups in the United States: a large multicenter study. Arch Intern Med 2003;163(3): 286–92.

[5] Sood A, Midha V, Sood N, et al. Increasing incidence of celiac disease in India. Am J Gastroenterol 2001;96(9):2804–5.

[6] Sood A, Midha V, Sood N, et al. Adult celiac disease in northern India. Indian J Gastroenterol 2003;22(4):124–6.

[7] Catassi C, Ratsch IM, Gandolfi L, et al. Why is coeliac disease endemic in the people of the Sahara? Lancet 1999;354(9179):647–8.

[8] Reza Akbari M, Mohammadkhani A, Fakheri H, et al. Screening of the adult population in Iran for coeliac disease: comparison of the tissue-transglutaminase antibody and anti-endomysial antibody tests. Eur J Gastroenterol Hepatol 2006;18(11):1181–6.

[9] Shahbazkhani B, Malekzadeh R, Sotoudeh M, et al. High prevalence of coeliac disease in apparently healthy Iranian blood donors. Eur J Gastroenterol Hepatol 2003;15(5): 475–8.

[10] Gursoy S, Guven K, Simsek T, et al. The prevalence of unrecognized adult celiac disease in Central Anatolia. J Clin Gastroenterol 2005;39(6):508–11.

[11] Remes-Troche JM, Ramirez-Iglesias MT, Rubio-Tapia A, et al. Celiac disease could be a frequent disease in Mexico: prevalence of tissue transglutaminase antibody in healthy blood donors. J Clin Gastroenterol 2006;40(8):697–700.

[12] Pereira MA, Ortiz-Agostinho CL, Nishitokukado I, et al. Prevalence of celiac disease in an urban area of Brazil with predominantly European ancestry. World J Gastroenterol 2006;12(40):6546–50.

[13] Elsurer R, Tatar G, Simsek H, et al. Celiac disease in the Turkish population. Dig Dis Sci 2005;50(1):136–42.

[14] Gomez JC, Selvaggio GS, Viola M, et al. Prevalence of celiac disease in Argentina: screening of an adult population in the La Plata area. Am J Gastroenterol 2001;96(9): 2700–4.

[15] Carlsson AK, Axelsson IE, Borulf SK, et al. Serological screening for celiac disease in healthy 2.5-year-old children in Sweden. Pediatrics 2001;107(1):42–5.

[16] Shamir R, Lerner A, Shinar E, et al. The use of a single serological marker underestimates the prevalence of celiac disease in Israel: a study of blood donors. Am J Gastroenterol 2002;97(10):2589–94.

[17] Henker J, Losel A, Conrad K, et al. Prevalence of asymptomatic coeliac disease in children and adults in the Dresden region of Germany [German]. Dtsch Med Wochenschr 2002;127(28–29):1511–5.

[18] Korponay-Szabo IR, Kovacs JB, Czinner A, et al. High prevalence of silent celiac disease in preschool children screened with IgA/IgG antiendomysium antibodies. J Pediatr Gastroenterol Nutr 1999;28(1):26–30.

[19] Menardo G, Brizzolara R, Bonassi S, et al. Population screening for coeliac disease in a low prevalence area in Italy. Scand J Gastroenterol 2006;41(12):1414–20.

[20] Hill I, Fasano A, Schwartz R, et al. The prevalence of celiac disease in at-risk groups of children in the United States. J Pediatr 2000;136(1):86–90.

[21] Kolho KL, Farkkila MA, Savilahti E. Undiagnosed coeliac disease is common in Finnish adults. Scand J Gastroenterol 1998;33(12):1280–3.

[22] West J, Logan RF, Hill PG, et al. Seroprevalence, correlates, and characteristics of undetected coeliac disease in England. Gut 2003;52(7):960–5.

[23] Catassi C, Fabiani E, Ratsch IM, et al. The coeliac iceberg in Italy: a multicentre antigliadin antibodies screening for coeliac disease in school-age subjects. Acta Paediatr Suppl 1996;412:29–35.

[24] Corrao G, Usai P, Galatola G, et al. Estimating the incidence of coeliac disease with capture-recapture methods within four geographic areas in Italy. J Epidemiol Community Health 1996;50(3):299–305.

[25] Cataldo F, Pitarresi N, Accomando S, et al. Epidemiological and clinical features in immigrant children with coeliac disease: an Italian multicentre study. Dig Liver Dis 2004;36(11):722–9.

[26] Riestra S, Fernandez E, Rodrigo L, et al. Prevalence of coeliac disease in the general population of northern Spain: strategies of serologic screening. Scand J Gastroenterol 2000;35(4):398–402.

[27] Schweizer JJ, von Blomberg BM, Bueno-de Mesquita HB, et al. Coeliac disease in the Netherlands. Scand J Gastroenterol 2004;39(4):359–64.

[28] Johnston SD, Watson RG, McMillan SA, et al. Coeliac disease detected by screening is not silent—simply unrecognized. Q J Med 1998;91(12):853–60.

[29] Jabri B, de Serre NP, Cellier C, et al. Selective expansion of intraepithelial lymphocytes expressing the HLA-E-specific natural killer receptor CD94 in celiac disease. Gastroenterology 2000;118(5):867–79.

[30] Fasano A. Systemic autoimmune disorders in celiac disease. Curr Opin Gastroenterol 2006;22(6):674–9.

[31] Green PH, Jabri B. Celiac disease. Annu Rev Med 2006;57:207–21.

[32] Forsberg G, Fahlgren A, Horstedt P, et al. Presence of bacteria and innate immunity of intestinal epithelium in childhood celiac disease. Am J Gastroenterol 2004;99(5):894–904. [Erratum in: Am J Gastroenterol. Jul 2004;99(7):following 1406].

[33] Sollid LM. Molecular basis of celiac disease. Annu Rev Immunol 2000;18:53–81.

[34] Freitag T, Schulze-Koops H, Niedobitek G, et al. The role of the immune response against tissue transglutaminase in the pathogenesis of coeliac disease. Autoimmun Rev 2004;3(2):13–20.

[35] Jabri B, Kasarda DD, Green PH. Innate and adaptive immunity: the yin and yang of celiac disease. Immunol Rev 2005;206:219–31.

[36] Murray JA, Herlein J, Mitros F, et al. Serologic testing for celiac disease in the United States: results of a multilaboratory comparison study. Clin Diagn Lab Immunol 2000;7(4):584–7.

[37] Leffler DA, Kelly CP. Update on the evaluation and diagnosis of celiac disease. Curr Opin Allergy Clin Immunol 2006;6(3):191–6.

[38] Rostami K, Kerckhaert J, Tiemessen R, et al. Sensitivity of antiendomysium and antigliadin antibodies in untreated celiac disease: disappointing in clinical practice. Am J Gastroenterol 1999;94(4):888–94.

[39] Rostom A, Dube C, Cranney A, et al. The diagnostic accuracy of serologic tests for celiac disease: a systematic review. Gastroenterology 2005;128(4 Suppl 1):S38–46.

[40] Marsh MN. The immunopathology of the small intestinal reaction in gluten-sensitivity. Immunol Invest 1989;18(1–4):509–31.

[41] Farrell RJ, Kelly CP. Celiac sprue. N Engl J Med 2002;346(3):180–8.

[42] Fasano A, Catassi C. Current approaches to diagnosis and treatment of celiac disease: an evolving spectrum. Gastroenterology 2001;120(3):636–51.

[43] Ventura A, Magazzu G, Greco L. Duration of exposure to gluten and risk for autoimmune disorders in patients with celiac disease. SIGEP Study Group for Autoimmune Disorders in Celiac Disease. Gastroenterology 1999;117(2):297–303.

[44] Halfdanarson TR, Litzow MR, Murray JA. Hematological manifestations of celiac disease. Blood 2006;109(2):412–21.

[45] Tikkakoski S, Savilahti E, Kolho KL. Undiagnosed coeliac disease and nutritional deficiencies in adults screened in primary health care. Scand J Gastroenterol 2007;42(1): 60–5.

[46] Fine KD. The prevalence of occult gastrointestinal bleeding in celiac sprue. N Engl J Med 1996;334(18):1163–7.

[47] Shamir R, Levine A, Yalon-Hacohen M, et al. Faecal occult blood in children with coeliac disease. Eur J Pediatr 2000;159(11):832–4.

[48] Logan RF, Howarth GF, West J, et al. How often is a positive faecal occult blood test the result of coeliac disease? Eur J Gastroenterol Hepatol 2003;15(10):1097–100.

[49] Mant MJ, Bain VG, Maguire CG, et al. Prevalence of occult gastrointestinal bleeding in celiac disease. Clin Gastroenterol Hepatol 2006;4(4):451–4.

[50] Bode S, Gudmand-Hoyer E. Symptoms and haematologic features in consecutive adult coeliac patients. Scand J Gastroenterol 1996;31(1):54–60.

[51] Dahele A, Ghosh S. Vitamin B12 deficiency in untreated celiac disease. Am J Gastroenterol 2001;96(3):745–50.

[52] Dickey W, Hughes DF. Histology of the terminal ileum in coeliac disease. Scand J Gastroenterol 2004;39(7):665–7.

[53] Clifford Lo. Micronutrient deficiencies. In: Buchman AL, editor. Clinical nutrition in gastrointestinal disease. Thorofare (NJ): SLACK Inc.; 2006.

[54] Holick MF. Vitamin D deficiency: what a pain it is. Mayo Clin Proc 2003;78(12): 1457–9.

[55] Kozanoglu E, Basaran S, Goncu MK. Proximal myopathy as an unusual presenting feature of celiac disease. Clin Rheumatol 2005;24(1):76–8 [Epub 2004 Sep 2].

[56] Wong M, Scally J, Watson K, et al. Proximal myopathy and bone pain as the presenting features of coeliac disease. Ann Rheum Dis 2002;61(1):87–8.

[57] Anthony AC. Megaloblastic anemias. In: Hoffman R, Benz EJ, Shattil SJ, et al, editors. Hematology: basic principles and practice. 3rd edition. New York: Churchill Livingstone; 2000. p. 460.

[58] Howard MR, Turnbull AJ, Morley P, et al. A prospective study of the prevalence of undiagnosed coeliac disease in laboratory defined iron and folate deficiency. J Clin Pathol 2002;55(10):754–7.

[59] Haapalahti M, Kulmala P, Karttunen TJ, et al. Nutritional status in adolescents and young adults with screen-detected celiac disease. J Pediatr Gastroenterol Nutr 2005;40(5): 566–70.

[60] Jameson S. Villous atrophy and nutritional status in celiac disease. Am J Clin Nutr 1999;69(3):573–5.

[61] Cousins RJ, Lee-Ambrose LM. Nuclear zinc uptake and interactions and metallothionein gene expression are influenced by dietary zinc in rats. J Nutr 1992;122(1):56–64.

[62] Fitzpatrick TB, Johnson RA, Wolf K, et al, editors. Color atlas and synopsis of clinical dermatology. 3rd edition. New York: McGraw Hill; 1997. p. 442.

[63] King JC. Assessment of zinc status. J Nutr 1990;120(Suppl 11):1474–9 [abstract].

[64] Turnlund JR. Copper. In: Shils ME, Olson JA, Shike M, et al, editors. Modern nutrition in health and disease. Philadelphia: Lippincott; 2000. p. 241.

[65] Goyens P, Brasseur D, Cadranel S. Copper deficiency in infants with active celiac disease. J Pediatr Gastroenterol Nutr 1985;4(4):677–80.

[66] Jameson S, Hellsing K, Magnusson S. Copper malabsorption in coeliac disease. Sci Total Environ 1985;42(1–2):29–36.

[67] Nagano T, Toyoda T, Tanabe H, et al. Clinical features of hematological disorders caused by copper deficiency during long-term enteral nutrition. Intern Med 2005;44(6):554–9.

[68] Gregg XT, Reddy V, Prchal JT. Copper deficiency masquerading as myelodysplastic syndrome. Blood 2002;100(4):1493–5.

[69] Salvatore S, Finazzi S, Radaelli G, et al. Prevalence of undiagnosed celiac disease in the parents of preterm and/or small for gestational age infants. Am J Gastroenterol 2006;102(1):168–73.

[70] Gasbarrini A, Torre ES, Trivellini C, et al. Recurrent spontaneous abortion and intrauterine fetal growth retardation as symptoms of coeliac disease. Lancet 2000;356(9227): 399–400.

[71] Sher KS, Mayberry JF. Female fertility, obstetric and gynaecological history in coeliac disease: a case control study. Acta Paediatr Suppl 1996;412:76–7.

[72] Ferguson R, Holmes GK, Cooke WT. Coeliac disease, fertility, and pregnancy. Scand J Gastroenterol 1982;17(1):65–8.

[73] Meloni GF, Dessole S, Vargiu N, et al. The prevalence of coeliac disease in infertility. Hum Reprod 1999;14(11):2759–61.

[74] Ludvigsson JF, Montgomery SM, Ekbom A. Celiac disease and risk of adverse fetal outcome: a population-based cohort study. Gastroenterology 2005;129(2):454–63.

[75] Ciacci C, Cirillo M, Auriemma G, et al. Celiac disease and pregnancy outcome. Am J Gastroenterol 1996;91(4):718–22.

[76] Robinson NJ, Glazier JD, Greenwood SL, et al. Tissue transglutaminase expression and activity in placenta. Placenta 2006;27(2–3):148–57.

[77] Dickey W, Kearney N. Overweight in celiac disease: prevalence, clinical characteristics, and effect of a gluten-free diet. Am J Gastroenterol 2006;101(10):2356–9.

[78] See J, Murray JA. Gluten-free diet: the medical and nutrition management of celiac disease. Nutr Clin Pract 2006;21(1):1–15.

[79] Brar P, Kwon GY, Holleran S, et al. Change in lipid profile in celiac disease: beneficial effect of gluten-free diet. Am J Med 2006;119(9):786–90.

[80] Ciacci C, Cirillo M, Giorgetti G, et al. Low plasma cholesterol: a correlate of nondiagnosed celiac disease in adults with hypochromic anemia. Am J Gastroenterol 1999; 94(7):1888–91 [abstract].

[81] Ciampolini M, Bini S. Serum lipids in celiac children. J Pediatr Gastroenterol Nutr 1991;12(4):459–60.

[82] West J, Logan RF, Smith CJ, et al. Malignancy and mortality in people with coeliac disease: population based cohort study. BMJ 2004;329(7468):716–9 [Epub 2004 Jul 21].

[83] Scott EM, Gaywood I, Scott BB. Guidelines for osteoporosis in coeliac disease and inflammatory bowel disease. British Society of Gastroenterology. Gut 2000;46(Suppl 1):i1–8.

[84] Ciacci C, Cirillo M, Mellone M, et al. Hypocalciuria in overt and subclinical celiac disease. Am J Gastroenterol 1995;90(9):1480–4.

[85] Corazza GR, Di Sario A, Cecchetti L, et al. Bone mass and metabolism in patients with celiac disease. Gastroenterology 1995;109(1):122–8.

[86] Fornari MC, Pedreira S, Niveloni S, et al. Pre- and post-treatment serum levels of cytokines IL-1beta, IL-6, and IL-1 receptor antagonist in celiac disease. Are they related to the associated osteopenia? Am J Gastroenterol 1998;93(3):413–8.

[87] Rea F, Polito C, Marotta A, et al. Restoration of body composition in celiac children after one year of gluten-free diet. J Pediatr Gastroenterol Nutr 1996;23(4):408–12.

[88] West J, Logan RF, Card TR, et al. Fracture risk in people with celiac disease: a population-based cohort study. Gastroenterology 2003;125(2):429–36.

[89] Vasquez H, Mazure R, Gonzalez D, et al. Risk of fractures in celiac disease patients: a cross-sectional, case-control study. Am J Gastroenterol 2000;95(1):183–9.

[90] Moreno ML, Vazquez H, Mazure R, et al. Stratification of bone fracture risk in patients with celiac disease. Clin Gastroenterol Hepatol 2004;2(2):127–34.

[91] Corazza GR, Di Stefano M, Maurino E, et al. Bones in coeliac disease: diagnosis and treatment. Best Pract Res Clin Gastroenterol 2005;19(3):453–65.

[92] Abenavoli L, Proietti I, Leggio L, et al. Cutaneous manifestations in celiac disease. World J Gastroenterol 2006;12(6):843–52.

[93] Zauli D, Grassi A, Granito A, et al. Prevalence of silent coeliac disease in atopics. Dig Liver Dis 2000;32(9):775–9.

[94] Corrao G, Corazza GR, Bagnardi V, et al. Mortality in patients with celiac disease and their relatives: a cohort study. Lancet 2001;358(9279):356–61.

[95] Green PHR, Stavropoulos SN, Panagi SG, et al. Characteristics of adult celiac disease in the USA: results of a national survey. Am J Gastroenterol 2001;96(1):126–31.

[96] Peters U, Askling J, Gridley G, et al. Causes of death in patients with celiac disease in a population-based Swedish cohort. Arch Intern Med 2003;163(13):1566–72.

[97] Askling J, Linet M, Gridley G, et al. Cancer incidence in a population-based cohort of individuals hospitalized with celiac disease dermatitis herpetiformis. Gastroenterology 2002;123(5):1428–35.

[98] Rostom A, Murray JA, Kagnoff MF. American Gastroenterological Association (AGA) institute technical review on the diagnosis and management of celiac disease. Gastroenterology 2006;131(6):1981–2002.

[99] Bazzigaluppi E, Roggero P, Parma B, et al. Antibodies to recombinant human tissue-transglutaminase in coeliac disease: diagnostic effectiveness and decline pattern after gluten-free diet. Dig Liver Dis 2006;38(2):98–102 [Epub 2005 Dec 28].

[100] Vahedi K, Mascart F, Mary JY, et al. Reliability of antitransglutaminase antibodies as predictors of gluten-free diet compliance in adult celiac disease. Am J Gastroenterol 2003;98(5):1079–87.

Gastroenterol Clin N Am 36 (2007) 109–121

GASTROENTEROLOGY CLINICS
OF NORTH AMERICA

Growth Factors in Short-Bowel Syndrome Patients

Palle Bekker Jeppesen, MD, PhD

Department of Medical Gastroenterology, CA-2121, Rigshospitalet, Blegdamsvej 9,
DK-2100 Copenhagen, Denmark

Malabsorption is a key finding in patients with short-bowel syndrome [1,2]. Malabsorption of nonessential and essential nutrients, fluids, and electrolytes, if not compensated for by increased intake, leads to diminished body stores and subclinical and (eventually) clinical deficiencies. By definition, intestinal failure prevails when parenteral support is necessary to maintain nutritional equilibrium [3]. Dependence on parenteral support significantly impairs the quality of life in short-bowel patients [4] and is associated with complications, such as recurrent infections, increased risk of venous thrombosis, and parenteral nutrition (PN)–associated liver failure [4–6]. After intestinal resection, adaptation (a spontaneous progressive recovery from the malabsorptive disorder) may be evident. In the past, research has mainly focused on optimizing remnant intestinal function through dietary interventions [7] and antidiarrheal and antisecretory agents [8], but in recent years pharmacologic hormonal therapy has been introduced. This article describes selected factors responsible for the morphologic and functional changes in the adaptive processes and presents results of clinical trials that use either growth hormone or glucagon-like peptide (GLP)–2 to facilitate a condition of hyperadaptation in short-bowel patients.

INTESTINAL ADAPTATION

The term "intestinal adaptation" may be applied to the progressive recovery from intestinal insufficiency or failure that follows a loss of intestinal length. Fig. 1 illustrates a purely theoretical graphic presentation of intestinal function in relation to time after intestinal resection. A spontaneous adaptation, or recovery of intestinal function, is generally described, reaching a plateau at a certain time. When trying to improve intestinal adaptation, therapies could either reach a higher plateau phase (hyperadaptation) or reduce the time period until the plateau was reached (accelerated adaptation or accelerated hyperadaptation). The time issue may be relevant in patients who are difficult to maintain

E-mail address: bekker@dadlnet.dk

0889-8553/07/$ – see front matter
doi:10.1016/j.gtc.2007.01.007

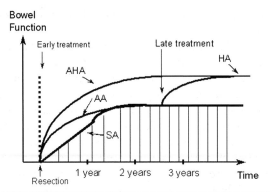

Fig. 1. Schematic presentation of intestinal adaptation. AA, accelerated adaptation; AHA, accelerated hyperadaptation; HA, hyperadaptation; SA, spontaneous adaptation.

on PN. The maximal increase in the functional absorptive capacity obtained by hyperadaptation, represented by the level of the plateau, however, is the aim when trying to wean stable patients from parenteral support.

Morphologic, biochemical, hormonal, and neural systems seem to be involved in intestinal adaptation. Data supporting this are mainly derived from animal studies in which the process of compensatory hyperplasia is extraordinary in some species. It is important to realize that an overall translation of these data to humans cannot be presumed. In the rat, the ileal villi grow to their fully adapted height within weeks. In humans, this process has been demonstrated in patients with jejunoileal bypass operations after which villus heights increased 80% and reached a plateau in 1 year [9]. In other studies, however, intestinal hypertrophy has not been found in humans [10,11]. Most animal and human resection studies describe jejunal changes in short bowels with colon-in-continuity. Conclusions drawn may not hold for patients with a jejunostomy.

The process of epithelial turnover is highly dynamic in the intestine. Within 3 to 6 days, the epithelial cells proliferate within the crypts at the base of the villi, mature, differentiate, and move upward toward the tip of a villus, from which they are shed into the bowel lumen [12]. Adaptation is characterized by cellular hyperplasia that increases the crypt depth and villus size [13–17]. The morphologic changes are more marked in the mucosal surface area, but changes are also seen in the submucosa or muscularis layers [18].

The intensity of the adaptive response seems to be proportional to the total length and to specific areas of the bowel resected. It is greater in the distal small bowel following proximal resection compared with the proximal bowel after distal resection [12,18,19]. A significant morphologic adaptive response is seen after proximal resection in the ileum in animal models [14,15,20,21]. Adaptive hyperplasia of colonic mucosa occurs after both jejunal and ileal resection [22–25]. The adaptive response also occurs in the jejunal remnant after ileal resection, but it is less dramatic, more variable, and may partly be related to adaptive changes in food intake [26]. Finally, ileal mucosa may also undergo hyperplasia after colectomy [27,28].

Only a few longitudinal studies have been performed in humans with respect to functional changes following intestinal resection. It is the clinical experience, however, that short-bowel patients with an intact colon show improved absorption with time, unlike patients with jejunostomy [1]. Althausen and colleagues [29] described diminished fecal water losses and increased absorption of glucose, galactose, amino acids, and fats during the time after extensive small bowel resection in two patients with preserved colons. The jejunal absorptive capacity of short-bowel patients has also been examined by segmental perfusion techniques, and the absorption of glucose, water, and sodium was increased per unit of length compared with that of control subjects [30,31]. Ileostomy adaptation does occur within a period of 6 months; however, this response is lacking in "ileostomists" who have had an ileal resection [32]. The preservation of the terminal ileum and the colon seems to be of importance in the adaptive response following intestinal resection. The time required to maximum adaptation is not certain. Studies of calcium absorption have suggested that it may continue for more than 2 years [33], although the main adaptive response seems to take place within a few months.

It seems that the increase in intestinal function with time following intestinal resection may simply be related to the morphologically demonstrated villus hyperplasia, because only minor changes in the activity of specific intestinal disaccharidases, hydrolases, enterokinase, and sodium-potassium-ATPase have been demonstrated [21,34,35]. The demonstration of an up-regulation of colonic PepT1 by Ziegler and colleagues [11] independent of changes in mucosal surface area also suggests a functional adaptation. Functional adaptation may also involve a trend toward normalization of gastric hypersecretion, gastric emptying, and rapid intestinal transit reported in the short-bowel syndrome [36].

The signals and precise mechanisms that trigger the hyperplastic adaptive response after small bowel resection are not completely understood. The main factors thought to influence intestinal adaptation are exposure of the remaining mucosa to luminal nutrients and nonnutritive components of the diet; various factors related to the provision of enteral feedings (eg, pancreatic-biliary secretions and enteric hormones); and possibly various growth factors and hormones not secreted from the intestine.

HORMONAL STIMULATION OF INTESTINAL ADAPTATION

Two major hormonal candidates (growth hormones and GLP-2) have been suggested and used in the treatment of patients with short-bowel syndrome. The studies described in this article are presented in Table 1. The Food and Drug Administration in the United States has approved both growth hormone and glutamine as drugs to be used for this indication. Hormonal therapy in short-bowel patients should be considered experimental, however, and is only recommended in research settings. The overall aim of any given treatment

Table 1
Summary of studies and results

Author [ref]	Drug/dose (mg/kg/d)	Days	Diet	Glutamine i.v./p.o	ORS	Pts with CD (N/total)	Remnant small bowel (cm)	Colon incontinuity (N/total)	ΔPN volume (kg/d)	Δwet weight Abs (kg/d)	Δsodium Abs (mmol/d)	ΔPN energy (kj/d)	Δenergy Abs (kj/d)	Δbody weight (kg)	Δlean body mass (kg)	ΔFat mass (kg)	Edema/swelling/fluid retention
Byrne, et al [37,38]	GH/0.14	21	HCLF	0.42 or 0.62 g/kg/d	Yes	1/8	37 ± 27	8/8	Fixed	0.7	39	Fixed	590	5.4 ± 1.2	NM	NM	NR
Scolapio, et al [40,48]	GH/0.14	21	HCLF	0 g/d and 0.63 g/kg/d	No	7/8	71 ± 23	2/8	Fixed	NR, NS	<5, P = .03	Fixed	NM	3 ± 0.7	4 ± 0.5	−1 ± 0.2	100%
Szkudlarek, et al [41], Jeppesen [49]	GH/0.12	28 (+5)	Habitual	5.2 ± 2.2 and 28 ± 2 g/d	No	6/8	104 ± 37	4/8	Fixed	−0.3 ± 0.2, NS	−18 ± 7, NS	Fixed	−300 ± 300, NS	1 ± 0.3	2.9 ± 0.4	−2.4 ± 0.5	100%
Byrne, et al [44]	a) Placebo	28	HCLF	0 and 30 g/d	Yes	1/9	62 ± 31	8/9	−0.54 ± 0.34	NM	NM	−1575 ± ?	NM	−0.7 ± ?	NM	NM	44%
	b) GH/0.10	28	HCLF	0 and 30 g/d	Yes	2/16	84 ± 50	15/16	−0.84 ± 0.54	NM	NM	−2594 ± ?	NM	1.2 ± ?	NM	NM	94%
	c) GH/0.10	28	HCLF	0 and 30 g/d	Yes	5/16	68 ± 33	13/16	−1.10 ± 0.46	NM	NM	−3439 ± ?	NM	1.8 ± ?	NM	NM	94%
	a) versus c)	—							−0.56 ± ?	NM	NM	−1864 ± ?, P<.001	NM	2.5 ± ?, NS	NM	NM	—
Seguy, et al [43]	GH/0.05	21	Habitual	0 and 0 g/d	No	3/12	48 ± 11	9/12	Fixed	NR, NS	NR	NM	1787 ± 339	2.4 ± ?	2 ± ?	0.0 ± ?, NS	0%
Ellegaard, et al [42]	GH/0.024	56	Habitual	0 and 0 g/d	No	8/8	125 ± 29	5/10	Fixed	NR, NS	NR, NS	Fixed	NR, NS	2.3 ± 0.8	2.5 ± ?	−0.1 ± ?	0%
Jeppesen, et al [46]	GLP-2/0.013	35	Habitual	No	No	6/8	30–180	0/8	Fixed	0.42 ± 0.48	33 ± 49, NS	Fixed	441 ± 634, P=.09	1.2 ± 1, P=.01	2.9 ± 1.9, P=.004	−1.8 ± 1.3, P=.007	0%
Jeppesen, et al [47]	Teduglutide/0.03–0.15	21	Habitual	No	No	11/16	25–150	6/16	Fixed	0.74 ± 0.48	53 ± 40, P<.001	Fixed	792 ± 2279, NS	0.9 ± 2.1, P=.12	NM	NM	44%

Abbreviations: GH, growth hormone; HCLF, high carbohydrate low fat; NM, not measured; NR, not reported; NS, not significant; ORS, oral rehydration solutions; Δ, compared with baseline; ?, Standard deviation not given.

in short-bowel patients is to improve their quality of life. Quality of life may be estimated by the use of standardized questionnaires; however, it is difficult to establish which numerical improvement on the disease-specific inflammatory bowel disease questionnaire or non–disease-specific sickness impact profile scales justifies the introduction of a new treatment.

The main focus of research performed in short bowel has been to increase the absolute intestinal absorption. In most studies assessing the effects of pharmacologic interventions, however, the dietary intake has been fixated during balance studies. In contrast to these physiologic studies, the effect on the dietary intake of these interventions, and thereby on the true spontaneous absolute absorption, has not been established in vivo in the everyday settings of the patients. For instance, pharmacologic agents could (ie, because of an effect on the gastric emptying) induce a sensation of satiety, thereby also reducing the overall dietary intake. Alternatively, pharmacologic agents could promote appetite and increase overall absorption merely by increasing oral intake.

Even in studies in which a true increase in the intestinal absorption has been established, the outcomes may differ in individual patients. It is possible that an improved energy and macronutrient balance in some patients may lead to changes in body weight and composition and, in others, to a change in basal metabolic rate, whereas some may increase their physical activity. Improved fluid and electrolyte balance may allow for increased perspiration and production of urine and sweat. To get a more precise picture of the individual short-bowel patient, each of these parameters ideally should be measured in long-term experiments. Because of the vast requirements and efforts to conduct such experiments, the ability to wean patients off from parenteral support has been used as a surrogate marker of an effect of given treatments. Unless the pretreatment need for parenteral support has been verified, such an end point is invalid. Most home PN patients can be reduced in parenteral support for shorter or longer periods, especially in patients with colon-in-continuity. They may even compensate for these changes in the energy, macronutrient, fluid, and electrolyte balances. Despite these difficulties, the search for factors to enhance bowel adaptation and increase the assimilation of macronutrients and absorption of wet weight, thereby decreasing the need for PN, is intensive. Although, the evidence-based knowledge is weak, a comparison of the results obtained in short-term clinical trials using growth hormone and GLP-2 is presented.

EFFECTS OF GROWTH HORMONE, GLUTAMINE, AND GLUCAGON-LIKE PEPTIDE 2 IN CLINICAL STUDIES

Wet-Weight Absorption

Byrne and colleagues [37,38] were the first to introduce the concept of bowel rehabilitation with the introduction of high-dose (0.14 mg/kg/d) growth hormone, glutamine, and a high-carbohydrate diet in the treatment of short-bowel patients. In the first study, published by Byrne and coworkers [37], the wet-weight absorption increased approximately 0.7 kg/d (from 1.7–2.4 kg/d), and sodium absorption increased approximately 40 mmol/d (from 74–113 mmol/d) over 4 weeks of treatment. From the baseline absorptive parameters, the actual need for parenteral fluid and sodium could be questioned in most patients in that study, according to the borderlines of intestinal failure defined by Jeppesen and Mortensen [39]. All eight patients in the Byrne and coworkers [37] study had a colon-in-continuity, and in addition to dietary changes toward a high-carbohydrate diet, they were also given oral rehydration solutions as a part of the rehabilitation. The effects may be related to dietary changes and rehydration solutions, rather than growth hormones and glutamine. Although significant, the effect of growth hormones (0.13 mg/kg/d) and oral glutamine on intestinal sodium and potassium absorption was less than 5 mmol/d in the placebo-controlled, double-blind study by Scolapio and colleagues [40]. No effect was described on wet-weight absorption. In contrast, growth hormone (0.11 mg/kg/d) and glutamine, both orally and parenterally administered, tended to decrease wet-weight absorption and increase fecal excretion of sodium and potassium, which reached significance ($P < .05$) in comparison with baseline values from the study of Szkudlarek and colleagues [41]. This was contrasted, however, by clinical findings of generalized edema, increased body weight, a need for diuretics, and a reduction in parenteral saline during treatment. The patients were probably in the process of excreting water and sodium accumulated during the treatment at the time of the posttreatment balance studies 5 days after termination of treatment. In the lower-dose studies from Ellegaard (growth hormone 0.024 mg/kg/d) [42] and Seguy (0.05 mg/kg/d) [43], no significant positive effects on either wet-weight or sodium absorption were seen. The efficacy data of somatotropin (0.1 mg/kg/d for 4 weeks) in a randomized, double-blind parallel group study of 41 patients with short-bowel syndrome (mainly with a preserved colon and stool volume less than 3 L/d) who were dependent on PN have recently been published by Byrne and colleagues [44]. The protocol for weaning from parenteral support was based on pre-established weaning criteria, mainly based on body weight; measurement of total body water by bioelectrical impedance; and measurements of serum sodium, potassium, and bicarbonate. A significant greater reduction from baseline in total parenteral volume occurred in recipients of somatropin (Zorptive) plus glutamine or somatropin alone than in placebo plus glutamine recipients (-7.7 and -5.9 versus -3.8 L/wk). The effect of somatropin and glutamine averages 0.5 to 0.6 L/d compared with the placebo group. In all groups, however, the oral fluid intake was approximately 0.5 L/d higher in relation to treatment at week 6 compared with baseline values at week 2. Balance studies on intestinal absorption were not performed and the results on urinary excretions are not given.

The effects of growth hormone are global and not specific for the intestine. It has recently been reported that growth hormone increase extracellular volume by stimulating sodium reabsorption in the distal nephron and preventing pressure natriuresis [45]. When using bioelectrical impedance in the weaning from parenteral support, it should be considered that the effects of growth hormone on fluid balance in short-bowel patients may be related to effects on the kidneys and the extracellular space rather than on the intestine.

In a study with native GLP-2 by Jeppesen and colleagues [46], eight patients were treated with 400 µg of GLP-2 twice a day, given subcutaneously for 35 days in an open-label study (corresponding to 0.013 ± 0.002 mg/kg/d, a range of 0.011–0.017 mg/kg/d). Four patients with a mean residual jejunum of 83 cm received home PN, whereas four patients with a mean ileum resection of 106 cm did not receive home PN. None of the patients had colon-in-continuity. Their average wet-weight absorption was 1.2 ± 1.7 kg/d at baseline, and the wet-weight absorption increased by approximately 0.4 ± 0.5 kg/d ($P = .04$).

In a subsequent open-label pilot study using a dipeptidyl peptidase IV–resistant GLP-2 analog, teduglutide, in doses 0.03 to 0.15 mg/kg/d, in 16 short-bowel patients (six with remnant parts of the colon), wet-weight absorption increased by approximately 0.7 ± 0.5 kg/d ($P < .001$), thereby significantly increasing urine weight by approximately 0.6 ± 0.5 kg/d ($P < .001$) and sodium excretion by approximately 50 ± 40 mmol/d ($P < .001$) [47].

Energy Absorption

In the initial study by Byrne and coworkers [37], the baseline dietary energy intake was 2692 kcal/d, and 1618 kcal/d ($\sim$6773 kJ/d; 60%) were absorbed. According to the borderlines that define intestinal failure suggested by Jeppesen and Mortensen [39], most of these patients did not need parenteral energy. After 3 weeks of treatment, the intake and absorption were 2367 and 1759 kcal/d ($\sim$7363 kJ/d; 74%), respectively, which was a significant improvement in percentage ($P < .003$) but only an increase of 141 kcal/d ($\sim$600 kJ/d) in absolute amounts. In this study by Byrne and coworkers [37], all eight short-bowel patients had a colon-in-continuity. As stated, the "rehabilitation" included a high-carbohydrate, low-fat diet, which in itself is known to increase the energy absorption in this segment of short-bowel patients. Supporting the hypothesis that diet alone resulted in this effect, intestinal fat absorption did not improve. In the study by Scolapio and colleagues [40], where only two of eight patients had colon-in-continuity, high-carbohydrate diets were provided in both the placebo and treatment arms. Energy absorption was not measured, but no changes were observed regarding nitrogen or fat absorption. In the studies by Ellegaard and colleagues [42] and Szkudlarek and colleagues [41], no changes were found in intestinal energy or in fat or nitrogen absorption. In the study by Seguy and colleagues [43], growth hormone (0.05 mg/kg/d, 9 of 12 patients with colon-in-continuity) and an unrestricted hyperphagic diet increased intestinal absorption of nitrogen by 14% ± 6% ($P < .040$), carbohydrates by 10% ± 4% ($P < .040$), and energy by 15% ± 5% ($P < .002$), which in absolute terms was approximately 400 kcal/d ($\sim$1800 kJ/d). Fat absorption was unaffected by the treatment. During growth hormone treatment the mean dietary energy intake was approximately 200 kcal/d (800 kJ/d) higher.

In the study on somatropin, the mean reductions from baseline in total parenteral calories were significantly greater in recipients of somatropin plus glutamine or somatropin alone than in recipients of placebo plus glutamine (5751 and 4338 versus 2633 kcal/wk) [44]. The effect of the combined therapy of somatropin plus glutamine corresponds to an effect of approximately 400 to 500 kcal/d (~1900 kJ/d). Although not statistically significant, the diet energy intake was 200 kcal/d (~800 kJ/d) higher during treatment with somatropin plus glutamine compared with baseline.

In the study with native GLP-2, the absolute energy absorption tended to increase by approximately 400 ± 600 kJ/d (~100 kcal/d; $P = .09$). The trend toward improvement in the absolute amount of energy absorbed was obtained despite a nonsignificant decrease in energy intake of approximately 200 kJ/d, which means that the reduction in the energy malabsorbed (equal to the stomal excretion) was proportionally larger, approximately 600 kJ/d.

In the study using the dipeptidyl peptidase IV–resistant GLP-2 analog teduglutide, in doses 0.03 to 0.15 mg/kg/d, in 16 short-bowel patients (six with remnant parts of the colon), fecal energy excretion was reduced by approximately 800 kJ/d ($P = .04$), but this only translated to a significant increase in intestinal absorption of approximately 1000 kJ/d in a post hoc defined subset of patients with high dietary compliance during balance studies. No significant changes were seen in the absorption of individual macronutrients [47].

Body Weight, Composition, and Urine Creatinine Excretion

In the growth-hormone study by Byrne and colleagues [37], a weight gain of 5.4 ± 1.2 kg was described in the eight patients after 21 days of treatment. Occurrence of edema was not reported, but increases in body weight of this size are difficult to explain considering the magnitude of the summarized effect of approximately 12 MJ (~600 kJ/d) on the energy balance over the 21 days of treatment. In the study by Byrne and colleagues [37], neither body composition nor urine creatinine excretion were measured. In the 8-week growth hormone (0.024 mg/kg/d) study by Ellegaard and colleagues [42], an increase in lean body mass of 2.5 kg and a decrease in fat mass of 0.1 kg were found. Total body potassium increased 4.7%, equivalent to 1.1 ± 0.4 kg of body cell mass, which was parallel to the 5.6% increase in lean body mass measured by dual energy x-ray absorptiometry (DXA). Ellegaard and colleagues [42] concluded that the increase in lean body mass was derived from both increased body cell mass and extracellular water. Using DXA measurements, Scolapio [48] found an increase in lean body mass of 3.96 ± 0.5 kg and a decrease in the percent of body fat of $2.51\% \pm 0.4\%$, which corresponded to approximately 1 kg compared with placebo. Scolapio [48] concluded that the increased body weight during treatment with high doses of growth hormone was mainly caused by the increase in extracellular water and the presence of peripheral edema, which was encountered in all eight patients treated. In the study by Jeppesen and colleagues [49], a weight gain of 1 ± 0.3 kg ($P < .050$) was measured daily for 5 days after 4 weeks of treatment. DXA evaluation indicated that lean body mass increased 2.9 kg ($P < .001$) and fat mass decreased 2.4 kg ($P < .001$) compared with baseline, whereas the changes were not significant in comparison with placebo. No changes were seen in urinary creatinine excretion. The most likely explanation of the rather modest weight gain and increase in lean body mass in the high-dose study of Jeppesen and colleagues [49] could be the timing of measurements. The patients had been off growth hormone and glutamine for 5 days when the DXA scan measurements were performed. At this time, generalized edemas, which occurred in all eight patients, were on the decline. In the other studies, lean body mass was measured while patients were still receiving treatment. In the study by Seguy and colleagues [43], body weight increased 2 kg ($P < .003$), and the lean body mass, measured by bioimpedance, increased 2.2 kg ($P < .006$). No adverse events to the growth hormone treatment were encountered.

In the study on somatropin, a weight loss of 5.2 kg of body weight was observed from week 2 (pretreatment) to week 18 (12 weeks posttreatment) in patients treated with the combined therapy of somatropin plus glutamine. This weight loss closely reflects the anticipated weight loss derived by calculation of the energy deficit obtained by reduction of the parenteral energy support of 1863 kJ/d [44].

In the 35-day study with native GLP-2 treatment, the overall increase in energy absorption of 15 MJ translated into a significant increase in body weight of 1.2 ± 1 kg ($P = .010$) [46]. Lean body mass improved with 2.9 ± 1.9 kg ($P = .004$), and fat mass decreased by 1.8 ± 1.3 kg ($P = .007$). The study demonstrated positive findings on urine creatinine excretion (0.7 ± 0.7 mmol/d; $P = .02$), which could suggest an increase in muscle mass in relation to GLP-2 treatment. An alternative hypothesis is, that GLP-2 improves hydrational status and thereby renal function and creatinine clearance in these patients, who often suffer from reversible renal impairment caused by intermittent dehydration [50].

In the 3-week study of the GLP-2 analog teduglutide, no changes were seen in the body weight (0.9 ± 2.1 kg; $P = .12$) [47].

SUMMARY

In recent years, increased attention has been addressed to the pharmacologic enhancement of bowel adaptation aimed at weaning patients with intestinal failure from parenteral support. In these patients, apart from posing a threat of causing line sepsis, thrombosis, and liver damage, the complex technology of home PN significantly impairs quality of life [4]. Although the initial trials using growth hormone and glutamine were positive, the subsequent controlled trials have demonstrated conflicting results.

Regarding improvements in wet-weight absorption, the largest effects seem to be seen in studies using the highest doses and mainly in short-bowel patients with a preserved colon. The maximum effect reported on wet-weight absorption is approximately 700 g/d, but it is not possible to determine if this effect is caused by the combination of growth hormone and glutamine and a high-carbohydrate low-fat diet, oral rehydration solutions, or the combination. The effect on wet-weight absorption in jejunostomy short-bowel patients without co-lon-in-continuity seems limited.

Regarding the intestinal energy absorption, the effects seem to be limited in the high-dose studies, whereas the low-dose study of Seguy and colleagues [43] demonstrated an impressive effect of approximately 400 kcal/d (~1800 kJ/d). This effect was, however, obtained at a higher dietary intake (~200 kcal/d; ~800 kJ/d), possibly reducing the true effect to around 200 kcal/d (~1000 kJ/d). The indirectly demonstrated effect on energy absorption by weaning from parenteral energy support in relation to somatropin treatment is approx-imately 450 kcal/d (~1900 kJ/d), but the 5.2-kg weight loss at week 18 after weaning from parenteral support raises concern.

The overall impression is that the effects of high doses of growth hormone are related to the wet-weight absorption (or fluid retention) and mainly in pa-tients with a preserved colon, whereas the effects on energy absorption are mi-nor. In the lower doses of growth hormone there may be an effect on energy absorption in short-bowel patients with a colon-in-continuity, whereas there is no effect on wet-weight absorption regardless of intestinal anatomy. This may restrict the benefit of this therapy, because most patients in a home PN popu-lation are jejunostomy patients without a colon-in-continuity. Because none of the studies have demonstrated ongoing effects after termination of treatment, there is a need for sustained treatment. The presence and severity of adverse events raises concern. The swelling, fluid retention symptoms, myalgia, arthral-gia, gynecomastia, carpal tunnel syndrome, nightmares, and insomnia reported in the high-dose growth hormone studies in short-bowel patients may jeopar-dize the positive effects on quality of life, which should be the ultimate goal of such treatment.

The physiologic effects of GLP-2 seem rather specific for the gut. This is con-cordant with the localization of the GLP-2 receptor. The peptide has intestino-trophic, antisecretory, and transit-modulating effects in the short-bowel patients, and the adverse events, even in supraphysiologic doses, seem limited. So far, the effects of GLP-2 are not clinically dramatic; an increase in wet-weight absorption of 420 g/d, but in the first human trial, the dose of GLP-2 and the duration of therapy were chosen arbitrarily. The GLP-2 analog teduglutide, which is more slowly degraded [51], doubled the effects seen in the study using native GLP-2, increasing the wet-weight absorption by approxi-mately 750 g/d [47]. Effects on energy absorption seem marginal (<1000 kJ/d). The optimal dosage and administration of this new treatment to short-bowel patients to induce beneficial effects on intestinal secretion, motility, morphol-ogy, and (most important) absorption are not known, but because the effect is seen in both short-bowel with and without a colon-in-continuity, it may even-tually result in long-term improvements in nutritional and fluid status and in-dependence of PN in a larger fraction of short-bowel patients.

Among the hormonal factors, teduglutide is the only agent that has been able to induce a significant intestinal growth in short-bowel patients as evaluated by intestinal biopsies. The increases in villus height of 38% ± 45% and crypt depths of 22% ± 18% in short-bowel patients with a jejunostomy are still significantly less, however, than the 80% increases in villus height demonstrated in patients with jejunoileal bypass operations [9] and the 2% to 300% increases in villus heights described in patients with enteroglucagonomas [52,53]. It remains to be demonstrated whether achieving intestinal growth of this magnitude is at all possible in patients with a jejunostomy, and in such case whether it benefits intestinal absorption. It may also require the combination of growth factors. Long-term treatment with any growth factor could be questioned, however, because of a theoretical risk of stimulating tumor growth [54]. It is recommended that treatment of short-bowel patients with intestinal growth factors be initiated in research settings only, and that a close surveillance and monitoring of the long-term effects be a part of the protocol.

References

[1] Nightingale JM, Lennard Jones JE. The short bowel syndrome: what's new and old? Dig Dis 1993;11(1):12–31.
[2] Buchman AL, Scolapio J, Fryer J. AGA technical review on short bowel syndrome and intestinal transplantation. Gastroenterology 2003;124(4):1111–34.
[3] Fleming CR, Remington M. Intestinal failure. In: Hill GL, editor. Nutrition and the surgical patient. New York: Churchill Livingstone; 1981. p. 219–35.
[4] Jeppesen PB, Langholz E, Mortensen PB. Quality of life in patients receiving home parenteral nutrition. Gut 1999;44(6):844–52.
[5] Jeppesen PB, Staun M, Mortensen PB. Adult patients receiving home parenteral nutrition in Denmark from 1991 to 1996: who will benefit from intestinal transplantation? Scand J Gastroenterol 1998;33(8):839–46.
[6] Ugur A, Marashdeh BH, Gottschalck I, et al. Home parenteral nutrition in Denmark in the period from 1996 to 2001. Scand J Gastroenterol 2006;41(4):401–7.
[7] Nordgaard I, Hansen BS, Mortensen PB. Colon as a digestive organ in patients with short bowel [see comments]. Lancet 1994;343(8894):373–6.
[8] Jeppesen PB, Staun M, Tjellesen L, et al. Effect of intravenous ranitidine and omeprazole on intestinal absorption of water, sodium, and macronutrients in patients with intestinal resection. Gut 1998;43(6):763–9.
[9] Friedman HI, Chandler JG, Peck CC, et al. Alterations in intestinal structure, fat absorption and body weight after intestinal bypass for morbid obesity. Surg Gynecol Obstet 1978; 146(5):757–67.
[10] O'Keefe SJ, Haymond MW, Bennet WM, et al. Long-acting somatostatin analogue therapy and protein metabolism in patients with jejunostomies. Gastroenterology 1994;107(2): 379–88.
[11] Ziegler TR, Fernandez-Estivariz C, Gu LH, et al. Distribution of the H+/peptide transporter PepT1 in human intestine: up-regulated expression in the colonic mucosa of patients with short-bowel syndrome. Am J Clin Nutr 2002;75(5):922–30.
[12] Eastwood GL. Gastrointestinal epithelial renewal. Gastroenterology 1977;72(5 Pt 1): 962–75.
[13] Dowling RH, Booth CC. Structural and functional changes following small intestinal resection in the rat. Clin Sci 1967;32(1):139–49.
[14] Obertop H, Nundy S, Malamud D, et al. Onset of cell proliferation in the shortened gut: rapid hyperplasia after jejunal resection. Gastroenterology 1977;72(2):267–70.
[15] Nygaard K. Resection of the small intestine in rats. 3. Morphological changes in the intestinal tract. Acta Chir Scand 1967;133(3):233–48.
[16] Booth CC, Evans KT, Menzies T, et al. Intestinal hypertrophy following partial resection of the small bowel in the rat. Br J Surg 1958;46:403–10.

[17] Porus RL. Epithelial hyperplasia following massive small bowel resection in man. Gastroenterology 1965;48(6):753–7.

[18] Hanson WR, Osborne JW, Sharp JG. Compensation by the residual intestine after intestinal resection in the rat. I. Influence of amount of tissue removed. Gastroenterology 1977;72(4 Pt 1):692–700.

[19] Hanson WR, Osborne JW, Sharp JG. Compensation by the residual intestine after intestinal resection in the rat. II. Influence of postoperative time interval. Gastroenterology 1977;72(4 Pt 1):701–5.

[20] Tilson MD, Wright HK. Adaptation of functioning and bypassed segments of ileum during compensatory hypertrophy of the gut. Surgery 1970;67(4):687–93.

[21] Weser E, Hernandez MH. Studies of small bowel adaptation after intestinal resection in the rat. Gastroenterology 1971;60(1):69–75.

[22] Tilson MD, Michaud JT, Livstone EM. Early proliferative activity in the left colon of the rat after partial small-bowel resection. Surg Forum 1976;27(62):445–6.

[23] Williamson RC, Bauer FL, Ross JS, et al. Proximal enterectomy stimulates distal hyperplasia more than bypass or pancreaticobiliary diversion. Gastroenterology 1978;74(1):16–23.

[24] Nundy S, Malamud D, Obertop H, et al. Onset of cell proliferation in the shortened gut: colonic hyperplasia after ileal resection. Gastroenterology 1977;72(2):263–6.

[25] Solhaug JH, Tvete S. Adaptative changes in the small intestine following bypass operation for obesity: a radiological and histological study. Scand J Gastroenterol 1978;13(4):401–8.

[26] Young EA, Weser E. Nutritional adaptation after small bowel resection in rats. J Nutr 1974;104(8):994–1001.

[27] Wright HK, Poskitt T, Cleveland JC, et al. The effect of total colectomy on morphology and absorptive capacity of ileum in the rat. J Surg Res 1969;9(5):301–4.

[28] Woo ZH, Nygaard K. Small-bowel adaptation after colectomy in rats. Scand J Gastroenterol 1978;13(8):903–10.

[29] Althausen TL, Doig RK, Uyeyama K, et al. Digestion and absorption after massive resection of the small intestine. II. Recovery of the absorptive function as shown by intestinal absorption tests in two patients and a consideration of compensatory mechanisms. Gastroenterology 1950;16(1):126–34.

[30] Dowling RH, Booth CC. Functional compensation after small-bowel resection in man: demonstration by direct measurement. Lancet 1966;2(7455):146–7.

[31] Weinstein LD, Shoemaker CP, Hersh T, et al. Enhanced intestinal absorption after small bowel resection in man. Arch Surg 1969;99(5):560–2.

[32] Hill GL, Mair WS, Goligher JC. Impairment of ileostomy adaptation in patients after ileal resection. Gut 1974;15(12):982–7.

[33] Gouttebel MC, Saint Aubert B, Colette C, et al. Intestinal adaptation in patients with short bowel syndrome: measurement by calcium absorption. Dig Dis Sci 1989;34(5):709–15.

[34] McCarthy DM, Kim YS. Changes in sucrase, enterokinase, and peptide hydrolase after intestinal resection: the association of cellular hyperplasia and adaptation. J Clin Invest 1973;52(4):942–51.

[35] Tilson MD, Wright HK. An adaptive change in ileal Na-K-ATPase activity after jejunectomy or jejunal transposition. Surgery 1971;70(3):421–4.

[36] Remington M, Malagelada JR, Zinsmeister A, et al. Abnormalities in gastrointestinal motor activity in patients with short bowels: effect of a synthetic opiate. Gastroenterology 1983;85(3):629–36.

[37] Byrne TA, Morrissey TB, Nattakom TV, et al. Growth hormone, glutamine, and a modified diet enhance nutrient absorption in patients with severe short bowel syndrome. JPEN J Parenter Enteral Nutr 1995;19(4):296–302.

[38] Byrne TA, Persinger RL, Young LS, et al. A new treatment for patients with short-bowel syndrome: growth hormone, glutamine, and a modified diet. Ann Surg 1995;222(3):243–54.

[39] Jeppesen PB, Mortensen PB. Intestinal failure defined by measurements of intestinal energy and wet weight absorption. Gut 2000;46(5):701–6.

[40] Scolapio JS, Camilleri M, Fleming CR, et al. Effect of growth hormone, glutamine, and diet on adaptation in short-bowel syndrome: a randomized, controlled study. Gastroenterology 1997;113(4):1074–81.

[41] Szkudlarek J, Jeppesen PB, Mortensen PB. Effect of high dose growth hormone with glutamine and no change in diet on intestinal absorption in short bowel patients: a randomised, double blind, crossover, placebo controlled study. Gut 2000;47(2):199–205.

[42] Ellegaard L, Bosaeus I, Nordgren S, et al. Low-dose recombinant human growth hormone increases body weight and lean body mass in patients with short bowel syndrome. Ann Surg 1997;225(1):88–96.

[43] Seguy D, Vahedi K, Kapel N, et al. Low-dose growth hormone in adult home parenteral nutrition-dependent short bowel syndrome patients: a positive study. Gastroenterology 2003;124(2):293–302.

[44] Byrne TA, Wilmore DW, Iyer K, et al. Growth hormone, glutamine, and an optimal diet reduces parenteral nutrition in patients with short bowel syndrome: a prospective, randomized, placebo-controlled, double-blind clinical trial. Ann Surg 2005;242(5):655–61.

[45] Johannsson G, Sverrisdottir YB, Ellegard L, et al. GH increases extracellular volume by stimulating sodium reabsorption in the distal nephron and preventing pressure natriuresis. J Clin Endocrinol Metab 2002;87(4):1743–9.

[46] Jeppesen PB, Hartmann B, Thulesen J, et al. Glucagon-like peptide 2 improves nutrient absorption and nutritional status in short-bowel patients with no colon. Gastroenterology 2001;120(4):806–15.

[47] Jeppesen PB, Sanguinetti EL, Buchman A, et al. Teduglutide (ALX-0600), a dipeptidyl peptidase IV resistant glucagon-like peptide 2 analogue, improves intestinal function in short bowel syndrome patients. Gut 2005;54(9):1224–31.

[48] Scolapio JS. Effect of growth hormone, glutamine, and diet on body composition in short bowel syndrome: a randomized, controlled study. JPEN J Parenter Enteral Nutr 1999; 23(6):309–13.

[49] Jeppesen PB, Szkudlarek J, Hoy CE, et al. Effect of high-dose growth hormone and glutamine on body composition, urine creatinine excretion, fatty acid absorption, and essential fatty acids status in short bowel patients: a randomized, double-blind, crossover, placebo-controlled study. Scand J Gastroenterol 2001;36(1):48–54.

[50] Lauverjat M, Hadj AA, Vanhems P, et al. Chronic dehydration may impair renal function in patients with chronic intestinal failure on long-term parenteral nutrition. Clin Nutr 2006;25(1):75–81.

[51] Drucker DJ, Shi Q, Crivici A, et al. Regulation of the biological activity of glucagon-like peptide 2 in vivo by dipeptidyl peptidase IV. Nat Biotechnol 1997;15(7):673–7.

[52] Gleeson MH, Bloom SR, Polak JM, et al. Endocrine tumour in kidney affecting small bowel structure, motility, and absorptive function. Gut 1971;12(10):773–82.

[53] Stevens FM, Flanagan RW, O'Gorman D, et al. Glucagonoma syndrome demonstrating giant duodenal villi. Gut 1984;25(7):784–91.

[54] Thulesen J, Hartmann B, Hare KJ, et al. Glucagon-like peptide 2 (GLP-2) accelerates the growth of colonic neoplasms in mice. Gut 2004;53(8):1145–50.

Gastroenterol Clin N Am 36 (2007) 123–144

ELSEVIER
SAUNDERS

Home Parenteral and Enteral Nutrition

John K. DiBaise, MD[a],*, James S. Scolapio, MD[b]

[a]Division of Gastroenterology and Hepatology, Mayo Clinic, 13400 East Shea Boulevard, Pablo Road, Scottsdale, AZ 85259, USA

[b]Division of Gastroenterology and Hepatology, Mayo Clinic, Jacksonville, FL 32224–1865, USA

Home parenteral and enteral nutrition (HPEN) has become a widely available nutrition support therapy for persons with intestinal and oral failure, respectively. Home enteral nutrition (HEN) is primarily for patients in whom there is a reduction in oral intake below the amount needed to maintain nutrition or hydration (ie, oral failure), whereas home parenteral nutrition (HPN) is used for patients when oral-enteral nutrition is temporarily or permanently impossible or absorption insufficient to maintain nutrition or hydration (ie, intestinal failure). Gastroenterologists are frequently asked to place enteral tubes and assist in the management of patients receiving HPEN. It is important to have a good knowledge of this area to provide safe, efficacious, and cost-effective support to the HPEN patient and other physicians participating in their care. This article describes the prevalence, indications, complications, outcomes, and costs associated with HPEN. Whereas some of the information in this article may be applicable to the pediatric patient, the focus is on the adult population.

HOME PARENTERAL AND ENTERAL NUTRITION PREVALENCE

In the United States, most information on the indications and outcomes relating to HPEN comes from the American Society of Parenteral and Enteral Nutrition information system and Medicare. In the United States between 1989 and 1992, the annual prevalence of HEN was 415 per 100,000 population versus 120 per 100,000 for HPN [1]. In most countries, there is approximately five times more HEN than HPN patients [1]. From the time of its initial description in the late 1960s, there are currently an estimated 40,000 HPN consumers in the United States. Although the number of long-term users of HPN (those on HPN greater than 1 year) has remained stable or declined over the years, the number of short-term users (those on HPN less than 1 year) has increased. There are an estimated 10,000 patients in the United States that are considered

*Corresponding author. E-mail address: dibaise.john@mayo.edu (J.K. DiBaise).

0889-8553/07/$ – see front matter
doi:10.1016/j.gtc.2007.01.008

long-term consumers. In contrast to the situation in Europe, where patients requiring HPN are managed in selected institutions, in the United States, more
than 80% of HPN patients seem to be managed by individual physicians or
small groups of physicians in community practice [2]. As a result, an understanding of the appropriate indications for HPN and the complications encountered with HPN is valuable for gastroenterologists.

HOME PARENTERAL AND ENTERAL NUTRITION INDICATIONS

Because HPN is associated with deterioration in intestinal integrity that may allow for bacterial translocation and systemic infection, a higher risk of complications, and is far more expensive than HEN [3–5], HEN is preferred over HPN
provided there are no contraindications and enteral access is attainable. HPN
is only absolutely necessary when the gut is unable to be used or is functionally
inadequate for absorption. Nevertheless, it is recognized that parenteral nutrition
is often used, particularly in the hospital setting, because of a variety of factors
including convenience, ease of delivery, and perceived comfort [6]. Medicare
Part B (prosthetic device benefit provision) and many private insurance providers require that patients needing HPEN have an anticipated duration of
use of at least 90 days. Medicare also requires detailed documentation in the
medical record of the confirmed diagnosis and, in the case of HPN, failure of enteral nutrition. Medicare coverage guidelines for HPEN are listed in Box 1 [7].

In some circumstances, the decision to withhold or withdraw HPEN remains
controversial and problematic [8]. It must be remembered that HPEN are active treatments and not simply supportive or comfort care. As such, they carry
the potential for discomfort and complication. Issues of starting and when to
stop should be discussed with the patient and the patient's family, particularly
the terminally ill patient, at the outset. This is critical for allowing them a sense
of control over the situation. In these difficult situations, seeking the opinion of
a hospital ethics committee should be considered [9]. Importantly, there is no
legal difference between withdrawing and withholding enteral or parenteral
feeding; however, its discontinuation is generally more emotional because it
will likely hasten death [10].

Home Enteral Nutrition

HEN is indicated in the patient who cannot or will not eat and has at least a partially functioning gut. The major indications for HEN are dysphagia and anorexia in cancer and neuromuscular disease patients (Box 2). Dysphagia is
the most common indication for HEN [1,11] and may result from acute cerebrovascular accident, treatment of head and neck or mediastinal cancer, or
rarely from refractory benign esophageal disease. In these instances, HEN
may be either temporary or permanent. Anorexia can be a significant problem
in those with increased energy needs, such as cancer and AIDS. Anorexia may
also occur in the elderly, demented, mentally ill, postsurgical patient, and those
in a persistent vegetative state. HEN is also occasionally used in patients with
small bowel malabsorptive conditions to supplement their limited gut.

Box 1: Medicare coverage guidelines for home parenteral and enteral nutrition

Enteral nutrition

Permanent (≥3 months) nonfunction or disease that prevents food from reaching the small bowel

Disease of the small bowel that impairs digestion or absorption of an oral diet

Tube feeding required to maintain weight and strength

Oral intake permissible but generally <30% of estimated total need

Total daily calorie intake of 20–35 kcal/kg/d

Use of a pump requires additional documentation

    Gravity feeding not possible because of to reflux or aspiration

    Severe diarrhea

    Dumping syndrome

    Erratic glycemic control

    Circulatory overload

    Administration rate <100 mL/h

    Jejunostomy feeding

Additional documentation required for any formula other than standard

Parenteral nutrition

Permanent (≥3 months) dysfunction of the gastrointestinal tract

Unable to maintain weight and strength on oral diet or a combination of oral, enteral, and parenteral

Nutrient requirements

    20–35 kcal/kg/d

    0.8–1.5 g protein/kg/d

    ≥10% dextrose concentration

    15 units of 20% or 30 units of 10% lipids per month (1 unit = 500 mL)

Specific disease criteria (and disease-specific supporting documentation)

    Short-bowel syndrome

    Pancreatitis

    Crohn's disease

    Proximal enterocutaneous fistula

    Complete small bowel obstruction

    Malabsorption

    Motility disorder

Box 2: Indications for home enteral nutrition

Cerebrovascular disease
Cerebral palsy
Motor neuron disease
Multiple sclerosis
Trauma
Crohn's disease
Parkinson's disease
Dementia
Esophageal cancer
Gastric cancer
Pancreatic cancer
Head and neck cancer
Congenital disorders
Cystic fibrosis
Failure to thrive
Motility disorders
Ischemic bowel disorders
Hyperemesis gravidarum
Pancreatitis
Chronic obstruction
AIDS

Mechanical obstruction is the only absolute contraindication to HEN; however, in the setting of chronic obstruction, HEN may be possible if the feeding tube can be placed distal to the site of obstruction. Severe diarrhea or vomiting, enterocutaneous fistulae, and intestinal dysmotility, although presenting significant challenges, are not absolute contraindications. Relative contraindications to HEN therapy include patients with an inability to adhere to a schedule because of either socioeconomic or psychosocial constraints. The occasional patient (eg, short-bowel syndrome) may benefit from a combination of both HPN and HEN to meet their nutritional needs and minimize the dependence on HPN.

Home Parenteral Nutrition

Candidates for HPN include those patients who otherwise require extended hospital stays and who cannot take sufficient calories orally or by an enteral feeding tube (Box 3) [1]. The most common diagnoses among HPN patients are cancer, short-bowel syndrome, Crohn's disease, ischemic bowel disease, and motility disorders [1]. Less common indications include AIDS, radiation

> **Box 3: Indications for home parenteral nutrition**
>
> Short-bowel syndrome
> Crohn's disease
> Ischemic bowel disorders
> Chronic intestinal pseudo-obstruction
> Chronic mechanical obstruction
> Nonterminal cancer
> Radiation enteritis
> Pancreatitis
> Refractory malabsorptive conditions
> Intestinal and pancreatic fistulae
> Hyperemesis gravidarum
> AIDS

enteritis, chronic pancreatitis, and hyperemesis gravidarum. It is very important that patients and their home health providers have the appropriate home situation and skills necessary safely to administer the HPN. Catheter infection is the most common complication of HPN therapy. If sterile catheter care cannot be completed by the patient or the home health care provider, the patient should not be discharged on HPN regardless of their diagnosis.

HOME PARENTERAL AND ENTERAL NUTRITION IMPLEMENTATION

Criteria for the successful provision of HPEN include proper patient selection, which involves not only an appropriate indication but also a clean and safe home environment and a patient or caregiver able to perform all the enteral procedures safely. Additional criteria are listed in Box 4. Although these criteria may seem obvious, patients are occasionally discharged on HPN without proper indications, education, or appropriate follow-up care arrangements. These problems can be prevented if a team of clinicians is designated to care for these patients.

A multidisciplinary nutrition support team competent in both HEN and HPN and consisting of a physician, nurse, dietitian, and pharmacist in close collaboration with the patient and his or her home care and primary care provider allows for a comprehensive and systematic approach to optimal nutrition support in these complex patients and is useful in the overall management of HPEN. This team serves to evaluate, educate, and monitor HPEN patients. Combined care from such a team has been suggested to result in improved care, decreased complications, and increased cost-effectiveness [12,13]. Before hospital discharge, this multidisciplinary team must evaluate the patient for appropriate indications and education and understanding about tube and catheter

Box 4: Guidelines for home parenteral and enteral nutrition

Appropriate candidate for HPEN

Stable medical condition

Home therapy more appropriate than inpatient care

Patient or caregiver able safely to administer HPEN independently

Monitoring available

   Nutrition intake and weight goals

   Laboratory studies

   Complications and tolerance

   Tube or catheter malfunction

Acceptable support system and follow-up availability

   Competent health professionals

   24-hour availability of home care company

   Family

   Adequate home situation (clean environment and adequate storage facilities)

Adequate education of the patient, caregiver, or family

care and HPEN administration. The hospital case manager needs to be actively involved several days before the anticipated hospital discharge date. Selection of a quality home care company can also be facilitated by the case manager. Although the patient is still in the hospital, a visit by the home care nurse can help to familiarize the patient with the HPEN routine, explain the process of HPEN administration, and emphasize the importance of sterile catheter technique.

The education of HPEN patients and their caregivers is of critical importance (Box 5). The main objective is to achieve a state of active independence on the part of the patient and caregiver. Sufficient education usually allows self-confidence and an improved relationship with the health care team. Models, booklets, lectures, videos, or a combination of these may be used. Patient support groups, such as the Oley Foundation (www.oley.org), are also important sources of information on practical topics (eg, body image, travel), education, and support and may reduce the risk of complications and enhance survival and the quality of life of the HPEN patient.

Home Enteral Nutrition

The stomach is the preferred route of enteral feeding when functioning normally. In contrast, intragastric feeding should be avoided and the patient fed directly into the jejunum when the stomach is not functioning normally or when there is significant risk for aspiration, although it is recognized that the latter indication is a subject of controversy [14,15]. Enteral tubes can be placed

Box 5: Components of home parenteral and enteral nutrition patient education

Understand illness and basic anatomy

Reason for HPEN

Identify necessary supplies

Use of equipment

   Tube

   Administration set

   Infusion pump

   Syringe

   Drip stand

   Tape

Care of access device

   Securing

   Flushing

   Cleaning

   Replacement

Safe preparation and administration of formula

Recognition and response to complications

Awareness of health care contacts

Understand financial responsibilities

transnasally; percutaneously (endoscopic or radiologic); or surgically. Advantages and disadvantages of the various approaches are summarized in Table 1. The optimal route of administration depends on the anticipated duration of use, adequacy of gut function, and risk of aspiration. Tube route options include nasogastric, nasojejunal, gastric, gastrojejunal, and jejunal. Physicians should be familiar with the advantages and limitations relative to the individual patient.

In patients with tubes expected to be used for less than 30 days, a nasoenteral tube is preferred. An exception is the patient who has been trained to insert and remove a nasogastric tube daily for nocturnal feedings. All others generally require percutaneously (eg, endoscopic or radiologic) or surgically placed gastrostomy or jejunostomy tubes. Because small differences in success rate and complication rate exist among these methods when used to place gastrostomy tubes, a decision to use one method over another largely depends on the availability of local expertise. Percutaneous methods to gastric access are generally preferred over surgery because the latter approach is more expensive and involves a longer recovery time. The major advantages of endoscopic placement compared with the other placement techniques are

Table 1
Advantages and disadvantages of the various methods of enteral access

	Advantages	Disadvantages
Transnasal	May be placed at the bedside Minimally invasive, short-term solution	Not for long-term use
Percutaneous Endoscopic	Done under conscious sedation	Not feasible if proximal obstruction
	Allows for direct visualization of esophagus, stomach, and duodenum	Procedure may fail if there is inadequate transillumination
Radiologic	Less sedation required than for a PEG, allowing for the procedure to be performed in sicker patients with respiratory or cardiovascular compromise	Diagnostic EGD not obtained in the same setting
	Usually possible even if there is a proximal obstruction	Smaller-diameter tubes are often used leading to higher rate of tube occlusion
Surgical	May be placed laparoscopically or at the time of surgery for another indication	General anesthesia required
	Large-diameter tube can be placed	A Foley catheter is usually used, which is prone to balloon malfunction or tube degradation

Abbreviations: EGD, esophagogastroduodenoscopy; PEG, percutaneous endoscopic gastrostomy.

the ability to visualize the upper gastrointestinal tract and the placement of larger-diameter tubes. Patients at high risk of aspiration, such as those with a history of tube feed-related aspiration, altered mental status, severe gastroesophageal reflux, gastroparesis, gastric outlet obstruction, unresectable gastric-pancreatic cancer, or insufficient stomach from prior resection should generally have a tube placed into the distal duodenum or jejunum [15]. The direct nonsurgical, percutaneous route of jejunostomy tube placement tends to be less successful and more likely to result in complications compared with this method's use to place gastrostomy tubes [16,17]. Although gastrojejunostomy tubes are an alternative and tend to be inserted with greater success and fewer complication than the direct jejunostomy approach, these tubes are prone to displacement back into the stomach and tube blockage [18]. As a consequence, the need for jejunal access should be considered in all patients planning to undergo surgery.

Enteral formulae are generally nutritionally complete emulsions of macronutrients and micronutrients that consist of intact protein, glucose polymers, and a mixture of long-chain and medium-chain triglycerides. These formulae may either supplement or completely replace a solid diet. Most are commercially prepared and are not palatable, and are suitable only for tube feeding. Most HEN patients, whether fed into the stomach or jejunum, tolerate standard formulations, which tend to be isotonic, lactose-free, 1 kcal/mL and meet most nutritional needs. Specialized formulations are also available including elemental (ie, chemically defined); fiber-containing; lactose-containing; organ-specific (eg, renal, pulmonary, hepatic); modular products; and immune-enhancing (eg, containing arginine, glutamine, nucleotides, omega-3 fatty acids). The benefits of most of these products over standard formulations remain insufficiently substantiated and they are considerably more expensive. In general, standard products are recommended and, if not tolerated, a specialty product can be tried. For example, in the setting of refractory malabsorptive conditions, anecdotal reports suggest that enteral feeding of an elemental formula may occasionally be successful and prevent the need of parenteral nutrition support. Care must always be taken to ensure proper mixing when contents are added to enteral products.

Methods of formula administration include bolus, gravity, and continuous. In bolus feeding, 300 to 400 mL is infused with a syringe over 5 to 10 minutes several times per day. Bolus feeding is reliable, easy to comprehend, and frees the patient from a mechanical device; however, it is limited by its propensity to generate high residual volumes and intolerance. Bolus feeding is preferred in active, alert patients with low aspiration risk. Gravity feeding provides an intermittent, continuous drip that requires a pole and a device to hold the formula while it is infusing. Closed enteral feeding systems allow delivery measured in a drip chamber, allowing whatever remains to be used later that same day. This contrasts with open systems in which the cans of formula are poured into a delivery system that is flushed and cleaned after each use. The rate of infusion with this method is not as precise and can predispose to gastroesophageal reflux and aspiration. Intermittent gravity feeding is sufficient for most patients with a gastrostomy or nasogastric tube and is typically used when the bolus method is not tolerated. Continuous infusion by pump is recommended for jejunostomy feeding and for gastrostomy feeding when a reduction in the risk of gastroesophageal reflux and aspiration is needed [19]. This method requires a pump and power source but provides accurate, controlled delivery. Too rapid delivery, particularly of a hyperosmolar solution, may cause abdominal distention, cramping, hyperperistalsis, and diarrhea as a consequence of fluid secretion into the lumen. There exists no well-defined process for the conversion from continuous to intermittent feeding. The overlapping of a gradual increase in intermittent feedings while maintaining continuous feeding at a gradually decreasing rate has been recommended [20]. Overnight feeding allows maximal use of the gut while enabling normal activities during the day.

Home Parenteral Nutrition

Once an appropriate indication for HPN is confirmed and the patient is ensured of having the appropriate education and means at home to administer HPN, certain steps need to be taken in the hospital before discharge. First, safe and accessible central venous access needs to be obtained. If the duration of HPN use is expected to be less than 90 days, a peripherally inserted central catheter is generally appropriate. If the use of HPN is anticipated to extend beyond 90 days, a tunneled (eg, Hickman or Groshong) or subcutaneously implanted (eg, infusaport or portocath) catheter should be placed. Placement of a single-lumen catheter is preferred because use of multilumen catheters is associated with an increased risk of catheter infection. The use of internal jugular or subclavian veins is preferred over femoral veins because of a lesser risk of infection. The tip of the catheter should generally be located in the superior vena cava near the cavo-atrial junction. In situations where the superior vena cava cannot be accessed, the inferior vena cava can be accessed using a long, tunneled femoral venous site. Uses of the hepatic vein and direct puncture of the right atrium have been described in desperate cases.

The pharmacist has an important role in making sure the volume and the formulation of the HPN are correct before hospital discharge. A 1.5- to 3-L parenteral nutrition solution is usually cycled to a nocturnal infusion before hospital discharge to allow the patient freedom from the infusion pump during the day and to minimize the potential risk of liver injury from the HPN [21]. When HPN is cycled, the patient receives more fluid in a shorter time, usually 10 to 14 hours including ramp up and taper down periods. The clinician must ensure that the patient can tolerate the rate of fluid infusion before discharge. Finally, because a 1-week supply of the HPN formula is usually delivered to the patient's home at one time by the home care company, it is important that the patient understand that the HPN preparation has to be refrigerated until used to prevent contamination and subsequent infection. Refrigeration space may be an issue for some patients.

In both HEN and HPN, an estimation of daily energy (eg, Harris-Benedict formula) and fluid needs is necessary before initiating feeding. In the occasional patient, use of nitrogen balance or indirect calorimetry after reaching the previously mentioned goal can provide further optimization of energy needs. Although daily caloric and fluid requirements vary, for a normally nourished adult, 25 to 35 kcal/kg/d and 25 to 35 mL/kg/d based on ideal body weight is a reasonable starting place. Because carbohydrates account for most of the calories (3.4 kcal/mL), blood glucose levels should be monitored daily; the addition of insulin to the HPN solution may be required in some patients. Intravenous lipids are usually administered as a three-in-one emulsion to provide 20% to 30% of the infused calories (usually <1 g/kg/d). Intravenous protein is supplied in the form of amino acids (usually 1–1.5 g/kg/d). The remainder of the HPN solution consists of electrolytes, vitamins, and trace elements. Common additives include insulin, histamine-receptor 2 antagonists, and heparin.

Perhaps the most important step before hospital discharge is to make sure the patient has follow-up care arranged with a physician who will also take responsibility for checking laboratory values and adjust the HPN formula as needed. This physician needs to work closely with a pharmacist and home care nurse when the patient finally goes home. Monitoring of routine blood chemistries is generally recommended weekly for the first month of HPN therapy and, if the patient's condition is stable, monthly or less often thereafter. For those patients on long-term HPN, multiple trace elements (chromium, selenium, zinc, copper, and manganese) and fat-soluble vitamins (A, D, E, and K) should be checked once or twice a year. A dietitian should also periodically monitor the patient's caloric intake because caloric intake, body weight, and amount of fluid losses ultimately determine when HPN can be discontinued [22].

HOME PARENTERAL AND ENTERAL NUTRITION COMPLICATIONS

Home Enteral Nutrition

Enteral feeding is a relatively safe procedure whose complications can usually be avoided or corrected. HEN complications resulting in hospitalization are infrequent, averaging about once every 3 years [1]. Rehospitalization for non–HEN-related causes has been shown to be less common for neuromuscular disease patients compared with those with cancer or malabsorptive process [23]. The overall complication rate of HEN is about 0.4 per patient per year with little difference between indications for HEN, approximately one half that of HPN [1]. Complications of enteral feeding are typically separated into those related to the tube and those related to its subsequent use (Box 6) [24,25]. The latter complications can be further divided into mechanical, infectious, gastrointestinal, and metabolic. Mechanical problems are often associated with aspects of the tube itself: size, material, pliability, or location within the gastrointestinal tract. Gastrointestinal complications usually occur in those receiving enteral feeding. Metabolic problems including a deficiency or excess of electrolytes, micronutrients, and water, although relatively uncommon, may occur when the tubes are used for either feeding or decompression. Finally, a variety of infectious problems can complicate the use of enteral tubes. In patients receiving HEN, specific complications that require monitoring include gastroesophageal reflux, aspiration, diarrhea, tube malfunction, feeding tolerance, metabolic derangements, and alterations in drug absorption and metabolism. Table 2 lists a selection of important potential complications of HEN and suggests interventions that may be used to manage them and prevent their occurrence.

Home Parenteral Nutrition

Complications are a greater concern with HPN compared with HEN and can be divided into those related to the central venous catheter and those related to

Box 6: Complications of enteral tubes

Insertion

Aspiration

Bleeding

Gastric wall or rectus sheath hematoma

Ileus

Fistulous tracts (eg, gastrocolocutaneous, jejunocolocutaneous, aortogastric, bronchoesophageal)

Asymptomatic pneumoperitoneum

Subcutaneous emphysema

Liver laceration

Gastric laceration

Perforation

Peritonitis

Skin site infection

Necrotizing fasciitis

Tumor implantation at skin site

Death

Subsequent use

Tube occlusion

Inadvertent removal

Skin site infection

Stomal leakage or skin irritation

Buried bumper

Bleeding

Subcostal neuralgia

Abdominal wall pain

Obstruction

Volvulus (intestinal, gastric)

Intestinal ischemia

the parenteral nutrition itself [26]. Catheter infection is the most common complication of HPN therapy, is most common reason for hospital readmission, and is usually the direct result of poor sterile technique. The rate of primary catheter infection has been reported to be between one and four infections per 1000 catheter-days [27–29]. Infection can occur in the bloodstream as a result of direct spread of bacteria from the catheter hub; at the catheter skin exit site; and along the subcutaneous tract of the catheter (ie, tunnel infection).

Table 2
Selected complications of enteral tube feeding

Complication	Prevention and Treatment
Mechanical	
Tube occlusion	Routine flushing with water; use liquid medications when possible; dissolve papain or sodium bicarbonate or alkalinized pancreatic enzymes; mechanical device
Tube displacement	Tube surveillance; adequate fixation
Bleeding	Prevent excessive traction on the tube; endoscopic assessment including under internal bolster; change of tube type
Leakage	Proper skin care; inspection of tube site for infection, fixation, side torsion, absence of external bolster; treat specific causative factor if identified; local measures; assistance from wound care nurse; avoid replacement with a larger-diameter tube
Metabolic	
Refeeding syndrome	Anticipate deficiencies; monitor electrolytes, weight, and fluid balance closely, particularly when initiating nutrition support; replete deficiencies
Fluid/electrolyte Imbalance	
Gastrointestinal	
Diarrhea	Systematic evaluation of potential causes, such as medications, infection, underlying disease, altered gut anatomy, formula; ensure proper formula handling; treat specific cause if identified; change rate or method of formula administration; add fiber to formula; use antidiarrheals; rarely change to specialized formula
Constipation	Maintain hydration and activity; minimize constipating medications; regular use of laxatives, suppositories, or enemas; add fiber to the formula (?)
Nausea/bloating/distention	Correct cause of ileus if present; evaluate medications; change feeding rate or method of administration; potential role of prokinetic medications (?)
Aspiration/reflux	Identify and modify risk factors if present; routinely assess feeding tolerance; elevate head of bed when infusing; monitor gastric residual volume (?); change method of administration; add a prokinetic medication; change to postpyloric feeding
Infectious	
Skin site infection	Recognize risk factors for infection; prevent excessive tension between bolsters; prophylactic antibiotic before tube placement; treat with oral antibiotic or by tube and local wound care; removal of the tube, intravenous antibiotics, and surgery

Symptoms and signs of a systemic catheter infection may include fever, lethargy, chills, rigors, and elevated white blood cell count and serum glucose. In contrast, an exit site infection may present with only discharge from the catheter skin site, whereas a tunnel infection may present with only redness and tenderness along the catheter tract.

If a bloodstream infection is suspected, blood cultures should be obtained immediately from the catheter and from a peripheral vein, and infusion of the HPN should be temporarily discontinued. Broad-spectrum antibiotics should be started empirically if the suspicion of infection is high. Commonly isolated organisms include *Staphylococcus aureus*, *Staphylococcus epidermis*, enterococci, pseudomonas, *Serratia marcescens*, *Klebsiella pneumoniae*, and *Escherichia coli*. Antibiotics can be adjusted depending on the organism isolated, antibiotic sensitivities, and the patient's clinical response. If the patient is stable, the infection can often be treated without removal of the catheter; however, if the patient is hemodynamically unstable, the catheter should be removed immediately. In the case of fungal infections, the catheter should always be removed and treatment with an antifungal agent begun. A 14-day course of antibiotic therapy is usually recommended followed by repeat cultures to make sure the infection has been cleared, particularly if placement of a new permanent catheter is needed. Persistently positive blood cultures may indicate an infected heart valve or thrombus.

In a suspected exit site or tunnel infection, cultures from the site are usually positive for staphylococcal organisms. Exit site infections can usually be managed with intravenous antibiotics without removal of the catheter, whereas tunnel infections usually require removal of the catheter and systemic antibiotics.

Catheter blockage is suspected when either flushing the catheter or drawing blood from the catheter is difficult. Nonthrombotic causes of catheter occlusion include a kinked or pinched catheter. A kinked catheter usually occurs at or near the skin site, whereas a pinched catheter generally occurs by compression of the catheter between the first rib and clavicle. Thrombus or precipitated HPN components can also cause catheter occlusion. If clinically suspected, venography should be performed to confirm the diagnosis.

Catheter-related venous thrombosis is a well-recognized complication affecting the subclavian vein with the potential for thromboembolization [30–32]. It often starts as a fibrin sheath that grows around the intravascular portion of the catheter. The incidence has been reported to range from 5% to 28% and is more likely to occur in patients with a coagulopathy or cancer. Although catheter-related venous thrombosis may go unrecognized, symptoms may include pain and swelling in the arm or neck during infusion and collateral vein formation of the chest wall. The diagnosis can be confirmed by ultrasonography or venography. If irrigation with normal saline is not successful, then irrigation with a thrombolytic agent (eg, tissue plasminogen activator, 1–2 mg) may dissolve the thrombus. If the thrombus cannot be cleared or if infection is suspected, the catheter should be removed. Blood cultures should be drawn from the catheter before removal. It is also recommended that systemic heparin be given followed by at least 4 months of anticoagulant therapy with warfarin. Efforts to prevent catheter-related venous thrombosis have yielded mixed results. The use of heparin flushes has shown some benefit in limiting thrombus formation, but the addition of heparin to the HPN preparation has not shown benefit. Minidose warfarin (2.5 mg every other day) may have prophylactic benefit in patients with hematologic malignancies.

Catheter fracture with subsequent catheter embolization can also occur. A chest radiograph should be obtained if clinically suspected and may demonstrate a catheter piece lodged in the right atrium, right ventricle, or pulmonary artery. The fractured catheter should be removed either by interventional radiology or surgery, because a mortality rate of 40% has been reported if it is not removed.

Liver test abnormalities occur commonly in HPN patients [33–37]. In a study by Luman and Shaffer [33], liver test abnormalities occurred in 47% of 107 patients receiving HPN. A raised alkaline phosphatase level was the most common abnormality noted. The pathogenesis is poorly understood and seems to be multifactorial. Caloric excess, choline deficiency, lack of stimulation by enteral feeding, and infection have all been implicated. The histopathology of HPN liver disease can vary from steatosis or cholestasis to steatohepatitis and cirrhosis. Steatosis is the most common finding in adults and can develop within 10 days of starting parenteral nutrition. In infants and children, cholestasis and cirrhosis are more common. Cavicchi and colleagues [34] demonstrated a 6.7% mortality rate from HPN liver disease. Liver failure was reported to be much less common in a recent retrospective study of adult HPN patients [37].

If HPN-induced cholestasis is suspected, ultrasonography should be completed initially to exclude extrahepatic causes, such as biliary sludge and gallstones, especially because about 35% of HPN patients develop gallstones. Medical management of HPN-related cholestasis should first center on improving oral or enteral nutrition intake, which stimulates bile output. The caloric content of the HPN solution should be reviewed to ensure the patient is not receiving excess calories (ie, >35 kcal/kg/d) or excess lipids (ie, >1 g/kg/d). Treatment of bacterial overgrowth when present and use of ursodeoxycholic acid may also be of benefit. Limited studies suggest that cyclical, as opposed to continuous, HPN may prevent liver disease over time. If, despite these treatments, the bilirubin level continues to increase or the patient has evidence of cirrhosis on liver biopsy, referral for consideration of transplantation is warranted. This point is highlighted by recent evidence showing that in HPN patients with a fatal outcome related to liver disease, the interval between the onset of jaundice and death was only 10 months [33].

Metabolic bone disease is also common in HPN patients [38–40]. In a study of 165 HPN patients, 81% were osteopenic and 41% had osteoporosis [40]. The cause of osteoporosis in HPN patients includes pre-existing disease, malabsorptive syndromes, corticosteroid therapy, inactivity, hypogonadism, and hypercalciuria. Calcium, phosphorus, and magnesium deficiency may play a role. Vitamin D deficiency or excess (by suppressing parathyroid hormone secretion) may also contribute. Current HPN formulations provide decreased vitamin D (200 IU/d), because higher levels are thought to worsen bone mineral density. Therapies to minimize bone mineral density loss for HPN patients include the use of bisphosphonates, calcitonin, and 1500 mg of daily oral calcium supplementation and vitamin D if deficient. Annual or biannual bone mineral density testing should be considered in all HPN patients.

Micronutrient deficiencies can lead to serious complications in the HPN patient. Fortunately, these deficiencies are much less common in the present day because of the routine addition of multivitamins and trace element preparations to the HPN formula. One exception is iron deficiency, because iron is not routinely in HPN. Trace element toxicity can also occur and result in serious lifethreatening complications. Manganese excess can accumulate in the basal ganglia and manifest as Parkinson's disease–like symptoms. Both manganese and copper are excreted by the liver and should be withheld from HPN in patients with cholestatic liver disease. Serum levels of trace elements should be checked at least twice a year and adjusted if necessary. Clinical guidelines, including recommendations on the frequency of laboratory testing, are available to help direct the management of HPN patients [41].

HOME PARENTERAL AND ENTERAL NUTRITION OUTCOMES
Home Enteral Nutrition
In a study from France, the overall probability of survival in HEN patients was 44% and 29% at 1 and 2 years, respectively [42]. The underlying diagnosis has the most predictable influence on HPEN outcome [1,23,43,44], the highest mortality being seen in cancer patients and those with amyotrophic lateral sclerosis and dementia and the lowest mortality in those with multiple sclerosis, cerebral palsy, and cystic fibrosis. A study from the United States found that 1 year after initiating HEN, 48% of neuromuscular disorder patients with dysphagia had died, whereas 25% remained on HEN and 19% had resumed full oral nutrition [1]. Fourteen percent of patients following a stroke were shown to resume full oral nutrition emphasizing the need periodically to reassess swallowing ability in these patients. Similarly, in cancer patients, data from the American Society of Parenteral and Enteral Nutrition registry found that at 1 year 59% had died, 6% were still receiving HEN, and 30% were on full oral nutrition [1,23]. In a large study involving head and neck cancer patients, a 30% 1-year survival was noted [45]. In another study of HEN patients with small bowel malabsorptive disease, it was demonstrated that 1 year after initiating HEN, 18% had died and 45% had resumed full oral nutrition [1,23].

Age also seems to influence survival in HEN patients, a finding related mainly to the different age-related causes of dysphagia [23,46]. In one study, only 46% of HEN patients older than 65 years were alive after 1 year compared with 89% of those less than 25 years of age. Stroke patients older than 75 years of age were shown to be three to four times more likely to die while receiving HEN than those younger than 65 [23]. The overall degree of rehabilitation has also been shown to be worse in older patients.

The few studies that have assessed the quality of life of HEN patients have generally described a poorer quality of life compared with the general population [46], usually because of their other physical disabilities (eg, in amyotrophic lateral sclerosis or stroke patients); however, most patients or their caregivers rate the feeding tube aspect of their care favorably [47]. There are no detailed studies of quality of life in HEN cancer patients and no formal quality of life studies in HEN patients with malabsorption.

Home Parenteral Nutrition

Because most HPN patients resume full oral nutrition and some die, less than 20% of patients who begin HPN ultimately require it long-term and most do not require HPN for more than 1 year [48,49]. A 94% probability of requiring HPN permanently has been demonstrated in those patients who are unable to be weaned within 2 years of its initiation [49]. Studies from both the United States and Europe have shown that the most important factor influencing home PN survival is the patient's underlying disease or primary diagnosis (Table 3) [21,48,49]. Death occurs relatively uncommonly as a consequence of an HPN complication, particularly in those requiring HPN for less than a year. In contrast, for those patients who require HPN for a longer time period (eg, nonmalignant causes of short-bowel syndrome), a 10% to 15% risk of mortality from an HPN-related complication (eg, line sepsis, liver failure, loss of vascular access) exists.

Younger HPN patients have a lower risk of mortality compared with older HPN patients. The length of remaining small bowel influences patient survival in short-bowel syndrome patients [49]. Those patients with a longer length of small bowel tend to have a better prognosis. The presence of chronic mechanical obstruction and subsequent increased risk of sepsis also increases the risk of mortality in HPN patients. Box 7 summarizes factors associated with improved HPN survival.

HPN is associated with a number of factors that, when combined with effects from their underlying disease process, may result in a restriction of activities

Table 3
Survival on home parenteral nutrition based on primary diagnosis

	% Survival		
Diagnosis	1 year	3 year	5 year
Crohn's disease	96	84	82
Mesenteric ischemia	87	84	56
Radiation enteritis	87	58	52
Motility disorder	87	62	—
Congenital bowel defects	94	80	—
Chronic bowel obstruction	83	40	—
Cancer	20	—	—

Data from Howard L. Home parenteral nutrition: survival, cost, and quality of life. Gastroenterology 2006;130:S53.

Box 7: Factors influencing improved survival in home parenteral nutrition

Primary diagnosis (eg, noncancer)

Younger age

Greater remnant small bowel length

Nonobstructed bowel

Greater experience of the supervising clinician

Absence of narcotic use

Social support

and deleteriously impact daily life (Box 8). The few studies investigating quality of life in HPN patients suggest a reduced quality of life in HPN patients compared with the general population [50,51]. With time and experience, patients on home PN can modify their lifestyles to minimize the impact of this therapy (eg, infuse parenteral nutrition overnight, travel with help from home health care company and support groups, modify diet and leisure activities). This is expected to be reflected as an improvement in quality of life. Quality of life seems to be better in younger HPN patients and worse in HPN patients with depression and narcotic dependence [50]. It is difficult to determine whether HPN itself or the underlying disease more affects quality of life.

HOME PARENTERAL AND ENTERAL NUTRITION COSTS

Although practice variations, patient heterogeneity, and uncertainty regarding outcomes pose methodologic problems, economic evaluations of HPEN have shown that providing nutrition support at home is up to 75% more cost-effective than keeping patients in the hospital. In the United States, the costs of HPEN are generally assumed by private insurance. Medicare covers about 48% of HEN patients and 27% of HPN patients [1]. In contrast, the costs of HPEN in Canada, France, and the United Kingdom are almost completely undertaken by the National Health Service.

Despite over five times the number of patients, the total national costs of HEN are about the same as HPN [1]. Annual costs associated with daily use of HEN in the United States in 2000 were estimated to be between $9000 and $25,000, with the variability primarily caused by the availability of different providers and competing commercial pharmacies. Direct costs associated with HPN include the nutrient solution, administration sets, infusion pump, and catheter dressing kits. In a report using 1992 dollars, these costs were estimated to range from $238 to $390 per day, which translated into $86,000 to $140,000 per year [1,21]. Importantly, these costs do not include fees associated with medical visits, laboratory monitoring, home nursing support, or hospitalizations for complications of PN. Although clearly an extremely expensive

Box 8: Factors affecting quality of life on home parenteral nutrition

Inconvenience

Expense

Interference with social and leisure activities

Altered body image or disfigurement

Parenteral nutrition–related complications

Emotional strain

Pain

Lack of employment or lowered status at work

Loss of income

Decreased social interaction

Loss of independence

Loss of control of bodily functions

Inability to eat normally

Sexual functioning

therapy, the cost of HPEN tends to be offset by its lifesaving nature and the likelihood of recovery of intestinal function. Periodic assessment of compliance, appropriateness of formulation, infusion regimen, and status of intestinal adaptation and ability to wean PN is critically important to provide the most cost-effective care for the HPEN patient [52].

SUMMARY

HPEN has evolved to become a very successful, lifesaving treatment in the management of patients with intestinal and oral failure. Although HPEN is associated with a number of factors that may result in a restriction of activities and deleteriously impact daily life, with time and experience HPEN patients can modify their lifestyles to minimize the impact of this therapy. Although clearly an extremely expensive therapy, the cost of HPEN tends to be offset by its lifesaving nature and the likelihood of recovery of intestinal function. The management of HPEN by a nutrition support team reduces HPEN-related morbidity and may reduce costs associated with its use. Because clinical expertise in the management of patients receiving HPEN is not widely available, the referral of these patients to experienced centers for periodic assessment is advised.

References
  [1] Howard L, Ament M, Fleming CR, et al. Current use and clinical outcome of home parenteral and enteral nutrition therapies in the United States. Gastroenterology 1995;109:355–65.
  [2] Howard L, Ashley C. Management of complications in patients receiving home parenteral nutrition. Gastroenterology 2003;124:1651–61.

[3] Sun X, Spencer AU, Yang H, et al. Impact of caloric intake on parenteral nutrition-associated intestinal morphology and mucosal barrier function. JPEN J Parenter Enteral Nutr 2006;30: 474–9.

[4] Alverdy J, Chi HS, Sheldon GF. The effect of parenteral nutrition on gastrointestinal immunity: the importance of enteral stimulation. Ann Surg 1985;202:681–4.

[5] McClave SA, Lowen CC, Snider HL. Immunonutrition and enteral hyperalimentation of critically ill patients. Dig Dis Sci 1992;37:1153–61.

[6] Scolapio JS, Picco MF, Tarraso VB. Enteral versus parenteral nutrition: the patient's preference. JPEN J Parenter Enteral Nutr 2002;26:248–50.

[7] Parver AK, Lubinski CA. Reimbursement issues in nutrition support. In: Merritt R, editor. The A.S.P.E.N. nutrition support practice manual. Silver Spring (MD): ASPEN; 1998. p. 36,1–36,18.

[8] Hebuterne X, Rampal P. Enteral nutrition of the elderly: an update. Nutrition Clinique et Metabolisme 1996;10:19–29.

[9] Kirby DF, Delegge MH, Fleming CR. American Gastroenterological Association Medical Position Statement: guidelines for the use of enteral nutrition. Gastroenterology 1995;108: 1280–301.

[10] Fairman RP. Withdrawing life-sustaining treatment: lessons from Nancy Cruzan. Arch Intern Med 1992;252:25–7.

[11] Elia M, Russell C, Shaffer J, et al. Annual report of the British Artificial Nutrition Survey (BANS) 1998. British Association of Parenteral and Enteral Nutrition. Available at: http://www.bapen.org.uk/pdfs/bans_reports/bans_98.pdf. Accessed March 1, 2007.

[12] Powers DA, Brown RO, Cowan GSM Jr, et al. Nutrition support team vs nonteam management of enteral nutrition support in a veteran's administration medical center teaching hospital. JPEN J Parenter Enteral Nutr 1986;10:635–8.

[13] Hamaoui E. Assessing the nutrition support team. JPEN J Parenter Enteral Nutr 1987;11: 412–21.

[14] Heyland DK, Dhaliwal R, Drover JW, et al. Canadian clinical practice guidelines for nutrition support in mechanically ventilated, critically ill adult patients. [see comment]. JPEN J Parenter Enteral Nutr 2003;27:355–73.

[15] Marik PE, Zaloga GP. Gastric versus post-pyloric feeding: a systematic review. Crit Care 2003;7:46–51.

[16] Maple JT, Petersen BT, Baron TH, et al. Direct percutaneous endoscopic jejunostomy: outcomes in 307 consecutive attempts. Am J Gastroenterol 2005;100:2681–8.

[17] Cosentini EP, Sautner T, Gnant M, et al. Outcomes of surgical, percutaneous, endoscopic, and percutaneous radiologic gastrostomies. Arch Surg 1998;133:1076–83.

[18] DiSario JA, Foutch PG, Sanowski RA. Poor results with percutaneous endoscopic jejunostomy. Gastrointest Endosc 1990;36:257–60.

[19] Ciocon JO, Galindo-Ciocon DJ, Tiessen C, et al. Continuous compared with intermittent tube feeding in the elderly. JPEN J Parenter Enteral Nutr 1992;16:525–8.

[20] Powers T, Cowan GSM, Deckard M, et al. Prospective randomized evaluation of two regimens for converting from continuous to intermittent feedings in patients with feeding gastrostomies. JPEN J Parenter Enteral Nutr 1991;15:405–7.

[21] Howard L. Home parenteral nutrition: survival, cost, and quality of life. Gastroenterology 2006;130:S52–9.

[22] DiBaise JK, Matarese LE, Messing B, et al. Strategies for weaning parenteral nutrition in adult patients with short bowel syndrome. J Clin Gastroenterol 2006;40(Suppl):S94–8.

[23] Howard L, Patton L, Scheib-Dahl R. Home enteral feeding: outcomes in long-term enteral feeding. Gastrointest Endosc Clin N Am 1998;8:705–22.

[24] McClave SA, Chang W-K. Complications of enteral access. Gastrointest Endosc 2003;58: 739–51.

[25] DiBaise JK, Decker GA. Enteral access options and management in the patient with intestinal failure. J Clin Gastroenterol, in press.

[26] DiBaise JK. Home parenteral nutrition: complications, survival, quality of life and costs. In: Langnas A, Goulet O, Quigley E, et al. editors. Intestinal failure: diagnosis, management and transplantation. Blackwell Publishing, in press.

[27] Bozzetti F, Mariani L, Bertinet DB, et al. Central venous catheter complications in 447 patients on home parenteral nutrition: an analysis of over 100,000 catheter days. Clin Nutr 2002;21:475–85.

[28] Mermel LA, Farr BM, Sherertz RJ, et al. Guidelines for the management of intravascular catheter-related infections. Clin Infect Dis 2001;32:1249–72.

[29] Ghabril MS, Aranda-Michel J, Scolapio JS. Metabolic and catheter complications of parenteral nutrition. Curr Gastroenterol Rep 2004;6:327–34.

[30] Steiger E. Dysfunction and thrombotic complications of vascular access devices. JPEN J Parenter Enteral Nutr 2006;30:S70–2.

[31] Grant J. Recognition, prevention and treatment of home total parenteral nutrition central venous access complications. JPEN J Parenter Enteral Nutr 2002;26:S21–8.

[32] Messing B, Joly F. Guidelines for management of home parenteral support in adult chronic intestinal failure patients. Gastroenterology 2006;130:S43–51.

[33] Luman W, Shaffer JL. Prevalence, outcome and associated factors of deranged liver function tests in patients on home parenteral nutrition. Clin Nutr 2002;21:37–343.

[34] Cavicchi M, Beau P, Crenn P, et al. Prevalence of liver disease and contributing factors in patients receiving home parenteral nutrition for permanent intestinal failure. Ann Intern Med 2000;132:525–32.

[35] Fulford A, Scolapio JS, Aranda-Michel J. Parenteral nutrition-associated hepatotoxicity. Nutr Clin Pract 2004;19:274–83.

[36] Kelly DA. Intestinal failure-associated liver disease: what do we know today? Gastroenterology 2006;130:S70–7.

[37] Salvino R, Ghanta R, Seidner DL, et al. Liver failure is uncommon in adults receiving long-term parenteral nutrition. JPEN J Parenter Enteral Nutr 2006;30:202–8.

[38] Seidner DL. Parenteral nutrition-associated metabolic bone disease. JPEN J Parenter Enteral Nutr 2002;26:S37–42.

[39] Cohen-Solal M, Baudoin C, Joly F, et al. Osteoporosis in patients on long term home parenteral nutrition: a longitudinal study. J Bone Miner Res 2003;18:1989–94.

[40] Pironi L, Tjellesen L, De Francesco A, et al. Bone mineral density in patients on home parenteral nutrition: a follow-up study. Clin Nutr 2004;23:1288–302.

[41] Guidelines for the use of parenteral and enteral nutrition in adult and pediatric patients. JPEN J Parenter Enteral Nutr 2002;26:20SA–1SA.

[42] Wehrlen –Martini S, Hebuterne X, Pugliese P, et al. 47 months activity of a center for home-enteral nutrition and long-term follow-up of the patients treated. Nutr Clin Metab 1997;11:7–17.

[43] North American Home Parenteral and Enteral Nutrition Patient Registry. Annual Reports 1985–1992. Albany, NY: Oley Foundation, 1987–1994.

[44] Van Gossum A, Bakker H, Bozzetti F, et al. Home parenteral nutrition in adults: a European multicenter survey in 1997. Clin Nutr 1999;18:135–40.

[45] Rabineck L, Wray NP, Petersen NJ. Long term outcomes of patients receiving percutaneous endoscopic gastrostomy tubes. J Gen Intern Med 1996;11:287–93.

[46] Parker T, Neale G, Elia M. Home enteral tube feeding in East Anglia. Eur J Clin Nutr 1996;50:47–53.

[47] Bannerman E, Pendlebury J, Phillips F, et al. A cross-sectional and longitudinal study of health-related quality of life after percutaneous endoscopic gastrostomy. Eur J Gastroenterol Hepatol 2000;12:1101–9.

[48] Scolapio JS, Fleming CR, Kelly DG, et al. Survival of home parenteral nutrition-treated patients: 20 years of experience at the Mayo Clinic. Mayo Clin Proc 1999;74:217–22.

[49] Messing B, Crenn P, Beau P, et al. Long-term survival and parenteral nutrition dependence in adult patients with the short bowel syndrome. Gastroenterology 1999;117:1043–50.

[50] Winkler MF. Quality of life in adult home parenteral nutrition patients. JPEN J Parenter Enteral Nutr 2005;29:162–70.

[51] Jeppesen PB, Langholz E, Mortensen PB. Quality of life in patients receiving home parenteral nutrition. Gut 1999;44:844–52.

[52] Baptista RJ, Lahey MA, Bistrian BR, et al. Periodic reassessment for improved, cost-effective care in HPN: a case report. JPEN J Parenter Enteral Nutr 1984;8:708–10.

Gastroenterol Clin N Am 36 (2007) 145–159

GASTROENTEROLOGY CLINICS
OF NORTH AMERICA

ELSEVIER
SAUNDERS

Intestinal Transplantation: Current Status

Jonathan P. Fryer, MD

Division of Transplantation, Department of Surgery, Feinberg School of Medicine,
Northwestern University, 675 North St. Clair Street, Galter, Pavilion Suite 17-200,
Chicago, IL 60611–2923S, USA

Transplantation of vascularized organs, such as the intestine, was first conceptualized at the turn of the century by Carrel [1], who recognized the potential for such procedures with the establishment of a reliable method of performing vascular anastomoses. The feasibility of intestinal transplantation was not demonstrated until 1959, however, when Lillihei and coworkers [2], at the University of Minnesota, reported success in a canine model. This inspired the first human intestinal transplants, which were performed by Deterling in Boston in 1964 (unpublished). The first reported human intestinal transplant was performed by Lillihei and coworkers [3] in 1967, and included the entire small bowel and right colon, with the superior mesenteric vessels being anastomosed to the left common iliac vessels. Unfortunately, these and other early attempts were uniformly unsuccessful [4].

When the effectiveness of cyclosporine was established in other organ transplants in the early 1980s, there was renewed interest in intestinal transplantation. Although the first intestinal transplant using cyclosporine, performed in 1985 by Cohen and coworkers [5] in Toronto, was also unsuccessful, in 1988 Deltz and coworkers [6] in Kiel, Germany, performed what is considered to be the first successful intestinal transplant. The recipient of this living-related allograft remained total parenteral nutrition (TPN)-free for 4 years before the graft was lost to chronic rejection. Soon after, other successful outcomes were reported by the groups headed by Goulet and coworkers [7] in Paris, and Grant and coworkers [8] in London, Canada, who had established the first intestinal transplant programs. The successes of these groups inspired other institutions to establish similar programs in the early 1990s [9]. There are now over 60 centers worldwide that have performed intestinal transplants, with over 1200 transplants performed to date [10].

E-mail address: jfryer@nmh.org

0889-8553/07/$ – see front matter
doi:10.1016/j.gtc.2007.01.001

INDICATIONS

The indication for intestinal transplant is intestinal failure. Intestinal failure results from obstruction, dysmotility, surgical resection, congenital defect, or disease-associated loss of absorption and is characterized by the inability to maintain protein-energy, fluid, electrolyte, or micronutrient balance [11] and is most commonly the result of previous extensive small bowel resections. The short-bowel syndrome is the consequence of insufficient functional small bowel and the inability to maintain protein-energy, fluid, electrolyte, or micronutrient balance despite administration of a normal diet. Short-bowel syndrome manifests as massive diarrhea or stomal output, electrolyte abnormalities, fat malabsorption, gastric hypersecretion, vitamin B_{12} deficiency, hyperbilirubinemia, and hepatic steatosis [12].

Although no specific disease entity, in and of itself, is an indication for intestinal transplant, in the intestinal transplants performed to date the primary diseases that have most commonly led to consideration of an intestinal transplant in adults are mesenteric thrombosis, Crohn's disease, trauma, volvulus, desmoid tumor, Gardner's syndrome, and familial polyposis; in children the list includes volvulus, gastroschisis, necrotizing enterocolitis, pseudo-obstruction, intestinal atresia, and Hirschsprung's disease [10].

Before the 1970s, intestinal failure was terminal, but with development of parenteral nutrition (PN), these patients can now be kept alive. Over the long term, PN support can be provided at home, and many individuals with intestinal failure have done very well for many years with home parenteral nutrition (HPN). HPN is a very expensive therapy, however, costing $250 to $500 a day. Furthermore, HPN can be associated with potentially life-threatening complications, including PN-associated liver disease (PNALD) [13], catheter-related sepsis, catheter-related thrombosis, severe dehydration, and metabolic derangements. Because central venous access is required for administration of TPN, and recurrent central line placements often lead to venous stenosis or occlusion, long-term HPN often results in a loss of sites for vascular access [14]. Although the prevalence of PNALD remains controversial, severe liver injury has been reported in up to 50% of intestinal failure patients receiving PN for greater than 5 years [15,16], and this is typically fatal [15–17]. Intestinal failure patients who are likely to be on PN for greater than 5 years and are at highest risk of developing severe, irreversible PNALD can be identified early based on their residual small intestinal anatomy. Generally, those with less than 50 cm of small intestine are at highest risk [15,16]. High-risk patients can be identified early and managed accordingly.

Unfortunately, the risk of PNALD is often not recognized early when intervention may be effective, and many intestinal failure patients are considered for intestinal transplantation only when PNALD is advanced. Approximately 75% of candidates listed for intestinal transplant also have needed to be listed for a liver transplant (N. Chungfal and colleagues, unpublished data, 2006). In addition to depleting the limited supply of donor livers, candidates that need to be listed for both intestine and liver transplants have a worse prognosis than those listed only for intestine. Waitlist mortality for liver-intestine candidates is higher than for any other organ transplant candidate population including those listed only for intestine. Furthermore, those who make it to transplant have inferior outcomes compared with recipients of intestine-only transplants.

High-risk intestinal failure patients need to be identified early, so that intestinal rehabilitation strategies and subsequent PN weaning efforts can be optimized. Patients successfully weaned from PN have the best prognosis and do not need intestinal transplantation, whereas those who cannot be weaned need to be considered for a transplant. Given the insidious nature of PNALD, the success of intestinal rehabilitation is incumbent on its early initiation in high-risk patients. The goal of intestinal rehabilitation is to facilitate PN withdrawal, but reasonable time lines for achieving this goal must be defined. If unsuccessful, subsequent decision making regarding the need to proceed with intestinal transplant must be done in a timely manner because intestinal transplant is usually considered too late.

Ideally, intestinal failure patients should be considered for transplantation when only an intestine is required. If severe PNALD has caused irreversible injury to the liver, however, a combined liver transplant must be performed. The criteria used to determine when a liver needs to be included have not been clearly defined. Although the presence of cirrhosis clearly mandates the inclusion of a liver, the indications for liver transplant with lesser degrees of PNALD remain controversial and seem to vary between transplant centers.

In addition to intestine-only and intestine-liver transplants, multivisceral transplants represent a third type of intestinal transplant. Unfortunately, consensus on what defines a multivisceral transplant is lacking. To maintain continuity of the portal venous system and bile duct, most intestine-liver transplants also include the pancreas, and some consider this to be a multivisceral transplant. United Network of Organ Sharing defines a multivisceral transplant as one that includes intestine, liver, and either pancreas or kidney [18]. Others define a multivisceral transplant as one that involves replacement of all organs dependent on the celiac and superior mesenteric arteries [19]. Using this definition, multivisceral transplants need to be considered if organs dependent on these two principle visceral arteries need replacement. Although this situation can exist in multiple scenarios, two potential examples include cirrhosis with complete mesenteric venous thrombosis and desmoid tumors involving the celiac and superior mesenteric axes. Unfortunately, the lack of consensus for what the definition of a multivisceral transplant is and what the indications for a multivisceral transplant are leads to some confusion in any discussion pertaining to the role of this type of transplant.

CONTRAINDICATIONS

Although circumstances can often dictate exceptions, in general intestinal transplants are contraindicated in individuals who have significant coexistent medical conditions that have no potential for improvement following transplantation, and negate any potential benefit provided by an intestinal transplant in terms of life expectancy or quality of life. If the patient has an active, uncontrolled infection or malignancy that is not eliminated by the transplant process, transplantation is contraindicated. If there is substantial evidence to indicate that a potential recipient or the primary care givers are not willing or able reliably to assume the responsibilities of the day-to-day management of the potential recipient following the transplant, transplantation is contraindicated.

PRETRANSPLANT RECIPIENT EVALUATION

All individuals under consideration for intestinal transplant should be seen and evaluated by a multidisciplinary intestinal failure team including transplant surgery, gastroenterology, nutritional services, psychiatry, social work, anesthesia, and financial services. Further consultation with other specialties (ie, cardiology, hematology, chest medicine, infectious disease, chemical dependency, dentistry, and so forth) is required in some cases. Baseline laboratory investigations including complete blood count, coagulation profile, complete metabolic panel, ABO blood group determination, HLA status, and panel reactive antibody status should be performed. Serologies for cytomegalovirus (CMV) and Epstein-Barr virus (EBV) should be obtained. If not done previously, the gastrointestinal (GI) tract should be assessed both radiologically and endoscopically to determine accurately the length and condition of the remaining bowel. If advanced liver disease is suspected, liver biopsy is useful in determining if there is severe fibrosis of cirrhosis. Using Doppler ultrasound or MR venography, it is important to establish which large veins are available for vascular access, because many of the patients have limited options. Living related donor transplantation can be discussed as an option if a potential living related donor is available [14].

If after these evaluations there is consensus that the patient is a good candidate for intestinal transplantation, the patient is listed. While waiting for a donor to become available, the stable patient should be reassessed every 3 months to determine whether there is any change is their medical status, such as deterioration in liver function or further loss of vascular access options. Furthermore, while waiting for intestine-only transplantation, the HPN administration should be monitored very closely to ensure that it does not contribute further to the development of PNALD. These patients also need ongoing maintenance of their central lines to minimize line-related complications, such as infections and thrombosis. Furthermore, while waiting for transplantation close attention must be paid to fluid and electrolyte disturbances, which are common because of the often excessive output from the residual GI tract.

DONOR EVALUATION AND MANAGEMENT

Cadaveric Donors

All cadaveric donors are potential intestine donors. The cadaveric donor needs to be ABO compatible with the recipient, and because of the risk of graft-versus-host disease ABO identical combinations should be used in most circumstances. In most cases, extensive prior bowel resection has significantly reduced the size of the recipient peritoneal cavity and a donor that is 50% to

75% the size of the recipient is often preferred. In certain circumstances, segments of the intestine from a larger donor may be considered.

Donors should have no previous history of significant intestinal pathology. As with all organ donors there should be no significant hemodynamic instability, sepsis, history of malignancy or chronic infection, severe hypoxia, or severe acidosis, and they must have negative serology for HIV and hepatitis B and C. Although it is generally believed to be unnecessary if a liver is included with the transplant, the role of a crossmatch with intestine-only transplants is unclear. Because of the need to minimize the intestinal cold ischemia time (<6 hours) [20,21] with intestine transplants, it may not always be possible to obtain the crossmatch results in time. Although HLA matching has not been studied extensively in small bowel transplantation, it may also be useful to know the HLA status of both donor and recipient, particularly if the recipient is known to be sensitized to certain HLA antigens.

Two other important considerations are the CMV and EBV serologic status of the donors and recipients. Transplantation of a serologically positive donor into a serologically negative recipient for either of these viruses can have serious consequences [22]. In addition to the risk of a systemic CMV infection, CMV enteritis can occur, which can lead to graft loss. A new EBV infection combined with posttransplant immunosuppression puts the patient at high risk for developing a posttransplant lymphoproliferative disorder (PTLD) [23].

Because the optimal cold ischemia time for intestinal grafts is less than 6 hours, careful attention must be given to the timing of the donor and recipient procedures to prevent prolonged cold ischemia. Consideration should also be given to what other organs are going to be procured, because this may influence the length of the donor procedure and the approach used by the small bowel procurement team.

Living Donors

If a living donor is being evaluated, it is important that the potential donor be evaluated by a multidisciplinary team that includes transplantation surgery, GI medicine, psychiatry, nutritional services, and social work. To avoid a conflict of interest, it is imperative that the physician in charge of working-up the donor not be an active part of the transplant team. As with any living donor procedure, possible complications should be explained in great detail to the potential donor on several occasions. It should also be made quite clear to the patient that other options besides using a living donor are available. Time must also be taken fully to understand the nature of the relationship between the donor and the recipient.

If a number of potential living donors are available, particularly among family members, then careful consideration should be given to the best available HLA match. The donor-recipient size discrepancy must also be considered, but because in a living donor only a segment of the intestine is transplanted, size limits are less restrictive. As with cadaver donors, the donor and recipient should be ABO identical, although in some circumstances ABO-compatible combinations can be considered.

As with cadaveric donors, living donors must be free of significant pathology involving the GI tract. Any potential living donor must be in good health with no previous significant medical problems, including diabetes, malignancy, or chronic infection. There should be no history of substance abuse or other high-risk activities in the donor, and no significant psychiatric history. Serology in the living donor must also be negative for HIV and hepatitis B and C. Obese donors should be avoided. As with cadaveric donors with CMV and EBV, status of the donor and recipient must be carefully considered and the combination of positive donors to negative recipients should be avoided. The living donor should be worked-up completely including complete blood count, electrolytes, liver function tests, EKG, and chest radiograph. The GI tract should be evaluated endoscopically and if any concerns exist, GI contrast studies should be performed. A mesenteric angiogram with selective study of the superior mesenteric artery and its venous phase should be performed to ensure that the terminal superior mesenteric artery and superior mesenteric vein, which are the vessels that the procured graft depends on, are adequate.

POSTOPERATIVE MANAGEMENT

Induction immunosuppression with monoclonal (alemtuzumab, basiliximab, daclizumab) or polyclonal (thymoglobulin) antibody preparations is often administered intraoperatively or preoperatively in the intestinal transplant recipient. Immediately following surgery, maintenance immunosuppression therapy is initiated by enteric administration. Tacrolimus is the mainstay drug for maintenance immunosuppression. Steroids are also included in the postoperative immunosuppressive regimen. Although some programs have included mycophenolate mofetil [24], others have avoided it because of its association with GI side effects. Sirolimus has been used in combination with tacrolimus and may help to prevent chronic rejection and thereby allow some reduction in the dependence on tacrolimus and steroids, because both drugs are associated with significant complications with long-term use. Prostaglandin E_1 is typically administered intravenously for the first several days posttransplant, both for its ability to improve the small bowel microcirculation and its potential immunosuppressive effects. Broad-spectrum intravenous antibiotics are typically continued for at least 1 week following the transplant.

Because CMV and EBV infections can be associated with significant morbidity and mortality in intestinal transplant recipients, it is imperative to initiate appropriate antiviral prophylaxis or regular polymerase chain reaction surveillance immediately following transplantation, particularly when the donor is positive for CMV or EBV and the recipient is negative. CMV prophylaxis is best accomplished with ganciclovir, although CMV immunoglobulin (Cytogam) has also been used. Acyclovir, which is less effective than ganciclovir for CMV, is effective prophylaxis for EBV. Intravenous immunoglobulin is also used by some centers as CMV or EBV prophylaxis.

In the immediate postoperative period, it is essential to check hemoglobin regularly for evidence of bleeding. It is also important to monitor serum pH and lactate levels to detect any evidence of intestinal ischemia or injury. When GI function is re-established, as indicated by decreasing G-tube returns and increasing gas and enteric contents in the ileostomy, a diet can be initiated and cautiously advanced as tolerated to provide full nutritional support. To avoid the development of chylous ascites, a consequence of the graft's severed lymphatics, a no-fat or low-fact diet can be used initially.

POSTOPERATIVE SURVEILLANCE

In the postoperative period several potential complications need to be closely watched for, as discussed next.

Rejection

Although hyperacute rejection can rarely occur immediately after transplantation, the more typical cellular allograft rejection is unlikely to occur within the first few days following the transplant, provided immunosuppression is adequate. Subsequently, rejection can occur at any time but is most common in the first year, particularly the first 6 months. There is currently no blood test that reliably detects an early rejection; therefore, surveillance biopsies are used. Suspicion of rejection is often based on clinical evaluation. No single clinical symptom or sign is entirely reliable, although in many instances rejection is associated with fever; a significant increase in stomal output; and GI symptoms, such as abdominal pain, cramping, nausea, vomiting, and diarrhea. A high index of suspicion for rejection should also be maintained whenever tacrolimus levels are found to be subtherapeutic.

Chromium ethylenediaminetetraacetic acid [25,26] or technetium diethylenetriamine pentaacetic acid [22] isotope studies have been useful in identifying increased intestinal permeability, which correlates well with, but is not specific for, rejection. Unfortunately, these studies are not often available in a timely manner. If rejection is suspected, endoscopic evaluation of the intestinal graft must be performed. The endoscopic evaluation should include as much of the small bowel as possible and biopsies from numerous sites (at least six) should be obtained, because rejection can often be segmental. The loop ileostomy greatly facilitates this type of assessment, and for that reason the ileostomy is usually kept in place for 6 months to a year following the transplant. Although the endoscopic appearance of rejecting small bowel is often abnormal with evidence of inflammation and ulceration, in early rejection it can be quite normal. The gold standard for diagnosing rejection is histologic evaluation of the biopsies. Typically, early rejection is associated with increased apoptotic figures (normal less than 2–3 per high power field); infiltration of activated lymphocytes in the lamina propria; loss of goblet cells; decrease in the villus:crypt ratio; and ulceration [27,28].

When a diagnosis of rejection is made, the patient should be treated with Solu-Medrol, 500 mg intravenously for 3 days. Prograf levels should be rechecked and doses increased accordingly. If there is persistent evidence of rejection following treatment with steroids, the patient should be treated with muromonab or thymoglobulin. If rejection episodes continue to occur, despite maintaining adequate immunosuppressive levels, consideration should be given to adding additional drugs to the immunosuppressive regimen, such as mycophenolate mofetil or sirolimus. Because escalation of immunosuppression can be complicated by life-threatening infections or malignancies, such patients should be carefully monitored.

Infection

Patients who undergo small bowel transplant are even more susceptible to infectious complications than other transplant recipients. There are primarily two reasons for this. First, the intestinal allograft is transplanted with a significantly higher load of microorganism than any other organ allograft. Any process that compromises the intestinal allograft influences the containment of these microorganisms within the graft and contributes to their spread to various areas of the body. Second, because intestinal rejection is difficult to detect and because severe rejection can often lead to life-threatening sepsis, these patients are maintained on higher degrees of immunosuppression than recipients of other organ transplants.

Bacterial infections

When bacteria translocate from the compromised intestinal allograft, there are commonly two places where they go initially. Because the lymphatics are divided in the procurement of the intestinal allograft, it is common that there is leakage of intestinal lymph into the peritoneal cavity. This often contains bacteria. Although typically the peritoneal cavity is capable of handling a moderate load of bacteria, in the immunocompromised state (particularly when significant ascites is present), bacterial peritonitis can occur. The second route by which bacteria can spread is by direct translocation into the portal circulation and subsequent dissemination to other sites. Particularly common infections resulting from bacterial translocation are central line infections and pneumonias. The typical organisms are consistent with those found in the GI tract and include *Escherichia coli, Klebsiella, Enterobacter*, staphylococci, and enterococci. Because of the degree of immunosuppression used, other typical and atypical postoperative infections are more likely to occur [29].

Viral infections

A primary concern with intestinal transplantation is the development of a CMV infection, which can manifest as CMV enteritis that can be severe and lead to graft loss. In general, transplantation of a graft from a CMV-positive donor to a CMV-negative recipient is avoided. Some centers are also cautious to transplant a CMV-positive graft into CMV-positive recipient. The clinical manifestations of CMV enteritis are not unlike that of rejection with fever, increased stomal output, and GI symptoms. Other important clues that may sway the clinical diagnosis more toward CMV enteritis include the CMV status of the donor and recipient, the degree of immunosuppression at the time symptoms developed, and a positive CMV antigenemia assay. Also with CMV infections, there is typically a decrease in the white blood cell count and flulike symptoms. Endoscopy should be performed and multiple biopsies taken if there is a clinical enteritis. Although the histologic picture of CMV can sometimes be similar to that of rejection, with CMV enteritis the presence of CMV inclusion bodies is diagnostic. If CMV is diagnosed, the patient should be treated with therapeutic doses of ganciclovir. If there is ganciclovir resistance, foscarnet or CMV immunoglobulin (Cytogam) should be considered. Furthermore, immunosuppression should be reduced until the CMV infection is controlled [30].

EBV-associated infection can initiate an entire spectrum of disease. Those particularly at risk are recipients who are EBV-negative and who receive an EBV-positive graft. An acute EBV virus infection is typically associated with severe malaise and fever and flulike symptoms (ie, infectious mononucleosis). Other evidence of EBV infection can include an increase of liver function tests, splenomegaly, and lymphadenopathy. In certain instances, an EBV infection can progress to a PTLD, which can develop into a malignant lymphoma.

Surveillance for PTLD should begin immediately following the transplant, particularly in EBV-negative recipients who have received EBV-positive grafts. Polymerase chain reaction has been used to monitor EBV replication semi-quantitatively by determining the amount of EBV-encoded RNA in the serum as an early warning of an impending PTLD [31]. Other approaches using in situ hybridization have also been described.

Although there is no standardized strategy for preventing PTLD, two basic approaches have evolved. One approach is to give long-term prophylaxis, with recipients maintained on ganciclovir or intravenous immunoglobulin for 3 to 12 months following the transplant. The other approach is to have a shorter period of prophylaxis (2–6 weeks) followed by surveillance, as described previously, and preemptive therapy should surveillance identify increased EBV replication.

POSTTRANSPLANT FUNCTION

Typically, the transplanted intestine initiates peristalsis immediately after reperfusion. In the process of procuring the donor intestine, however, all extrinsic innervation to the bowel is disrupted. This and other factors contribute to a less orderly peristalsis than is seen in a normal intestine. Often, a more significant problem is the dysfunction of residual native intestine in a patient with a primary dysmotility syndrome. In some instances the stomach, duodenum, and colon, are left in place to approximate best the re-establishment of normal GI continuity. Sometimes these retained native segments function adequately, whereas in other instances they do not. It remains controversial whether such patients are best served by isolated intestinal transplants, or by multivisceral transplants, which provide a new stomach, duodenum, and colon if necessary.

The absorptive capacity of the transplanted intestine is typically good. Although there may be some initial malabsorption of carbohydrates, for the most part carbohydrate absorption seems to normalize within the first several months as determined by d-xylose absorption [32]. Clearly, absorption of immunosuppressive drugs, particularly Prograf, is instantaneous and some transplant programs initiate oral immunosuppressive drugs immediately following surgery. Although drug malabsorption has been described [33], difficulty in obtaining levels is often associated with inability to retain ingested drugs because of nausea or vomiting, or noncompliance. Although very little has been done to measure amino acid absorption in intestinal transplantation, this also seems to be adequate quite early as determined by nonspecific markers of protein nutrition, such as prealbumin. Fat absorption, however, is impaired for several months following intestinal transplantation. Because the intestinal lymphatics are unavoidably disrupted in the procurement process, intestinal lymphatic drainage is not re-established for several months following the transplant. Absorption of dietary lipids, which primarily are made up of long-chain triglycerides, depends on lymphatic drainage. Medium-chain triglycerides (ie, those consisting of 8–12 carbon fatty acids) can be absorbed directly into the portal circulation. For these reasons, it is essential to supplement enteral feeds with medium-chain triglycerides for several months following transplantation. Use of more complex fatty acids leads to malabsorption of fat, with increased ileostomy output and possible dehydration. To avoid an essential fatty acid deficiency, it may be necessary intermittently to supplement with intravenous fats, until the intestinal lymphatics are re-established. Because of the obligatory fat malabsorption, there can also be malabsorption of the fat-soluble vitamins (vitamin D, E, A, and K). Despite this, 72% of adults and 93% of children gain weight, and essentially all achieve their ideal body weight range [34].

Because of the abnormal intestinal motility and malabsorption associated with the early posttransplant period, the ileostomy output can be unpredictable and often excessive. Even in the best of circumstances, high ileostomy output can be anticipated early once full enteral nutrition has been established. Close attention must be made to the overall fluid and electrolyte balance to prevent severe dehydration or electrolyte imbalances. It is imperative, in addition to accurate monitoring of daily in and outs, to follow daily weights and electrolytes. Once enteral nutrition is found to be providing all nutritional requirements, TPN is discontinued. If weight is maintained or weight gain occurs, and there is no significant evidence for protein malnutrition, TPN can be permanently discontinued. After a brief period of adjustment, ostomy output should become quite predictable over a given period of time. Dramatic changes in ostomy output should be investigated, because this can be an early indicator of rejection or other pathology. Overall, 70% to 80% of patients who undergo successful transplantation can be completely removed from TPN [10].

PATIENT AND GRAFT SURVIVAL

Because most intestines have been transplanted in combination with a liver, posttransplant graft and patient survivals should be evaluated based on whether or not a liver was also transplanted. One-year graft and patient survival for transplants where an intestine only (ie, no liver) was included are 73.8% and 85.7%, respectively. For transplants where both intestine and liver were transplanted, 1-year intestine graft and patient survivals are 65.7% and 66.7%, respectively. For comparison, 1-year graft and patient survivals after liver transplant are 82.2% and 86.8%, respectively (Table 1). Although longer-term outcomes with intestinal transplants remain inferior to those of most other organs transplants, they have demonstrated the most significant improvement over the last 10 years [18], and are likely to improve further if recent improvements in 1-year survival can be extrapolated.

MORBIDITY

Acute rejection has occurred in 79% of patients undergoing intestine-only transplants. The liver, and perhaps other organs, may have a protective effect because the acute rejection rates for liver-intestine and multivisceral transplants have been 71% and 56%, respectively. Similarly, chronic rejection, which has been demonstrated in 13% of intestine-only transplants, has been uncommon in liver-intestine (3%) and multivisceral transplants (0%). Despite the fact that most centers avoid transplanting intestinal grafts from CMV-positive donors, CMV infections occurred in 24% of intestine-only grafts, 18% of liver-intestine grafts, and 40% of multivisceral grafts.

PTLDs have been seen in 7% of intestine-only, 11% of liver-intestine, and 13% of multivisceral grafts [10]. PTLDs often manifest as fever and lymphadenopathy or lymphoproliferation in either donor or recipient tissue. Lymphoma can also manifest with GI symptoms, including nausea, vomiting, diarrhea, bowel obstruction, GI bleeding, or perforation.

The incidence of PTLD in intestinal transplant recipients is higher than in other organ transplant recipients. The occurrence of PTLD clearly correlates with the intensity of immunosuppression. Significant increases in the incidence of PTLD are noted in patients who receive OKT3 or ATGAM, especially if their total antibody course exceeds 21 days. Although PTLD tends first to manifest between 2 weeks and 6 months after a transplant, it can appear at any time.

The diagnosis of PTLD usually requires a biopsy. Often this is most easily obtained from an enlarged superficial lymph node or from clinically or radiologically involved tissue. If the suspected organ is the intestine graft itself, it can

Table 1				
Graft and patient survival after transplantation				
		1 Year	3 Years	5 Years
Liver only (deceased donor only)	Graft survival %	82.2	73.2	66.9
	Patient survival %	86.8	79.1	73.1
Intestine only	Graft survival %	73.8	46.7	37.6
	Patient survival %	85.7	60.6	53.5
Liver and intestine	Graft survival %	65.7	49.7	44.1
	Patient survival %	66.7	56.6	47.2

sometimes be difficult to differentiate PTLD from rejection or CMV infection. When this is the case it is often useful to obtain further studies including EBV-encoded RNA staining of suspicious tissue. It is often also useful to evaluate the serum for a typical monoclonal or polyclonal immunoglobulin band, which can sometimes be present. Gene studies are often helpful to identify abnormal karyotypes, which can aid in diagnosis and prognosis (C-myc, N-ras, p53). It should also be determined whether the abnormal lymphocytes sites are primarily B cells or T cells. T-cell lymphomas are less common than B-cell lymphomas in PTLDs.

If the diagnosis of PTLD is made, immunosuppression should be reduced to approximately half of what it had been. In approximately one third of cases, this results in a remission of the PTLD. If after 2 weeks there is no evidence of improvements, all immunosuppression should be discontinued and serious consideration should be given to additional therapeutic measures, including chemotherapy, monoclonal antibody administration, or adoptive immunotherapy. If necessary, an intestine-only graft can also be removed.

MORTALITY

Overall, the most significant cause of morbidity and mortality has been infectious complications. Approximately one half (47%) of the deaths in intestinal transplant patients have been clearly attributed to sepsis, whereas another 26% have been attributed to multiorgan failure to which sepsis was likely a contributing factor. Other causes of death have included graft thrombosis (10%), PTLD (10%), and rejection (4%) [10].

FUTURE DIRECTIONS

Intestinal transplantation provides unique and difficult challenges. Because of the delicate balance that must be maintained to provide adequate immunosuppression without overimmunosuppression, it is imperative that a simple marker be developed that alerts clinicians that an early rejection is brewing. Another goal is to develop strategies that eliminate or minimize the risk of rejection. Many researchers are attempting to develop strategies for inducing tolerance. Several groups have attempted to induce a state of microchimerism and tolerance by transplanting bone marrow along with the intestinal allograft [35]. To date, this approach has not been shown to be effective. Other groups have administered donor-specific transfusions simultaneous with implantation of the intestinal graft [36]. Although there are some preliminary animal studies suggesting that this approach might be effective, its benefit has not yet been proved in humans. Another approach, which has been effective in kidney transplantation, is HLA matching. Although because of time constraints this may not always be practical in the realm of cadaveric intestinal transplantation, it is possible with living related donors. Although the experience with living related donor intestinal transplantation has been very limited to date, some of the longest surviving intestinal grafts from the pre-cyclosporine era were achieved when living related donors were used. More recent experiences with modern immunosuppression have shown that graft survival with living donors is at least comparable with that achieved with cadaveric donors [10,37]. The potential advantages of using living donors are the opportunity for better HLA matching, and better control over ischemia times. The potential disadvantages are that the donor, who does not need a surgical procedure, is put at risk, and the allograft consists of a shorter segment of bowel with smaller blood vessels.

SUMMARY

Intestinal transplantation is a viable option for individuals who are otherwise committed to a life of HPN because of intestinal failure. As with kidney transplantation and dialysis decades earlier, intestinal transplantation must prove to be superior to the established, default strategy of long-term PN before it can be considered the treatment of choice. Through national and international registries, outcomes with intestinal transplant are accurately monitored. Unfortunately, similar population-based data on long-term outcomes in intestinal failure are scare, but existing data suggest that serious life-threatening complications can occur in subpopulations of patients who require long-term PN therapy [15–17]. Intestinal transplant is currently being used as a last resort for intestinal failure patients who develop life-threatening complications (Medicare criteria). UNOS waitlist data suggest that most patients listed for transplant have already developed irreversible complications. Intestinal transplants are being performed in significantly sicker populations of intestinal failure patients than those receiving long-term PN therapy. This must be considered in any comparison between long-term PN patients and recipients of intestinal transplants using existing data. Existing data clearly warrant early consideration of intestinal transplantation in high-risk intestinal failure patient populations and only randomized controlled trials in this patient population will determine which therapy is associated with better outcomes.

References
[1] Carrel A. The transplantation of organs: a preliminary communication. JAMA 1905;45: 1645.
[2] Lillehei R, Goott B, Miller F. The physiological response of the small bowel of the dog to ischemia including prolonged in vitro preservation of the bowel with successful replacement and survival. Ann Surg 1959;150:543.
[3] Lillehei RC, Idezuki Y, Feemster JA, et al. Transplantation of stomach, intestine, and pancreas: experimental and clinical observation. Surgery 1967;62:721.
[4] Margreiter R. The history of intestinal transplantation. Transplant Rev 1997;11(1):9.
[5] Cohen Z, Silverman R, Wassef R, et al. Small intestine transplantation using cyclosporine: report of a case. Transplantation 1986;42:613.
[6] Deltz E, Schroeder P, Gebhardt H, et al. Successful clinical small bowel transplantation: report of a case. Clin Transplant 1989;3:89.
[7] Goulet O, Revillon Y, Jan D, et al. Two and one-half-year follow-up after isolated cadaveric small bowel transplantation in an infant. Transplant Proc 1992;24:1224.
[8] Grant D, Wall W, Mimeault R, et al. Successful small-bowel liver transplantation. Lancet 1990;335:181.
[9] McAllister VC, Grant DR. Clinical small bowel transplantation. In: Grant DR, Woods RFM, editors. Small bowel transplantation. Kent, Great Britain: Edward Arnold; 1994. p. 121.

[10] Grant D, Abu-Elmagd K, Reyes J, et al. 2003 Report of the Intestine Transplant Registry. A new era has dawned. Ann Surg 2005;241(4):607–13.

[11] O'Keefe SJ, Buchman AL, Fishbein TM, et al. Short bowel syndrome and intestinal failure: consensus definitions and overview. Clin Gastroenterol Hepatol 2006;4(1):6–10.

[12] Nightingale J. The short bowel syndrome. Eur J Gastroenterol Hepatol 1995;7(6):514.

[13] Buchman AL, Iyer K, Fryer J. Parenteral nutrition associated liver disease and the role for isolated intestine and intestine/liver transplantation. Hepatology 2006;43:9–19.

[14] Howard L, Ament M, Fleming R, et al. Current use and clinical outcomes of home parenteral and enteral nutrition therapies in the United States. Gastroenterology 1995;109:355.

[15] Messing B, Crenn P, Beau P, et al. Long term survival and parenteral nutrition dependence in adult patients with short bowel syndrome. Gastroenterology 1999;117:1043–50.

[16] Cavicchi M, Beau P, Crenn P, et al. Prevalence of liver disease and contributing factors in patients receiving home parenteral nutrition for permanent intestinal failure. Ann Intern Med 2000;132:525–32.

[17] Chan S, McCowen KC, Bistrian BC, et al. Incidence, prognosis, and etiology of end-stage liver disease in patients receiving home total parenteral nutrition. Surgery 1999;126: 28–34.

[18] United Network for Organ Sharing. Available at: http://www.UNOS.org. Accessed March 23, 2007.

[19] Tzakis AG, Kato T, Levi DM, et al. 100 multivisceral transplants at a single center. Ann Surg 2005;242(4):480–90.

[20] Schweizer E, Gassel A, Deltz E, et al. A comparison of preservation solutions for small bowel transplantation in the rat. Transplantation 1994;57(9):1406.

[21] Scholten E, Manek G, Green C. A comparison of preservation solutions for long term storage in rat small bowel transplantation. Acta Chirurgica Austriaca 1992;24:5.

[22] Kusne S, Manez R, Frye B, et al. Use of DNA amplification for diagnosis of cytomegalovirus enteritis after intestinal transplantation. Gastroenterology 1997;112(4):1121.

[23] Reyes J, Green M, Bueno J, et al. Epstein Barr virus associated posttransplant lymphoproliferative disease after intestinal transplantation. Transplant Proc 1996;28(5):2768.

[24] Tzakis A, Weppler D, Khan M, et al. Mycophenolate mofetil as primary and rescue therapy in intestinal transplantation. Transplant Proc 1998;30(6):2677.

[25] Grant D, Lamont D, Zhong R, et al. 51Cr-EDTA: a marker of early intestinal rejection in the rat. J Surg Res 1989;46(5):507.

[26] D'Alessandro AM, Kalayoglu M, Hammes R, et al. Diagnosis of intestinal transplant rejection using technetium-99m-DTPA. Transplantation 1994;58(1):112.

[27] Lee RG, Nakamura K, Tsamandas AC, et al. Pathology of human intestinal transplantation. Gastroenterology 1996;110(6):1820.

[28] Ruiz P, Bagni A, Brown R, et al. Histological criteria for the identification of acute cellular rejection in human small bowel allografts: results of the pathology workshop at the VIII international small bowel transplant symposium. Transplant Proc 2004;36:335–7.

[29] Kusne S, Furukawa H, Abu-Elmagd K, et al. Infectious complications after small bowel transplantation in adults: an update. Transplant Proc 1996;28(5):2761.

[30] Bueno J, Green M, Kocoshis S, et al. Cytomegalovirus infection after intestinal transplantation in children. Clin Infect Dis 1997;25(5):1078.

[31] Rowe DT, Qu L, Reyes J, et al. Use of quantitative competitive PCR to measure Epstein-Barr virus genome load in the peripheral blood of pediatric transplant patients with lymphoproliferative disorders. J Clin Microbiol 1997;35(6):1612.

[32] Kim J, Fryer J, Craig RM. Absorptive function following intestinal transplantation. Dig Dis Sci 1998;43(9):1925–30.

[33] Fryer J, Kaplan B, Lown K, et al. Low bioavailability of cyclosporine microemulsion and tacrolimus in a small bowel transplant recipient. Transplantation 1999;67(2):333.

[34] Abu-Elmagd, Todo S, Tzakis A, et al. Three years clinical experience with intestinal transplantation. J Am Coll Surg 1994;179(4):385.

[35] Todo S, Reyes J, Furukawa H, et al. Outcome analysis of 71 clinical intestinal transplantations. Ann Surg 1995;222(3):270.
[36] Gruessner RW, Nakhleh RE, Harmon JV, et al. Donor-specific portal blood transfusion in intestinal transplantation: a prospective, preclinical large animal study. Transplantation 1998;66(2):164.
[37] Gruessner RW, Sharp HL. Living-related intestinal transplantation: first report of a standardized surgical technique. Transplantation 1997;64(11):1605.

Gastroenterol Clin N Am 36 (2007) 161–190

GASTROENTEROLOGY CLINICS
OF NORTH AMERICA

Metabolic Bone Disease in Gastrointestinal Illness

Susan E. Williams, MD, MS, RD, CNS*,[1],
Douglas L. Seidner, MD, FACG

Department of Gastroenterology and Hepatology, Cleveland Clinic Foundation,
9500 Euclid Avenue, A 30, Cleveland, OH 44195, USA

P rimary metabolic bone disease (MBD), like many silent but serious diseases, often remains undiagnosed and can lead to devastating consequences because of low bone mass and fragility fractures [1]. By far the most common MBD is osteoporosis, and contrary to common belief, osteoporosis is not part of normal aging. Osteoporosis and low bone mass are currently estimated to be a major public health threat for more than 44 million American women and men aged 50 and older [2]. At least one resource has estimated that another 18 million people have undiagnosed low bone mass. About 1.3 million osteoporotic fractures occur each year in the United States [3]. Of those patients who suffer a hip fracture, only 40% fully regain their prefracture level of independence, whereas most others experience chronic pain, disability, and a 10% to 20% excess mortality within 1 year [2,3].

Secondary MBD results from a variety of chronic conditions that compromise achieving optimal peak bone mass or contribute to bone mineral loss, such as malnutrition, malabsorption, or the long-term use of certain medications. First reported over 25 years ago, disorders of the gastrointestinal (GI) tract and liver have a strong association with osteoporosis, and a high prevalence of osteopenia [4,5]. Of particular concern is that many patients with GI diseases are stricken in their youth, when adult height potential and peak bone mass are being achieved. Potentially modifiable risk factors, such as poor dietary habits, protein-calorie malnutrition, malabsorption of essential nutrients, such as calcium, prolonged use of corticosteroids, and a sedentary lifestyle can lead to low peak bone mass, an increased rate of bone loss, and debilitating bone disease if left untreated [2]. Causes of MBD seen in GI illness are listed in Box 1 [4,6–11].

[1]Present address: Wright State University School of Medicine, 3640 Col. Glenn Highway, Dayton, OH 45435-0001.

*Corresponding author. *E-mail address:* Susan.E.Williams@wright.edu (S.E. Williams).

0889-8553/07/$ – see front matter
doi:10.1016/j.gtc.2007.01.005

Box 1: Causes of metabolic bone disease in gastrointestinal illness

Gastrointestinal disease and surgery
- Gastroesophageal reflux disease[a]
- Achlorhydria[b]
- Lactase deficiency
- Gastrectomy
- Bariatric surgery
- Inflammatory bowel disease
- Gluten-sensitive enteropathy (celiac disease)

Chronic liver disease
- Alcoholic liver disease
- Autoimmune hepatitis
- Chronic viral hepatitis
- Primary biliary cirrhosis
- Primary sclerosing cholangitis

Organ failure and transplantation
- Liver
- Intestine[c]

Medical interventions
- Glucocorticoids
- Methotrexate
- Aluminum-containing antacids
- Total parenteral nutrition

Nutritional disorders of insufficient intake or malabsorption
- Protein-calorie malnutrition
- Calcium
- Magnesium
- Vitamin B_{12}
- Vitamin D
- Vitamin K

Nutritional disorders of excess
- Alcohol
- Caffeine
- Phosphorus

- Protein
- Sodium
- Vitamin A (retinol)

[a]Associated with the development of hypophosphatemia when treated with aluminum-containing antacids.
[b]Known to decrease calcium bioavailability; the relationship to MBD remains unclear.
[c]Associated with risks for the development of MBD; prevalence is unknown at this time.

METABOLIC BONE DISEASE
Osteoporosis

Osteoporosis is a disease of low bone mass with significant change in bone architecture that results in fractures caused by minimal trauma, or fragility fractures [5]. Primary osteoporosis is perhaps best recognized as a disease of post-menopausal women and is classified into two types. Type I osteoporosis occurs when the protective effects of estrogen are lost, daily calcium losses increase, and an accelerated loss of mainly trabecular bone results, caused by a relative increase in bone resorption over formation. Type II osteoporosis results from factors related to age, begins to occur around age 30, affects both trabecular and cortical bone, and does not have a period of accelerated loss [2,5].

It is important to note that men are also affected by osteoporosis, although between 50% and 70% of cases of osteoporosis in men is secondary to another disease process [12]. Men account for about 20% of all osteoporosis, 25% of hip fractures, and typically have a worse prognosis than women after sustaining a hip fracture.

Secondary MBD occurs as a result of a wide variety of diseases, including many chronic GI illnesses [7]. The resulting malabsorption, malnutrition, interruption of essential metabolic pathways, and chronic use of glucocorticoids in the treatment of these illnesses leads to bone loss that can be equally as severe and debilitating as primary bone disease.

Although osteoporosis is a treatable disease, prevention needs to be the primary approach. Identifying patients at risk, pursuing diagnostic evaluation, addressing risk factor reduction, and starting appropriate therapeutic interventions must become core components of clinical gastroenterology practice [2,4,5].

Osteopenia

Osteopenia, or low bone mass, is more common in women than in men, typically occurs in people age 50 and over, and is considered a risk factor for osteoporosis and for fractures. Individuals typically become osteopenic either because of bone loss as an adult, or as a result of a failure to attain peak bone mass during growth and development.

Acquisitional osteopenia is a failure to achieve peak bone mass due to inadequate calcium and vitamin D during growth, development, and skeletal consolidation. This type of osteopenia is common in patients who develop chronic GI illness in their childhood or teenage years. Common GI illnesses in which osteopenia should be suspected include inflammatory bowel disease (IBD) and gluten-sensitive enteropathy [1,5,13].

Whether osteopenia is as a result of bone loss or failure to achieve peak bone mass, it can progress to osteoporosis and result in fragility fractures. Diagnosing MBD in the patient suspected of having osteopenia is the same as for patients at risk for osteoporosis: identify those patients at risk, address risk factor reduction, pursue diagnostic evaluation, and institute therapeutic interventions as appropriate [2].

Osteomalacia

Osteomalacia is caused by abnormal mineralization of cartilage and bone. The most commonly recognized cause of osteomalacia is vitamin D deficiency. Vitamin D deficiency can occur as a result of inadequate intake of vitamin D, inadequate exposure to sunlight, or malabsorption of vitamin D. Those patients who develop secondary hyperparathyroidism following gastrectomy, small bowel resection, or bariatric bypass procedures also likely have osteomalacia [4,5,14].

Clinically, these patients can present with complaints of bone pain and proximal muscle weakness; however, distinguishing osteomalacia from osteoporosis can be difficult. Unlike osteoporosis and osteopenia, osteomalacia affects primarily cortical bone; bone densitometry testing with dual x-ray absorptiometry (DXA) is unlikely to confirm the diagnosis. The gold standard for the diagnosis of osteomalacia is a transcortical bone biopsy of the rib or iliac crest; however, this test is painful and not commonly done. Similarly, the effects of secondary hyperparathyroidism may be seen on plain radiographs in the form of subperiosteal resorption of the fingers or pseudofractures of the hands, but these findings are often not evident despite the presence of osteomalacia. Therefore, it is recommended that diagnosis and treatment be guided by biochemical indices including 25-hydroxyvitamin D (25[OH]D), calcium, phosphate, alkaline phosphatase, parathyroid hormone (PTH), and urine calcium and phosphate in the at-risk patient [5,15].

Osteodystrophy

The term "hepatic osteodystrophy" refers to the abnormalities of decreased bone density that occurs in the presence of advanced liver disease [9,15]. It is characterized by low serum 25(OH)D and 1,25-dihydroxyvitamin D $(1,25[OH]_2D_3)$, decreased production of albumin, and decreased production of vitamin D binding protein required for transport of 25(OH)D to the kidneys. This is typically not a true vitamin D deficiency, but rather a combination of malabsorption and protein-calorie malnutrition [5]. In chronic liver disease, as in many other causes of secondary MBD, preventive strategies including early diagnosis and correction of all reversible factors remain the cornerstone of treatment.

Diagnosis and Treatment

The most widely accepted study to quantify bone mineral density (BMD) is DXA. DXA results quantify absolute bone density and define the standard deviation of the density from that of a young adult with peak bone mass and density (T score). The World Health Organization (WHO) has defined normal bone density, osteopenia, and osteoporosis based on the T score that has become the industry standard for quantifying fracture risk. DXA results also quantify the standard deviation from that of an age- and gender-matched control, reported as the Z score. If bone loss is exclusively caused by the normal process of aging, the Z score is near zero. Secondary disease should be suspected when there is a significant negative deviation of the Z score [2,16–18]. The WHO T-score definitions and a clinical approach to the diagnosis and management of MBD in GI illness are included in Table 1 [2,4,9,17–19].

Once the diagnosis has been made and the cause of the disease has been defined to the degree possible, patient-specific treatment goals should be established and appropriate interventions implemented. When considering treatment options, modifiable risk factors, severity of disease, and the patient's willingness and ability to participate in their care must all be carefully considered. Modifiable risk factors for progression of bone disease must be identified and effectively addressed with all patients at risk. It is also important to identify those patients at high risk for falls because of poor visual acuity, frailty, neuropathy, or dementia and risk management strategies implemented to the degree possible [2].

Nutritional inadequacies can often be corrected through improved dietary habits and appropriate supplementation; however, in the presence of malabsorption, patients may require larger doses, and more readily absorbable forms, such as chewable or liquid supplements. Parenterally administered supplements may also be required. Before recommending supplementation, the patient's nutrition history, including the use of homeopathic medications, herbal preparations, and supplements, must be carefully reviewed. There are many over-the-counter and over-the-internet supplements targeting bone health, and whereas some may indeed be beneficial, others can be detrimental. Table 2 provides a review of many common foods, supplements, and over-the-counter products often cited in the lay literature [20–32].

Prescribed medications for the prevention and treatment of osteoporosis should also be an integral part of the treatment plan for at-risk patients. As with any medication, the decision to prescribe an antiresorptive or bone-forming medication must take into consideration the patient's risk-benefit profile, including the ability and willingness to follow drug-specific dosing recommendations. Drugs currently approved by the Food and Drug Administration for the prevention and treatment of osteoporosis are discussed in Table 3 [3,33,34].

GASTROINTESTINAL DISEASE AND SURGERY
Gastroesophageal Reflux Disease
Gastroesophageal reflux disease does not share a causal relationship with MBD; however, the clinician should maintain a healthy degree of suspicion when reviewing patients' over-the-counter medications. Specifically, chronic overuse of antacids containing aluminum hydroxide can lead to phosphorus deficiency and osteomalacia [35,36]. Hypophosphatemia results in increased

Table 1
Metabolic bone disease in gastrointestinal illness: approach to diagnosis and management

Risk factors	Who should be tested	Interventions based on DXA[a]

Primary diagnosis:
• Postgastrectomy
• Postbariatric surgery
• Inflammatory bowel disease
• Gluten-sensitive enteropathy
• Severe liver disease
• Liver transplant
Medical interventions
• Glucocorticoid use >3 months or multiple courses
• Excess antacids containing aluminum
• Methotrexate
• Total parenteral nutrition
Past medical history
• Female >age 65[b]
• Fragility fractures
• Postmenopausal
• Weight <127 lb
• Malnutrition
• Malabsorption
Family history
• First degree relative with fragility fracture
Social and lifestyle history
• Current smoking
• Alcohol in excess of two drinks daily
• Little or no weight-bearing exercise
• Poor dietary habits
	Pursue testing based on
	• Patient risk profile
	• If the test results influence treatment decisions
	Recommend bone mineral density testing
	• All women >65 years
	• Younger women with one or more risk factors
	• Any patient with a fragility fracture
	• Transplant candidates
	Consider bone mineral density testing for
	• Postgastrectomy patients
	• All bariatric surgery patients
	  • baseline
	  • annual
	• High-risk patients with inflammatory bowel disease
	• Patients with celiac disease
	• Patients with chronic liver disease
	• Patients with chronic malnutrition or malabsorption resistant to treatment
	• Patients on long-term corticosteroid therapy
	• Patients starting and maintained on long-term parenteral nutrition
	Is osteomalacia suspected?
	• Bone density is not a reliable indicator
	• Consider biochemical testing to determine the underlying cause
		T-Score >−1
		Normal bone density
		• Counsel all patients on risk factor reduction including
		• Adequate consumption of calcium and vitamin D
		• Regular weight-bearing and muscle-strengthening exercise
		• Smoking cessation
		• Limiting alcohol intake to <2 drinks daily
		• Discontinue or substitute high-risk medications when clinically appropriate
		• Initiate therapy for patients on long-term steroids
		T-Score between −1 and −2.5
		Low bone mass (osteopenia)
		• Counsel the patient on risk factor reduction
		• Initiate therapy for women with T scores below −2
		• Initiate therapy for women with one or more risk factors and a T score below −1.5
		• Initiate therapy for any patient with a history of fragility fracture
		• Initiate therapy for patients on long-term corticosteroids

(continued on next page)

Table 1 (continued)		
Risk factors	Who should be tested	Interventions based on DXA[a]
		T-Score ≤ -2.5 Osteoporosis • Counsel the patient on risk factor reduction • Initiate therapy • Schedule routine follow-up appointments to assess compliance and effectiveness of prescribed interventions • Repeat DXA no sooner than 12–24 mo • Requires lifelong management

[a]World Health Organization established definitions based on bone mass measurement at the spine, hip, and wrist in white, postmenopausal women. T scores are to be used to assist the clinician in determining the diagnosis and appropriate treatment options, and can be misleading in younger women, men, and nonwhites.

[b]All women age 65 and older, regardless of additional risk factors, should have a DXA. Women who are considering therapy for osteoporosis should also have a DXA to facilitate the decision.

levels of $1,25(OH)_2D_3$, increased calcium absorption, hypercalciuria, and increased bone resorption. Known as "antacid-induced osteomalacia," symptomatic patients may admit to diffuse bone pain, proximal muscle weakness, difficulty climbing stairs, and rising from a chair [6]. Discontinuation of the over-the-counter antacid, treatment of the gastroesophageal reflux disease with an appropriately dosed antisecretory agent, and proper diet in most cases alleviates the problem [35].

Achlorhydria

Decreased stomach acid, which occurs in otherwise healthy elderly, achlorhydria, and autoimmune gastritis, reduces the solubility of calcium salts, such as calcium carbonate and calcium phosphate, when consumed in a fasting state [37,38]. The result is decreased absorption of calcium, which can be easily corrected by instructing the patient to take calcium supplements with meals. Although the effects of achlorhydria on the bioavailability of calcium are well documented, the relationship to MBD remains unclear. Similarly, patients who have undergone acid-reducing procedures, such as vagotomy, do not seem to have an increased risk of developing MBD [37].

Lactase Deficiency

Adult lactase deficiency is a common autosomal-recessive condition resulting in a relative inability to hydrolyze lactose into galactose and glucose [8,39].

Table 2
Rating of foods, supplements, and over-the-counter products used in the prevention and treatment of osteoporosis

Product	Current knowledge	Rating
Antioxidant vitamins		
Vitamin A (betacarotene)	Vitamin A: essential for bone growth; deficiency and excess is known to be detrimental to bone. Best sources of betacarotene include carrots, sweet potatoes, spinach, cantaloupe, and kale.	Vitamin A: optimal dose is unknown.
Vitamin C	Vitamin C: important in the formation of collagen; deficiency has been associated with loss of bone density. Studies in animals have demonstrated vitamin C >2000 mg/day may accelerate bone loss.	Vitamin C: intake of 100–125 mg/day, along with adequate calcium, may increase bone mineral density in postmenopausal women.
Vitamin E	Vitamin E: limited studies suggest a possible benefit in bone strength.	Vitamin E: supplementation is not recommended at this time.
Boron	No established recommended daily intake. Benefit has been seen in postmenopausal women taking 3 mg/day. Sources include fruits, vegetables, nuts, milk, eggs, and legumes.	Possible benefit; may enhance calcium absorption but studies are lacking.
Calcium	Choose a supplement from a respected manufacturer. Avoid supplements that include dolomite, bone meal, and unrefined oyster shell.	Beneficial. Daily adequate intake: ages 19–50, 1000 mg; ages ≥51, 1200 mg. The upper limit of safe daily intake is 2500 mg.
Copper	Essential as an enzyme cofactor required for normal bone metabolism and bone strength.	Present in most foods and true deficiency is very rare. Safe intake range is 2–3 g/day. Excess intake interferes with absorption of zinc.
Fluoride	Required for normal growth of teeth and bone. Studies in adults note brittle bone formation and no decrease in fracture risk.	Not recommended for prevention or treatment of osteoporosis.

(continued on next page)

Table 2
(continued)

Product	Current knowledge	Rating
Iron	Acts as a coenzyme involved on collagen synthesis. Bone mass and iron status is currently being studied. The best sources of iron include red meats and poultry. Other sources include dark green vegetables, fortified grain products, and fruits.	Adequate intake of iron is recommended. Iron absorption is impaired when consumed concurrently with calcium.
Lycopene	A carotenoid abundant in tomatoes. Preliminary studies in animals suggest it may inhibit bone resorption.	No current recommendations.
Manganese	An essential enzyme cofactor required for the formation of healthy cartilage and bone. Found in legumes, nuts, and whole grains.	Adequate dietary intake may prevent bone loss in adults. Adequate intake: men, 2.3 mg/day; women, 1.8 mg/day.
Milk	Milk consumption has been shown to protect against osteoporosis. Bone integrity may be further enhanced by other components in milk, such as protein.	Beneficial.
Omega-3 fatty acids	Beneficial effect on bone mass in animals. Human studies have failed to demonstrate a similar benefit. Dietary sources include soy products, flaxseed, walnuts, mackerel, trout, salmon, and tuna.	No current recommendation.
Oxalate, oxalic acid	The most potent inhibitor of calcium absorption. Present in spinach and rhubarb, sweet potatoes, and dried beans. When consumed with milk, the absorption of calcium is decreased.	If overall calcium intake is adequate, intake of oxalate-rich foods is unlikely to have a significant effect.
Phosphorus	Excess phosphorus interferes with calcium absorption. Phosphorus deficiency reduces calcium absorption. The amount of phosphorus consumed in the typical American diet likely has no adverse effect on bone health.	RDA is 700 mg for adults >30 years old. Daily intake >4000 mg is not recommended.
Phytic acid (phytate)	Found in outer husks of cereal grains, extruded wheat bran, dried beans, and high-fiber vegetables. A modest inhibitor of calcium absorption.	If overall calcium intake is adequate, intake of phytic acid–rich foods is unlikely to have a significant effect.

(continued on next page)

Table 2
(continued)

Product	Current knowledge	Rating
Phytoestrogens Isoflavones Lignans Coumestans	Plant compounds with mild estrogenic or antiestrogenic effects. Isoflavones are derived from soy. Lignans are found in flaxseed, bran, and legumes. Coumestans are found in alfalfa and clover.	Recent studies continue to suggest that consumption of >50 mg/day of isoflavones may be beneficial; however, the effectiveness in decreasing fractures remains unknown.
Protein	Essential for bone health. Low-protein diets result in decreased calcium absorption. High-protein diets result in increased calciuria. The literature remains unclear as to whether animal or vegetable sources might be more beneficial.	Consuming 1–1.5 g protein/kg body weight daily seems to be optimal for bone health.
Strontium	Studies in humans suggest a positive effect on bone density. Sources include seafood, whole milk, meat, poultry, and wheat bran.	Excess intake has been associated with bone fragility, impaired bone mineralization, and vitamin D metabolism.
Vitamin A (retinol)	Unlike betacarotene, excess retinol is well known to reduce bone mass and increase the rate of fractures.	Vitamin A obtained from sources rich in betacarotene is recommended.
Vitamin D	Vitamin D is essential for calcium absorption, bone mineralization, and involved in bone turnover. Casual sunlight exposure is the best source. Excellent food sources include butter, margarine, liver, and eggs. Additional sources include fortified milk, juices, and cereals.	Beneficial. Daily adequate intake: ages 19–50, 200 IU (5 μg); ages 51–69, 400 IU (10 μg); ≥70: 600 IU (15 μg). NOF recommends 800 IU daily for those at risk of deficiency. Safe upper limit is 2000 IU daily.
Vitamin K	Functions as a coenzyme that enhances calcium incorporation into bone. Epidemiologic data showed an increased incidence of hip fractures with lower dietary vitamin K intake.	Adequate intake through the consumption of broccoli, cabbage, spinach, Brussels sprouts, lettuce, and turnip greens is recommended.
Zinc	Functions as a coenzyme essential for bone structure and strength. Low serum levels of zinc have been related to osteoporosis. Excess intake of zinc interferes with copper absorption.	Adequate intake through the consumption of animal protein, legumes, nuts, whole grains, and milk is recommended.

Abbreviations: NOF, National Osteoporosis Foundation; RDA, recommended dietary allowance.

Patients may complain of bloating, flatulence, cramps, and diarrhea in response to the osmotic load and the fermentation by the gut flora producing hydrogen gas, carbon dioxide, and lactic and other organic acids.

Secondary lactase deficiency can develop as a result of disruption of the mucosal cells of the small intestine, such as in small bowel surgery, celiac disease, and Crohn's disease; and as a result of infections, such as giardiasis and transient viral gastroenteritis. Prolonged disuse of the GI tract can also result in secondary lactase deficiency. Typically, when the gut returns to normal function, secondary lactase deficiency eventually resolves [8].

Several studies have demonstrated a strong correlation with adult lactase deficiency and the development of osteoporosis. Interestingly, regardless of the ability to biochemically validate the subjective complaints, patient avoidance of milk and other dairy products resulted in an increased incidence of osteoporosis and bone fracture [8,39]. Although it was once believed that lactose was essential for optimal calcium absorption, it is now known that calcium absorption from various dairy products is equivalent, regardless of the lactose content or the chemical form of calcium.

A very common misconception is that a lactose-restricted diet requires strict avoidance of all dairy products. In fact, most lactase-deficient patients can tolerate small quantities of milk and other lactose-rich products. Judicious use of these products, inclusion of low-lactose products, and use of lactase enzyme replacements can assist in symptom management while promoting adequate calcium consumption.

Gastrectomy

Essentially all postgastrectomy patients have an increased risk of fracture and should be routinely evaluated for the presence of MBD. The incidence of osteomalacia in this population is estimated to be 10% to 20%, and although the incidence of osteoporosis in this patient population is unknown, it is estimated to be as high as 32% to 42% [4].

The more common surgical approaches have been examined to correlate degree of risk associated per procedure. Current literature, including the American Gastroenterological Association technical review on MBD and GI illnesses, concurs with the fact that there is no difference in risk for postgastrectomy bone disease between a Billroth I and a Billroth II procedure, or between a partial gastrectomy and total gastrectomy [4,17].

Bariatric Surgery

Morbid obesity has historically been viewed as having a protective effect against the development of MBD. However, recent research has revealed that many obese individuals have inadequate nutrition status, vitamin D deficiency, elevated PTH levels, and are at risk for low bone mass presumably as a result of chronic dieting [40–42]. Studies attempting to define the presurgical prevalence of vitamin D deficiency have identified rates in excess of 60% among patients selected to undergo weight loss surgery [14,40]. Similarly, the prevalence of preoperative elevated intact PTH in this population ranged from 25% to 48% [40,41].

Table 3
FDA-approved pharmacologic therapy for the treatment of osteoporosis

Drug	Brand name	Approved indications and dosing	Notes
Antiresorptive medications			
Alendronate sodium	Fosamax	Approved for prevention (5 mg daily or 35 mg once a week) and treatment (10 mg daily or 70 mg once a week) of postmenopausal osteoporosis. Also approved for treating glucocorticoid-induced osteoporosis and for treating osteoporosis in men.	Class: bisphosphonate. Reduces bone loss; increases bone density; and reduces the risk of vertebral, wrist, and hip fractures.
Alendronate Sodium plus 2800 IU vitamin D_3	Fosamax Plus D	Approved for the treatment of osteoporosis in postmenopausal women (70 mg once a week), and for treatment in men with osteoporosis.	Class: bisphosphonate. Reduces bone loss; increases bone density; and reduces the risk of vertebral, wrist, and hip fractures
Calcitonin-Salmon (recombinant)	Fortical Miacalcin	Approved for treating osteoporosis in postmenopausal women who are at least 5 years beyond menopause. Available as a 200-IU daily nasal spray or 50-100 IU daily injection.	Class: calcitonin. Slows bone loss, increases vertebral bone density, may relieve pain associated with fractures. Reduces the risk of vertebral fractures, but has not been shown to decrease risk of nonvertebral fractures.
Estrogen therapy	Many available including Climara Estrace Estraderm Estratab Premarin Vivelle	Approved for the prevention of osteoporosis. Available in low-dose tablet or transdermal patch (0.3 mg daily), or standard dose tablet (0.625 mg daily).	Class: estrogens. Reduces bone loss, increases bone density in the spine and hip, and reduces the risk of hip and vertebral fractures in postmenopausal women. Effective even when started after age 70. Because of multiple significant health risks, the FDA recommends women first consider other osteoporosis medications.

Hormone therapy	Many available including Activella Femhrt Premphase Prempro	Approved for preventing osteoporosis in postmenopausal women. Available as a combination tablet taken daily. Conjugated estrogen dose range: 0.3–0.625 mg; with medroxyprogesterone, dose range: 1.5–5 mg.	Class: hormone replacement. The Woman's Health Initiative study confirmed that Prempro reduced the risk of hip and other fractures. The FDA recommends women first consider other osteoporosis medications.
Ibandronate sodium	Boniva	Approved for the prevention and treatment of postmenopausal osteoporosis. Dosed as a once-a-month (150 mg) pill or as an intravenous injection administered once every 3 months.	Class: bisphosphonate. Should be taken on the same day each month. Reduces bone loss, increases bone density and reduces the risk of vertebral fractures.
Raloxifene hydrochloride	Evista	Approved for the prevention and treatment of postmenopausal osteoporosis. Taken daily as a 60-mg tablet.	Class: selective estrogen receptor modulators. Raloxifene increases bone mass and reduces the risk of vertebral fractures; and has been shown to decrease the risk of estrogen-dependent breast cancer by 65% over 4 years.
Risedronate sodium	Actonel	Approved for the prevention and treatment of postmenopausal osteoporosis, and for preventing and treating glucocorticoid-induced osteoporosis in women and men. Taken daily (5-mg dose) or weekly (35-mg dose).	Class: bisphosphonate. Slows bone loss, increases bone density, and reduces the risk of spine and nonspine fractures.
Risedronate sodium with 500 mg calcium carbonate	Actonel with calcium	Approved for the prevention and treatment of postmenopausal osteoporosis, and for preventing and treating glucocorticoid-induced osteoporosis in women and men. Dosed 35 mg weekly.	Class: bisphosphonate. Slows bone loss, increases bone density, and reduces the risk of vertebral and nonvertebral fractures.

(continued on next page)

Table 3
(continued)

Drug	Brand name	Approved indications and dosing	Notes
Bone-forming medication			
Teriparatide (rhPTH[1-34])	Fortéo	Approved for the treatment of osteoporosis in postmenopausal women, and men who are at high risk for fracture. Taken daily as a self-administered 20-μg injection for up to 24 months.	Class: parathyroid hormone. Stimulates new bone formation and significantly increases bone mineral density. In postmenopausal women, fracture reduction occurs in the spine, hip, foot, ribs, and wrist. In men, fracture reduction occurs in the spine.

Abbreviation: FDA, Food and Drug Administration.

Postsurgically, significant weight loss, severely restricted oral intake, calcium malabsorption, and concomitant vitamin D deficiency place these patients at extremely high risk for the development of MBD [42]. With excess weight loss after combination restrictive-malabsorptive procedures, such as a bilio-pancreatic diversion with duodenal switch, 25(OH)D levels decrease, PTH levels increase, and corrected calcium levels remain within normal limits [42,43]. Numerous case reports in the literature further emphasize the ever-present risk of MBD, noting occurrences of significant bone disease from 8 weeks to 32 years after bariatric surgery [44–48].

Although there are many, varying current recommendations in the literature, to date there are no established guidelines for perioperative management of MBD in bariatric patients [14,49–51]. The literature remains inconclusive on key issues such as preoperative and postoperative DXA, use and frequency of biochemical indices, use and effectiveness of supplements, and prophylactic use of bisphosphonates.

Inflammatory Bowel Disease

Patients with IBD have a high prevalence of decreased BMD and an increased rate of vertebral fractures when compared with healthy subjects [52]. Crohn's disease and ulcerative colitis carry similar risks for osteoporosis and fragility fracture [17]. Three key mechanisms for the development of osteoporosis in IBD are (1) the presence of proinflammatory cytokines, (2) low body mass index, and (3) the use of glucocorticoids [18,52–54].

Because the development of MBD in patients with IBD is the result of both impaired bone formation and increased bone resorption, treatment strategies have included calcium and vitamin D supplementation, risk factor reduction, and trials of bone-stimulating and antiresorptive drugs. Perhaps of foremost importance is the observation that there is a strong correlation with the activity of IBD and the severity of bone loss [18,52,53]. Effective treatment of the underlying disease, and avoiding the use of glucocorticoids when possible, are equally important aspects in the prevention and treatment of MBD. Although appropriate diagnostic and therapeutic regimens addressing BMD in IBD patients is essential, a standard treatment strategy has yet to be defined [52,53].

Gluten-Sensitive Enteropathy (Celiac Disease)

Celiac disease is an autoimmune disorder of varying severity, characterized by small bowel enteropathy caused by ingesting gluten in genetically susceptible individuals, and is seen frequently in patients presenting with osteoporosis [7,13,55]. It is estimated that celiac disease affects nearly 1% of the population and of those affected, approximately 50% of patients will not have clinically significant diarrhea; however, stooling frequency may be greater than normal [55]. Decreased BMD has been described in up to 25% of patients with celiac disease [56]. Patients with osteoporosis have been found to have an incidence of celiac disease of 1.2%, however patients with concurrent gastrointestinal symptoms have a reported rate as high as 3.9% [57].

Malabsorption secondary to villous atrophy contributes to iron deficiency anemia and calcium and vitamin D deficiency in untreated patients. An abnormal stooling history, low or low-normal hemoglobin, and low urine calcium should raise the suspicion of malabsorption. Further testing will likely reveal low serum 25(OH)D in affected patients. Although the research to date remains somewhat controversial, DXA testing should be considered in adults with celiac disease approximately 1 year after initiation of a gluten-free diet [4,58].

Previous claims of bone disease being cured in adult patients following a gluten-free diet are again being challenged in the medical literature [59]. A research group in Italy recently found reduced spine and femoral bone mass in adults following a gluten-free diet long-term [13]. It remains clear, however, that if BMD is going to improve, it typically does so within the first year after initiation of a gluten-free diet [4].

Effective treatment of celiac disease requires not just gluten restriction but often iron, calcium, and vitamin D supplements. Celiac patients also need education and counseling on risk factor reduction regarding osteoporosis, followed by serial testing to determine the efficacy of the prescribed treatment plan. Consideration of the inclusion of an antiresorptive agent, such as a bisphosphonate, in this population is also supported in the literature [60,61].

LIVER DISEASE

MBD, specifically osteopenia and osteoporosis, is a common clinical problem associated with liver disorders [9,15]. Osteoporosis affects patients with a broad spectrum of liver diseases including cholestatic disease, autoimmune hepatitis, chronic viral hepatitis, and alcoholic liver disease [9]. In fact, osteoporosis can be one of the first clinical manifestations of cholestatic disease [4]. Advanced chronic cholestatic disorders, such as primary sclerosing cholangitis, place the patient at significant risk of developing osteopenia [9]. The relationship between cholestasis and MBD remains controversial. Patients with advanced liver disease, high serum bilirubin levels, and muscle wasting classically have reduced BMD. The development of MBD in most reports has been directly related to the duration and severity of the underlying disease, and the intensity and duration of jaundice [9,15].

The term "hepatic osteodystrophy" refers to abnormal bone metabolism that occurs in the presence of advanced liver disease. The cause of hepatic osteodystrophy remains unclear and difficult to determine because patients with chronic liver disease often have other risk factors for MBD, such as alcohol abuse, chronic glucocorticoid use, malnutrition, weight loss, hypogonadism, and vitamin D deficiency [9,15,62]. Patients with alcoholic cirrhosis tend to develop low-turnover osteoporosis [9,15]. Patients with autoimmune hepatitis or primary biliary cirrhosis frequently require long-term treatment with glucocorticoids, which further increases the risk of MBD and fragility fractures. Additional medications used in the treatment of advanced liver disease, such as loop diuretics, anticoagulants, and chemotherapy, also have deleterious effects on bone [7,10].

Vitamin D levels are typically low in patients with alcoholic liver disease, autoimmune hepatitis treated with glucocorticoids, and primary biliary cirrhosis, thereby increasing the risk of osteoporosis and osteomalacia [9,12,15]. Persistently low vitamin D increases the risk of osteomalacia, which can present clinically with complaints of bone pain and proximal muscle weakness; however, distinguishing osteomalacia from osteoporosis can be difficult. It is recommended that diagnosis and treatment be guided by biochemical indices including 25(OH)D, calcium, phosphate, alkaline phosphatase, PTH, and urine calcium and phosphate in the at-risk patient [5,15]. In chronic liver disease, as in other causes of secondary MBD, preventive strategies including early diagnosis and aggressive correction of all reversible factors remains the cornerstone of treatment [9].

ORGAN FAILURE AND TRANSPLANTATION
Liver Transplantation
Transplantation is the established therapy for end-stage diseases of the kidney, heart, liver, and lung [10]. The severity and cause of the liver disease leading up to transplantation constitute the main risk factors for developing MBD (see previous section on liver disease) [10,63]. The success of organ transplantation is related to advances in immunosuppressive therapy; however, these medications are also associated with complications, including bone damage [10,64].

Liver transplant recipients experience rapid bone loss and high fracture rates, especially during the early posttransplant period [65,66]. There are no clinical factors that reliably predict posttransplant bone loss and fractures in an individual patient; all transplant candidates and recipients should receive a thorough evaluation and early preventive therapy for MBD. Although active metabolites of vitamin D and bisphosphonates have both shown efficacy, data from clinical trials suggest that bisphosphonates are the safest and most consistently effective agents for the prevention and treatment of pretransplantation and posttransplantation MBD [66].

Intestinal Transplant
In the face of intestinal failure and complications associated with long-term parenteral nutrition (PN), intestinal transplant offers hope to patients who would otherwise succumb because of intestinal disease, secondary liver failure, and frank malnutrition [67]. As outcomes continue to improve, intestinal transplant is becoming an established therapy for intestinal failure [11]. The risk of MBD in intestinal transplant candidates is speculative at this time, but likely is related to the severity and cause of the underlying disease, the length of time on PN, medications used in treatment of underlying disease, and posttransplant immunosuppressive medications.

MEDICAL INTERVENTIONS
Glucocorticoids
The most common cause of secondary osteoporosis, and the second most common cause of osteoporosis overall, is the chronic use of glucocorticoids

[5,12,68]. Glucocorticoid-induced bone loss generally ensues following sustained systemic doses greater than 5 mg per day of prednisone or its equivalent [5]. There is also evidence that potent inhaled glucocorticoids may have deleterious effects on the skeleton [68]. Those individuals who require maintenance corticosteroid replacement because of adrenal insufficiency do not seem to be at increased risk [5].

The cumulative dose of glucocorticoids correlates with the severity of the bone disease and the incidence of fracture. The mechanism by which glucocorticoids negatively affect bone includes blunting of intestinal calcium absorption even in the presence of adequate vitamin D, calciuria, increased osteoclast activity, osteoblast suppression, and the development of secondary hyperparathyroidism [5,7,68].

Budesonide is a corticosteroid used in the treatment of Crohn's disease that is known for its high topical activity, low systemic activity, and fewer adverse effects when compared with prednisone [69]. Two recent studies compared the effects of budesonide with prednisone on BMD. The first study concluded that budesonide-treated patients were likely to lose bone mass, particularly in the lumbar spine, during the first year of treatment, and conferred no advantage over prednisone [69]. The second study noted that budesonide caused fewer corticosteroid side effects, but bone mass was better preserved only in corticosteroid-naive patients [70]. It is important to note that both studies identified some degree of bone loss in budesonide-treated patients, but neither study was sufficiently powered to detect differences in fracture rate.

The response to therapies currently available for established bone disease remains suboptimal; therefore, prevention of glucocorticoid-induced bone disease is the first-line approach, either by limiting exposure or finding alternate treatments [17]. When chronic steroid treatment is initiated, bisphosphonates such as alendronate and risedronate, have been approved for use in patients taking glucocorticoids, and should be prescribed prophylactically [2]. Taking 1500 mg of supplemental calcium and 400 IU of vitamin D daily can reduce bone remodeling. Other modifiable risk factors previously discussed remain an essential component of treatment, and of particular importance is the avoidance of immobilization, which further precipitates bone loss.

Methotrexate

The term "methotrexate osteopathy" was first used to name a syndrome of bone pain, fragility fractures, and radiographic osteopenia first reported predominantly in children placed on long-term treatment for acute lymphoblastic leukemia in the 1970s [71,72]. Methotrexate is also used in high doses in the treatment of a variety of malignancies including gastric carcinoma, bladder tumors, and occasionally in colorectal carcinomas [73]. The negative effects of high-dose methotrexate on bone appear to be due to increased bone resorption in the presence of inhibited bone formation, resulting in a massive uncoupling of bone turnover [73–75].

Prescribed in lower doses in the treatment of IBD, methotrexate has many anti-inflammatory and cytokine-modulating properties likely resulting in its beneficial effect in the treatment of chronic inflammatory conditions and does not seem to cause accelerated bone loss [76–78].

Enteral and Parenteral Nutrition Support

Enteral nutrition support has many advantages over parenteral nutrition (PN), and early initiation of enteral feeding in the course of trauma, surgery, or severe illness has been advocated not only to establish and maintain adequate nutrition status but also to maintain the GI mucosa, prevent bacterial transmigration, promote immunocompetence, decrease the incidence of sepsis, and decrease the length of hospital stay [79,80].

Unlike PN, a thorough review of the literature failed to identify a relationship between enteral nutrition support and MBD. Although enteral nutrition should be considered first, honoring the mantra "if the gut works, use it," in the presence of severe intestinal obstruction or severe malabsorption, PN support is the only remaining option.

MBD has been recognized as a complication of PN for more than 25 years and its cause appears to be to be multifactorial [81–83]. Early studies found intravenous nutrition solutions to contain excess vitamin D and aluminum, but despite newer PN formulations that strictly limit these elements, MBD continues to occur [83]. A longitudinal study recently conducted in Denmark noted an absence of accelerated bone lost but found the BMD of many long-term PN patients substantially reduced, making them susceptible to fragility fractures and in need of interventions to prevent osteoporosis [84]. Both the Denmark study and a more recent report from Canada point out that a significant part of the MBD in long-term PN patients is related to the underlying disease for which the PN was indicated [84,85].

Guidelines for the prevention and management of PN-associated MBD have yet to be established. The PN formula should be optimized, however, to reduce the risk of MBD in the stable patient as follows: provide at least 15 mEq of calcium gluconate daily to promote a positive calcium balance, give phosphorus in a dose approximating a calcium to phosphorus ratio of 1:2, and add sufficient magnesium (usually 15 mEq or more daily) to replace fecal losses; limit amino acids to maintenance levels; match sodium to daily losses; include sufficient acetate to maintain normal serum bicarbonate; and provide daily trace elements and multivitamins for injection that includes vitamin D as cholecalciferol [83,86,87].

NUTRITIONAL DISORDERS OF INSUFFICIENT INTAKE OR MALABSORPTION

Protein-Calorie Malnutrition

Protein-calorie malnutrition occurs as a result of many chronic GI diseases and left uncorrected, results in MBD. In the NHANES 1 study, hip fractures were associated with low energy intake, low serum albumin, and decreased muscle strength, all reflecting protein and caloric deficit [88]. In the large Nurses Health Study, hip fracture incidence was inversely related to protein intake [89].

There is a strong correlation with body weight and BMD. The occurrence of MBD has been well established in both men and women with eating disorders, particularly anorexia nervosa, and pathologic fractures can be seen 7 to 15 years after onset of the disorder [23]. A 10% decrease in body weight typically results in a 1% to 2% bone loss, and more severe weight loss and malnutrition are considered risk factors for osteoporosis, which likely due to low protein intake [23].

High-protein diets have been shown to increase urinary calcium losses (see section on nutritional disorders of excess) [23,90]. There is growing evidence, however, that a low-protein diet has a detrimental effect on bone [91]. A study examining the effects of a low-protein (0.7 g protein/kg body weight) diet noted an increase in biochemical markers of bone turnover when compared with a diet containing 2.1 g/kg of protein [92]. In two interventional trials examining graded levels of protein intake of 0.7, 0.8, 0.9, and 1 g protein/kg body weight on calcium homeostasis, decreased calcium absorption and an acute rise in PTH was noted by day 4 of the 0.7 and 0.8 g/kg diets, but not during the 0.9 or 1 g/kg diets [93,94]. A systematic review of the literature addressing protein and bone health concluded that diets containing moderate protein levels (approximately 1–1.5 g/kg) are probably optimal for bone health [23]. This is particularly worrisome, in that these studies suggest the current recommended dietary allowance of 0.8 g protein/kg is inadequate to promote calcium homeostasis.

Protein-calorie malnutrition is often a multifactorial disease and can include cognitive, emotional, and environmental factors in addition to physical malady and physiologic abnormalities. Effectively addressing protein-calorie malnutrition is challenging, whether it is in the inpatient or outpatient setting, and requires establishing the cause of the malnutrition before effective treatment can be prescribed.

Calcium

The duodenum is the major site of active calcium uptake, although the remainder of the small intestine and possibly the colon seem to absorb some calcium passively [95]. In the healthy GI tract approximately one third of total ingested calcium is absorbed [6,31]. Despite the evidence supporting the beneficial effects of dietary calcium, its availability in the food supply, and numerous public awareness campaigns, population studies continue to report inadequate calcium intake across all age groups [23,26,96]. In GI illnesses malabsorption of calcium is common, further compounding the problem [4].

Calcium deficiency is a well-established risk factor for the development of osteoporosis and fragility fractures. Supplemental calcium should be prescribed for all patients who fall short of meeting their defined dietary reference intake [2,26]. Patients who have lost absorptive surface area because of surgery or disease should also have their calcium intake optimized through diet and supplements. Absorption of calcium in the form of an oral supplement can be problematic for some patients; judicious monitoring to assess efficacy is essential. Although there are several formulations and a variety of doses available, the quantity of calcium required to prevent and treat deficiency in the absence of a functioning duodenum remain unknown [50,53,97]. Vitamin D also needs to be a consideration, because both active and passive absorption of calcium is enhanced by vitamin D [2,97].

Magnesium

Magnesium is mainly absorbed in the distal small intestine both by carrier mediated and paracellular routes, although absorptions studies suggest that magnesium is absorbed along the entire intestinal tract [97]. When the distal small intestine has either become chronically diseased or surgically removed, magnesium deficiency occurs because of reduced absorption and chelation with unabsorbed fatty acids in the bowel lumen [98].

Magnesium appears to affect bone remodeling and strength, has a positive association with hip BMD in both men and women, and plays an important role in calcium and bone metabolism [23,29,98]. Hypomagnesemia blunts PTH activity resulting in altered calcium metabolism, hypocalcemia, vitamin D abnormalities, and further decreased jejunal magnesium absorption [19,23,98].

Few well-designed studies have investigated the effect of magnesium intake on bone health, and although there is evidence demonstrating benefit in postmenopausal women, studies looking at magnesium supplementation in GI diseases are lacking [29,99]. Current recommendations from the British Society of Gastroenterology for achieving and maintaining normal magnesium levels include correcting sodium depletion, oral or intravenous magnesium supplements, and occasionally adding vitamin D [98].

Vitamin B_{12} (Cobalamin)

Vitamin B_{12} is an essential nutrient obtained from the diet by consuming animal proteins [100,101]. At acidic pH vitamin B_{12} has a high affinity for R protein, which is produced predominantly by salivary glands [100,101]. Once exposed to trypsin, R protein is cleaved and vitamin B_{12} binds with intrinsic factor produced by gastric parietal cells. Intrinsic factor protects cobalamin from degradation, allowing it to reach the terminal ileum where it binds with enterocyte receptor sites. Once within the enterocyte, intrinsic factor is cleaved and the free form of vitamin B_{12} leaves the cell and enters the plasma [101].

Malabsorption of vitamin B_{12} is commonly the result of abnormal gut function at three key sites. First, gastric pathology can result in decreased production of intrinsic factor resulting in an inability to absorb vitamin B_{12}. Next is the result of pancreatic insufficiency, which can lead to persistent R protein–cobalamin complexes that are unabsorbable. Finally, but perhaps of greatest importance, is that vitamin B_{12} malabsorption uniformly occurs when more than 100 cm of terminal ileum has been resected [98].

An association between vitamin B_{12} deficiency and increased fracture risk has been documented in patients with pernicious anemia, and may be an important modifiable risk factor for the development of osteoporosis [100,102,103]. A study of over 3500 participants from the Framingham Off-spring Cohort demonstrated an association between low vitamin B_{12} and low BMD in men, and confirmed this association in women [100].

Questions have been raised concerning the long-term use of proton pump inhibitors and vitamin B_{12} malabsorption. It seems that over the course of many years of antisecretory therapy, subnormal vitamin B_{12} levels may occur, but whether clinical B_{12} deficiency develops as a result of long-term acid suppression remains unclear [103,104].

Supplementation is recommended for patients who are deficient in vitamin B_{12}. Some patients with relatively mild GI disease are able to restore and maintain B_{12} levels by taking oral supplements; however, most patients require repletion and lifelong maintenance by subcutaneous injections [14,51,98,100,101].

Vitamin D

Vitamin D is one of the principle hormonal regulators of calcium homeostasis in the body. Vitamin D is essential for calcium and phosphate absorption in the gut, stimulation of osteoblast activity, calcium reabsorption in the renal tubules, and normal bone mineralization throughout the life span [9,105]. Absorption of vitamin D occurs mainly by passive diffusion in the proximal and mid small intestine and is highly dependant on bile salts [5,85,105,106]. Whether consumed in the diet or obtained from sunlight (UVB radiation), vitamin D undergoes hydroxylation in the liver and the kidneys on the way to becoming the active form of the hormone [5,32,105].

Vitamin D deficiency is increasingly common in the general population and very common among the elderly [5,105]. Chronic vitamin D deficiency is the principle cause of osteomalacia. The clinical symptoms of osteomalacia include bone pain and proximal muscle weakness. Biochemically, patients have low $25(OH)D$, normal or low $1,25(OH)_2D_3$, high PTH, high indices of bone turnover including alkaline phosphatase, and low urinary calcium [5,106]. The consequences of untreated osteomalacia include insufficiency-type stress fractures of the ribs, pelvis, scapulae, femoral neck, and the shaft of long bones [5,105,106].

Of the six levels at which vitamin D metabolism can be affected, GI-associated diseases play an integral part in three [106]. The first and most common defect in vitamin D metabolism is extrinsic depletion caused by inadequate oral intake seen in many malnourished patients with anorexia caused by underlying GI disease [4,106]. Intrinsic vitamin D depletion, caused by malabsorption, can also result in osteomalacia, and the most common disorders associated with this condition include celiac disease, gastric bypass surgery, postgastrectomy states, chronic pancreatitis, IBD, and biliary cirrhosis [106]. Impaired 25-hydroxylation of vitamin D is the third level at which vitamin D metabolism is affected, and this occurs frequently in end stage liver disease, alcoholic liver disease, and primary biliary cirrhosis [4,106].

Patients with vitamin D deficiency require immediate and aggressive therapy. Repletion with over-the-counter multivitamins is ineffective and not recommended because of the risk of concomitant vitamin A excess. Repletion can be achieved by giving oral pharmacologic doses (50,000 IU of vitamin D_2 or 15,000 IU of vitamin D_3) once weekly for 8 weeks. Efficacy of the treatment should be determined by repeat serum level, and an additional 8-week course prescribed if needed [105]. For patients who are chronically deficient, after the initial 8-week course, twice-per-month maintenance dosing is recommended. For patients who are unable to tolerate or adequately absorb oral supplements, exposure to sunlight (UVB radiation) is still the best source of vitamin D and is an effective alternative [105,106].

Vitamin K
Vitamin K deficiency is associated with an abnormal activation of bone matrix, altered osteocalcin, blunted osteoblast function and resulting impaired bone formation, and an increased risk of fracture [9]. Vitamin K affects bone quality at the level of the microarchitecture. DXA is unlikely to detect suspected disease. Vitamin K supplementation has been found to prevent new fractures in patients with osteoporosis, and may have a protective effect against vertebral fractures in patients with steroid-induced osteoporosis [9,23].

NUTRITIONAL DISORDERS OF EXCESS
Alcohol
Alcohol use is an independent risk factor for the development of MBD [107]. Alcoholic bone disease results from chronic excessive alcohol consumption and is characterized as a disease of decreased bone formation, deficient bone repair, and delayed fracture healing [108].

Daily alcohol consumption of 50 g (four standard drinks) results in a dose-dependant decrease in osteoblast activity; daily consumption of greater than 100 g eventually results in an osteopenic skeleton and increased risk for the development of osteoporosis [9,105,108]. Modest intake of alcohol does not seem to be deleterious to bone [12].

Caffeine
Caffeine is known to increase urinary calcium losses and may have harmful effects on bone. A recent prospective study demonstrated that intake of greater than 300 mg daily accelerated bone loss at the spine in elderly women [109]. Further investigations demonstrated that bone loss occurred in those women who had both low calcium intake and high caffeine intakes [110]. Overall, the evidence indicates that the deleterious effects of caffeine on bone can be negated by consuming adequate calcium [12,109,111].

Phosphorus
Phosphorus is absorbed most efficiently in the duodenum and ileum, and is plentiful in the food supply predominantly because of the increased use of phosphate salts in food additives and cola beverages [23,26,27,112]. Although

phosphorus is an essential nutrient, the current literature notes that both phosphorus deficiency and excess intake interferes with calcium absorption and leads to bone loss [23,113]. The need for daily supplementation as a result of GI surgery or disease has not been specifically addressed in the literature.

Protein

Dietary protein is required to maintain bone structure; however, studies have shown a positive association between excess protein intake and urinary excretion of calcium, contributing to a negative calcium balance [114]. A link between high protein intake and an increased risk of fracture has also been demonstrated, regardless of whether it was of animal or vegetable origin [90,114]. When high protein intake is coupled with adequate calcium intake, the potentially harmful effects of protein appear to be ameliorated [115–117].

Sodium

The evidence of a detrimental effect of high salt intake on bone health is primarily limited to short-term effects of sodium on calcium metabolism [118]. There is strong evidence in support of the fact that high salt intake produces a calciuretic effect, but investigations attempting to define the association of sodium with bone loss and BMD have produced conflicting results [118,119]. Individual differences in sensitivity to salt, such as that seen in blood pressure control, has been well documented but the long-term impact of salt-sensitivity and sodium restriction on MBD is unknown [118]. Acid-base balance, protein, and potassium also affect the relationship between sodium and calcium absorption in the kidney, making it difficult to establish the unique effects of sodium separate from the overall diet. The current recommendations to reduce the average salt intake from the Scientific Advisory Committee on Nutrition [120] are based on cardiovascular disease data. There are insufficient data to make similar recommendations regarding bone health.

Vitamin A

Vitamin A (retinol) taken in excess causes osteoporosis and can also lead to hypercalcemia. This noted toxic effect, previously ascribed only to the ingestion of large doses, also occurs in smaller doses and has been identified as a risk factor for hip fractures. Vitamin A as betacarotene does not seem to be associated with increased fracture risk; however, this fact is still being argued [30].

SUMMARY

MBD is often silent, often undiagnosed, and occurs frequently in patients with chronic GI illnesses. Disorders of the GI tract and liver have a strong association with osteoporosis, and a high prevalence of osteopenia. Potentially modifiable risk factors, such as poor dietary habits, protein-calorie malnutrition, malabsorption, prolonged use of glucocorticoids, and a sedentary lifestyle, can lead to low peak bone mass, an increased rate of bone loss, and debilitating bone disease if left untreated.

Although MBD is treatable, prevention must be the primary approach. Identifying patients at risk, pursuing diagnostic evaluation, addressing risk factor reduction, and starting appropriate therapeutic interventions must be essential components of the practice of gastroenterology.

Acknowledgments

S.E.W. acknowledges Dr. Douglas Seidner, and offers sincere thanks for providing the opportunity to write this article, and for his attention to detail in proofreading and editing the work. S.E.W. also thanks her family - her true co-authors - for providing support, encouragement, and enthusiasm without which this would not have been possible.

References

[1] Dennisson E. Osteoporosis. In: Pinchera A, Bertagna X, Fischer J, editors. Endocrinology and metabolism. London: McGraw-Hill International (UK); 2001. p. 271–82.

[2] National Osteoporosis Foundation. Physician's guide to prevention and treatment of osteoporosis. Available at: http://www.nof.org/physguide. Accessed October 21, 2006.

[3] Skugor M, Licata A. The Cleveland Clinic Disease Management Project: osteoporosis. The Cleveland Clinic Foundation. Available at: http://www.clevelandclinicmeded.com/diseasemanagement/2005. Accessed October 21, 2006.

[4] Bernstein CN, Leslie WD, Leboff M. AGA technical review: osteoporosis in gastrointestinal diseases. Gastroenterology 2003;124(3):795–841.

[5] Shoback D, Marcus R, Bilke D. Metabolic bone disease. In: Greenspan FS, Gardner DG, editors. Basic and clinical endocrinology. 7th edition. New York: McGraw-Hill; 2004. p. 295–361.

[6] Weaver CM, Heaney RP, et al. Calcium. In: Shils ME, Olsen JA, Shine M, editors. Modern nutrition in health and disease. 9th edition. Philadelphia: Lippincott Williams & Wilkins; 1999. p. 141–55.

[7] National Osteoporosis Foundation. The many faces of secondary osteoporosis. Osteoporosis Clinical Updates 2002;vol. III(3). p. 2–7.

[8] Obermayer-Pietsch BM, Bonelli CM, Walter DE, et al. Genetic predisposition for adult lactose intolerance and relation to diet, bone density, and bone fractures. J Bone Miner Res 2004;19(1):42–7.

[9] Sanchez AJ, Aranda-Michel J. Liver disease and osteoporosis. Nutr Clin Pract 2006;21: 273–8.

[10] Cohen A, Ebeling P, Sprague S, et al. Transplantation osteoporosis. In: Favus M, editor. Primer on the metabolic bone diseases and disorders of mineral metabolism. 6th edition. Washington, DC: American Society for Bone and Mineral Research; 2006. p. 302–9.

[11] Fryer JP. Intestinal transplant: an update. Curr Opin Gastroenterol 2005;21(2):162–8.

[12] Licata AA. Osteoporosis in men: suspect secondary disease first. Cleve Clin J Med 2003;70(3):247–54.

[13] Fiore CE, Pennisi P, Ferro G, et al. Altered osteoprotegerin/RANKL ratio and low bone mineral density in celiac patients on long-term treatment with gluten-free diet. Horm Metab Res 2006;38:417–22.

[14] Mason EM, Jalagani H, Vinik AI. Metabolic complications of bariatric surgery: diagnosis and management issues. Gastroenterol Clin North Am 2006;34:25–33.

[15] Cijevschi C, Mihai C, Zbranca E, et al. Osteoporosis in liver cirrhosis. Rom J Gastroenterol 2005;14(4):337–41.

[16] Licata A. Diagnosing primary osteoporosis: it's more than a T score. Cleve Clin J Med 2006;73(5):473–6.

[17] American Gastroenterological Association medical position statement: guidelines on osteoporosis in gastrointestinal disease. Gastroenterology 2003;124(3):791–4.

[18] Lichtenstein GR, Sands BE, Paziansa M. Prevention and treatment of osteoporosis in inflammatory bowel disease. Inflamm Bowel Dis 2006;12(8):797–813.

[19] Nightingale JMD. Hepatobiliary, renal and bone complications of intestinal failure. Best Pract Res Clin Gastroenterology 2003;17(6):907–29.

[20] U.S. Department of Health and Human Services. Bone health and osteoporosis: a report of the Surgeon General. Rockville (MD): U.S. Department of Health and Human Services, Office of the Surgeon General; 2004. p. 166–70.

[21] Higdon J. Manganese. Linus Pauling Institute, Oregon State University; 2001. Available at: http://lpi.oregonstate.edu. Accessed October 24, 2006.

[22] Higdon J. Lignans. Linus Pauling Institute, Oregon State University; 2005. Available at: http://lpi.oregonstate.edu. Accessed October 26, 2006.

[23] Ilich JZ, Kerstetter JE. Nutrition in bone health revisited: a story beyond calcium. J Am Coll Nutr 2000;19(6):715–37.

[24] Maggio D, Polidori MC, Barabani M. Low levels of carotenoids and retinol in involutional osteoporosis. Bone 2006;38:244–8.

[25] Marie JP, Ammann P, Boivin G, et al. Mechanisms of action and therapeutic potential of strontium in bone. Calcif Tissue Int 2001;69:121–9.

[26] National Academy of Sciences Executive Summary: dietary reference intakes for calcium, phosphorus, magnesium, vitamin D, and fluoride. Washington, DC. 1997. Available at: http://niams.nih.gov.

[27] National Institutes of Health Osteoporosis and Related Bone Diseases–National Resource Center. Health topics: other nutrients and bone health. Bethesda (MD). 2004.

[28] National Institutes of Health Osteoporosis and Related Bone Diseases–National Resource Center. Health topics: phytoestrogens and bone health. Bethesda (MD). 2005.

[29] National Osteoporosis Foundation. Over-the-counter products and osteoporosis: case discussions. Osteoporosis Clinical Updates 2002;vol. III(2). p. 1–7.

[30] Penniston KL, Tanumihardjo SA. The acute and chronic toxic effects of vitamin A. Am J Clin Nutr 2006;83:191–201.

[31] Gueguen L, Oiubtukkart A. The bioavailability of dietary calcium. J Am Coll Nutr 2000;19(2):119S–36S.

[32] Holick MF, Garabedian M. Vitamin D: photobiology, metabolism, mechanism of action, and clinical applications. In: Favus MJ, editor. Primer on the metabolic bone diseases and disorders of mineral metabolism. 6th edition. Washington, DC: American Society for Bone and Mineral Research; 2006. p. 106–14.

[33] National Institute of arthritis and musculoskeletal and skin diseases. Medications to prevent and treat osteoporosis. Available at: http://www.niams.nih.gov/. Accessed October 26, 2006.

[34] National Osteoporosis Foundation. Pharmacologic options (2005 update). In: Physician's guide to prevention and treatment of osteoporosis. Washington, DC; National Osteoporosis Foundation: 1998.

[35] Chines A, Pacifici R. Antacid and sucralfate-induced hypophosphatemic osteomalacia: a case report and review of the literature. Calcif Tissue Int 1990;47(5):291–5.

[36] Neumann L, Jensen BG. Osteomalacia from Al and Mg antacids. Report of a case of bilateral hip fracture. Acta Orthop Scand 1989;60(3):361–2.

[37] Recker RR. Calcium absorption and achlorhydria. N Engl J Med 1985;313:70–3.

[38] Drinka PJ, Moore J, Boushon MC. Severe hypercalcemia after transition from calcium carbonate to calcium citrate in an elderly woman treated with ergocalciferol 50,000 IU per day. Am J Geriatr Pharmacother 2006;4:70–4.

[39] Newcomer AD, Hodgson SF, McGill DB, et al. Lactase deficiency: prevalence in osteoporosis. Ann Intern Med 1978;89(2):218–20.

[40] Carlin AM, Rao DS, Meslemani AM, et al. Prevalence of vitamin D depletion among morbidly obese patients seeking gastric bypass surgery. Surg Obes Rel Dis 2006;2(2):98–103.

[41] Puzziferri N, Blankenship J, Wolfe BM. Surgical treatment for obesity. Endocrine 2006;29(1):11–9.

[42] Hamoui N, Anthone G, Crookes F. Calcium metabolism in the morbidly obese. Obes Surg 2004;14(1):9–12.

[43] Newbery L, Dolan K, Hatzifotis M, et al. Calcium and vitamin D depletion and elevated parathyroid hormone following biliopancreatic diversion. Obes Surg 2003; 13(6):893–5.

[44] Haria DM, Sibonga JD, Taylor HC. Hypocalcemia, hypovitaminosis D osteopathy, osteopenia, and secondary hyperparathyroidism 32 years after jejunoileal bypass. Endocr Pract 2005;11(5):335–40.

[45] Goldner WS, O'Dorisio TM, Dillon JS, et al. Severe metabolic bone disease as a long-term complication of obesity surgery. Obes Surg 2002;12:685–92.

[46] De Prisco C, Levine SN. Metabolic bone disease after gastric bypass surgery for obesity. Am J Med Sci 2005;329:57–61.

[47] Atreja A, Abacan C, Licata A. A 51-year-old woman with debilitating cramps 12 years after bariatric surgery. Cleve Clin J Med 2003;70:417–26.

[48] Collazo-Clavell ML, Jimenez A, Hodgson SF, et al. Osteomalacia after Roux-en-Y gastric bypass. Endocr Pract 2004;10:287–8.

[49] Hensrud DD, McMahon MM. Bariatric surgery in adults with extreme (not morbid) obesity. Mayo Clin Proc 2006;81(10 Suppl):S3–4.

[50] McGlinch BP, Que FG, Nelson JL, et al. Perioperative care of patients undergoing bariatric surgery. Mayo Clin Proc 2006;81(10 Suppl):S25–33.

[51] Brethauer SA, Chand C, Schauer PR. Risks and benefits of bariatric surgery: current evidence. Cleve Clin J Med 2006;73(11):993–1007.

[52] Klaus J, Brueckel J, Steinkamp M, et al. High prevalence of vertebral fractures in patients with Crohn's disease. Gut 2002;51:654–8.

[53] von Tirpitz C, Reinshagen M. Management of osteoporosis in patients with gastrointestinal diseases. Eur J Gastroenterol Hepatol 2003;15(8):869–76.

[54] Lashner B. Inflammatory bowel disease. The Cleveland Clinic Disease Management Project. The Cleveland Clinic Foundation. Available at: http://www.clevelandclinicmeded.com/diseasemanagement/2005. Accessed October 21, 2006.

[55] Lee SK, Green PHR. Celiac sprue (the great modern-day imposter). Curr Opin Rheumatol 2006;18:101–7.

[56] Vasquez H, Mazure R, Gonzalez D, et al. Risk of fractures in celiac disease patients: a cross-sectional, case-control study. Am J Gastroenterol 2000;95(1):183–9.

[57] Sanders DS, Patel D, Khan FB, et al. Case-finding for adult celiac disease in patients with reduced bone mineral density. Dig Dis Sci 2005;50(3):587–92.

[58] Lewis NR, Scott BB. Should patients with celiac disease have their bone mineral density measured? Eur J Gastroenterol Hepatol 2005;17:1065–70.

[59] Kemppainen T, Kroger H, Janatuinen E, et al. Bone recovery after a gluten-free diet: a 5-year follow-up study. Bone 1999;25:355–60.

[60] Bianchi ML, Bardella MT. Bone and celiac disease. Calcif Tissue Int 2002;71:465–71.

[61] Pazianas M, Butcher GP, Subhani MJ, et al. Calcium absorption and bone mineral density in celiacs after long term treatment with gluten-free diet and adequate calcium intake. Osteoporos Int 2005;16:56–63.

[62] DiCecco SR, Francisco-Zeller N. Nutrition in alcoholic liver disease. Nutr Clin Pract 2006;21:245–54.

[63] Monegal A, Navasa M, Guanabens N, et al. Bone disease after liver transplantation: a long-term prospective study of bone mass changes, hormonal status and histomorphometric characteristics. Osteoporos Int 2001;12(6):484–92.

[64] Ramsey-Goldman R, Dunn JE, Dunlop DD, et al. Increased risk of fracture in patients receiving solid organ transplants. J Bone Miner Res 1999;14:456–63.

[65] Ninkovic M, Skingle SJ, Bearcroft PW, et al. Incidence of vertebral fractures in the first three months after orthotopic liver transplantation. Eur J Gastroenterol Hepatol 2000;12(8): 931–3.

[66] Cohen A, Sambrook P, Shane E. Management of bone loss after organ transplantation. J Bone Miner Res 2004;19:1919–32.

[67] Abu-Elmagd KM. Intestinal transplantation for short bowel syndrome and gastrointestinal failure: current consensus, rewarding outcomes, and practical guidelines. Gastroenterology 2006;130:S132–7.

[68] Lipworth BJ. Systemic adverse effects of inhaled corticosteroid therapy: a systematic review and meta analysis. Arch Intern Med 1999;159:941–55.

[69] Cino M, Greenberg GR. Bone mineral density in Crohn's disease: a longitudinal study of budesonide, prednisone, and nonsteroid therapy. Am J Gastroenterol 2002;97(4): 915–21.

[70] Schoon EJ, Bollani S, Mills PR, et al. Bone mineral density in relation to efficacy and side effects of budesonide and prednisolone in Crohn's disease. Clin Gastroenterol Hepatol 2005;3:113–21.

[71] O'Regan S, Melhorn DR, Newman AJ. Methotrexate induced bone pain in childhood leukemia. Am J Dis Child 1973;126:448–50.

[72] Ragab AH, Fresh RS, Vietti TJ. Osteoporosis fractures secondary to methotrexate therapy of leukemia in remission. Cancer 1970;25:580–5.

[73] Pfeilschifter J, Diel IJ. Osteoporosis due to cancer treatment: pathogenesis and management. J Clin Oncol 2000;28:1570–93.

[74] May KP, West SG, McDermott MT. The effect of low dose methotrexate on bone metabolism and histomorphology in rats. Arthritis Rheum 1994;37:201–6.

[75] Wheeler DL, Vander Griend RA, Wronski TJ, et al. The short and long-term effects of methotrexate on the rat skeleton. Bone 1995;16:215–21.

[76] Carbone LD, Kaeley G, McKown KM, et al. Effects of long-term administration of methotrexate on bone mineral density in rheumatoid arthritis. Calcif Tissue Int 1999;64: 100–1.

[77] Di Munno O, Mazzantini M, Sinigaglia L, et al. Effect of low dose methotrexate on bone density in women with rheumatoid arthritis: results from a multicenter cross-sectional study. J Rheumatol 2004;31:1305–9.

[78] Minaur NJ, Kounali SV, Compston JE, et al. Methotrexate in the treatment of rheumatoid arthritis: II. In vivo effects on bone mineral density. Br J Rheumatol 2002;41:741–9.

[79] McClave S. Critical care nutrition: getting involved as a gastrointestinal endoscopist. J Clin Gastroenterol 2006;40(10):870–90.

[80] Taylor SJ, Fettes SB, Jewkes C, et al. Prospective, randomized, controlled trial to determine the effect of early enhanced enteral nutrition on clinical outcome in mechanically ventilated patients suffering head injury. Crit Care Med 1999;27(11):2525–31.

[81] Cohen-Solal M, Baudoin C, Joly F, et al. Osteoporosis in patients on long-term home parenteral nutrition: a longitudinal study. J Bone Miner Res 2003;18(11):1989–94.

[82] Hise ME, Compher C, Harlan L, et al. Inflammatory mediators and immune function are altered in home parenteral nutrition patients. Nutrition 2006;22:97–103.

[83] Seidner DL, Licata A. Parenteral nutrition-associated metabolic bone disease: pathophysiology, evaluation, and treatment. Nutr Clin Pract 2000;15:163–70.

[84] Haderslev KV, Tjellesen L, Haderslev PH, et al. Assessment of the longitudinal changes in bone mineral density in patients receiving home parenteral nutrition. JPEN J Parenter Enteral Nutr 2004;28(5):289–94.

[85] Raman M, Aghdassi E, Baum M, et al. Metabolic bone disease in patients receiving home parenteral nutrition: a Canadian study and review. JPEN J Parenter Enteral Nutr 2006;30(6):492–6.

[86] Seidner DL. Parenteral nutrition-associated metabolic bone disease. JPEN J Parenter Enteral Nutr 2002;26:S37–42.

[87] Houghton LA, Veith R. The case against ergocalciferol (vitamin D₂) as a vitamin supplement. Am J Clin Nutr 2006;84:694–7.

[88] Huang Z, Himes JH, McGovern PG. Nutrition and subsequent hip fracture risk among a national cohort of white women. Am J Epidemiol 1996;144:124–34.

[89] Feskanich D, Willett WC, Stampfer MJ, et al. Protein consumption and bone fractures in women. Am J Epidemiol 1996;143:472–9.

[90] Rizzoli R, Ammann P, Chevalley T, et al. Protein intake and bone disorders in the elderly. Joint Bone Spine 2001;68:383–92.

[91] Greenspan SL, Resnick NM. Geriatric endocrinology. In: Greenspan FS, Gardner DG, editors. Basic and clinical endocrinology. 7th edition. New York: McGraw-Hill; 2004. p. 842–66.

[92] Rizzoli R, Bonjour JP. Dietary protein and bone health. J Bone Miner Res 2004;19(4): 527–31.

[93] Kerstetter J, Svastisalee C, Caseria D, et al. A threshold for low-protein-diet-induced elevations in parathyroid hormone. Am J Clin Nutr 2000;72:168–73.

[94] Giannini S, Nobile M, Sartori L, et al. Acute effects of moderate dietary protein restriction in patients with idiopathic hypercalciuria and calcium nephrolithiasis. Am J Clin Nutr 1999;69:267–71.

[95] Krejs GJ, Nicar MJ, Zerwekh JE, et al. Effect of 1, 25-dihydroxyvitamin D on calcium and magnesium absorption in the healthy human jejunum and ileum. Am J Med 1983;75: 973–81.

[96] Heaney RP. Calcium, dairy products and osteoporosis. J Am Coll Nutr 2000;19:83S–99S.

[97] Shils ME, et al. Magnesium. In: Shils ME, Olsen JA, Shine M, editors. Modern nutrition in health and disease. 9th edition. Philadelphia: Lippincott Williams & Wilkins; 1999. p. 169–92.

[98] Nightingale JMD, Woodward JM. Guidelines for management of patients with a short bowel. Gut 2006;55:1–12.

[99] Stendig-Lindenberg G, Tepper R, Leicher I. Trabecular bone density in a two year controlled trial of personal magnesium in osteoporosis. Magnes Res 1993;155–63.

[100] Tucker KL, Hannan MT, Qiao N, et al. Low plasma vitamin B₁₂ is associated with lower BMD: the Framingham osteoporosis study. J Bone Miner Res 2005;20(1):152–8.

[101] Weir DG, Scott JW, et al. Vitamin B12 Cobalamin. In: Shils ME, Olsen JA, Shine M, editors. Modern nutrition in health and disease. 9th edition. Philadelphia: Lippincott Williams & Wilkins; 1999. p. 447–58.

[102] Goerss JB, Kim CH, Atkinson EJ, et al. Risk of fractures in patients with pernicious anemia. J Bone Miner Res 1992;7:573–9.

[103] Eastell R, Vieira NE, Yergey AL, et al. Pernicious anemia is a risk factor for osteoporosis. Clin Sci 1992;82:681–5.

[104] Laine L, Ahnen D, McClain C, et al. Review article: potential gastrointestinal effects of long-term acid suppression with proton pump inhibitors. Aliment Pharmacol Ther 2000;14: 651–68.

[105] Holick MF, et al. Vitamin D. In: Shils ME, Olsen JA, Shine M, editors. Modern nutrition in health and disease. 9th edition. Philadelphia: Lippincott Williams & Wilkins; 1999. p. 329–46.

[106] Rosen CJ. Vitamin D and bone health in adults and the elderly. In: Holick MF, editor. Vitamin D: physiology, molecular biology, and clinical applications. Totowa (NJ): Humana Press; 1999. p. 287–306.

[107] Turner RT. Skeletal response to alcohol. Alcohol Clin Exp Res 2000;24:1693–701.

[108] Chakkalakal DA. Alcohol-induced bone loss and deficient bone repair. Alcohol Clin Exp Res 2005;29(12):2077–90.

[109] Rapuri PB, Gallagher JC, Kinyamu HK. Caffeine intake increases the rate of bone loss in elderly women and interacts with vitamin D receptor genotypes. Am J Clin Nutr 2001;74:694–700.

[110] Harris SS, Dawson-Hughes B. Caffeine and bone loss in healthy postmenopausal women. Am J Clin Nutr 1994;60:573–8.

[111] Massey LK. Is caffeine a risk factor for bone loss in the elderly? Am J Clin Nutr 2001;74: 569–70.

[112] Knochel JP, et al. Phosphorus. In: Shils ME, Olsen JA, Shine M, editors. Modern nutrition in health and disease. 9th edition. Philadelphia: Lippincott Williams & Wilkins; 1999. p. 157–68.

[113] Heaney RP, Nordin BEC. Calcium effects on phosphorus absorption: implications for the prevention and co-therapy of osteoporosis. J Am Coll Nutr 2002;21(3):239–44.

[114] Munger RG, Cerhan JR, Chiu BC. Prospective study of dietary protein intake and risk of hip fracture in postmenopausal women. Am J Clin Nutr 1999;69:147–52.

[115] Weikert C, Walter D, Hoffmann K, et al. The relation between dietary protein, calcium and bone health in women: results from the EPIC-Potsdam cohort. Ann Nutr Metab 2005;49: 312–8.

[116] Whiting SJ, Boyle JL, Thompson A. Dietary protein, phosphorus and potassium are beneficial to bone mineral density in adult men consuming adequate dietary calcium. J Am Coll Nutr 2002;21:402–9.

[117] Teegarden D, Lyle RM, McCabe GP, et al. Dietary calcium, protein, and phosphorus are related to bone mineral density and content in young women. Am J Clin Nutr 1998;68: 749–54.

[118] Teucher B, Fairweather-Tait S. Dietary sodium as a risk factor for osteoporosis: where is the evidence? Proc Nutr Soc 2003;62:859–66.

[119] Harrington M, Cashman KD. High salt intake appears to increase bone resorption in postmenopausal women but high potassium intake ameliorates this adverse effect. Nutr Rev 2003;61(5):179–83.

[120] Scientific Advisory Committee on Nutrition: report on salt and health. Available at: http://www.sacn.gov.uk2003. Accessed November 4, 2006.

Gastroenterol Clin N Am 36 (2007) 191–210

GASTROENTEROLOGY CLINICS
OF NORTH AMERICA

Obesity Management

Robert F. Kushner, MD

Department of Medicine, Northwestern University Feinberg School of Medicine, Wellness Institute, 150 East Huron Street, Suite 1100, Chicago, IL 60611, USA

C ompetency training in diet and nutrition for the gastroenterologist has traditionally centered on the specialized nutrition support modalities of total parenteral nutrition and enteral tube feedings, diets for malabsorptive syndromes, and management of patients with chronic liver disease. It is clear that nutritional competency must now extend to the management of patients who are overweight or obese. This shift in focus is caused by the rapidly escalating prevalence of the condition (over 65% of United States adults and 17% of children and adolescents currently categorized as overweight or obese [1]) and the increasing number of obesity-related symptoms and medical conditions that patients present with to their health care provider. Obesity is a multiple organ disorder, affecting nine organ systems involving over 40 conditions (Table 1) [2]. For the gastroenterologist, these include gastroesophageal reflux disease [3–10], nonalcoholic fatty liver disease [15–22], cholelithiasis [23,24], umbilical and incisional hernias, and colon cancer [11–14]. Although not identified as a diagnostic criterion, nonalcoholic fatty liver disease is now considered a component of the metabolic syndrome related to insulin resistance [15,16,25–27]. Most patients with nonalcoholic fatty liver disease present with a constellation of other factors of the metabolic syndrome, including abdominal obesity, type 2 diabetes, and hyperlipidemia. Although not all patients with nonalcoholic fatty liver disease are obese, obesity is considered the most important risk factor, both for its occurrence and for its progression to fibrosis and cirrhosis [28]. Data from the Third National Health and Nutrition Examination Survey showed that 69% of cases of aminotransferase elevations are unexplained and strongly associated with central adiposity and related features including dyslipidemia, higher insulin levels, diabetes, and hypertension [29]. Obesity is also considered an independent risk factor for nonresponse to antiviral treatment in chronic hepatitis C [30–33].

Because obesity is associated with an increased risk of multiple health problems, it is important for gastroenterologists and all health care providers routinely to identify, evaluate, and treat patients for obesity in the course of daily practice. The importance of screening for overweight and obesity by periodic measurement

E-mail address: rkushner@nmh.org

0889-8553/07/$ – see front matter
doi:10.1016/j.gtc.2007.01.004

Table 1 Obesity-related organ systems review	
Cardiovascular	Respiratory
Hypertension	Dyspnea
Congestive heart failure	Obstructive sleep apnea
Cor pulmonale	Hypoventilation syndrome
Varicose veins	Pickwickian syndrome
Pulmonary embolism	Asthma
Coronary artery disease	
Endocrine	Gastrointestinal
Metabolic syndrome	Gastroesophageal reflux disease
Type 2 diabetes	Non-alcoholic fatty liver disease
Dyslipidemia	Cholelithiasis
Polycystic ovarian syndrome/angrogenicity	Hernias
Amenorrhea/infertility/menstrual disorders	Colon cancer
Musculoskeletal	Genitourinary
Hyperuricemia and gout	Urinary stress incontinence
Immobility	Obesity-related glomerulopathy
Osteoarthritis (knees and hips)	Chronic kidney disease
Low back pain	Hypogonadism (male)
Psychologic	Breast and uterine cancer
Depression/low self esteem	Pregnancy complications
Body image disturbance	Neurologic
Reduced quality of life	Stroke
Integument	Idiopathic intracranial hypertension
Striae distensae (stretch marks)	Meralgia paresthetica
Stasis pigmentation of legs	
Lymphedema	
Cellulitis	
Intertrigo, carbuncles	
Acanthosis nigricans/skin tags	

Adapted from Kushner RF, Roth JL. Assessment of the obese patient. Endocrinol Metab Clin North Am 2003;32:924; with permission.

of height and weight along with recording of the body mass index (BMI) is recommended by multiple organizations, including the US Preventive Services Task Force [34] and the National Institutes of Health [35,36]. This article reviews the assessment process, and then describes in more detail the treatment of the overweight and obese adult patient.

ASSESSMENT

Similar to other medical conditions commonly seen in practice, a thorough history, physical examination, and laboratory evaluation based on the patient's risk factors needs to be performed before discussing and initiating treatment for obesity. The weight history should include an assessment of physiologic (medical illness, drug-induced) and environmental (social and psychologic) factors that may contribute to weight gain. A family history is important to identify a potential genetic predisposition for obesity-associated comorbid conditions. A history of weight loss attempts, including a patient's insight as to why attempts were or were not successful, is particularly useful. Lastly, it is valuable to ascertain the patient's level of nutritional knowledge along with eating, activity, and coping lifestyle patterns.

Physical assessment of the patient should include the evaluation of BMI; waist circumference (for BMI <35 kg/m^2); and overall medical risk. BMI can be conveniently and routinely documented on all patients with use of a BMI height-weight table (Table 2). Alternatively, BMI can be calculated as [(weight in kg)/(height in m)^2]. Waist circumference should be measured (at the end of normal expiration) around the abdomen at the level of the iliac crest. The importance of measuring and documenting waist circumference in patients with a BMI less than 35 kg/m^2 is because of the independent contribution of visceral fat to the development of comorbid diseases [37]. BMI is used to define weight status, with healthy weight BMI 18.5 to 24.9, overweight BMI 25 to 29.9, and obesity BMI greater than or equal to 30. Obesity can be further classified as class I, class II, and class III (Table 3). For a more thorough discussion of the obesity evaluation process, readers are referred to other current resources [2,38,39].

TREATMENT

Information obtained from the history, physical examination, and diagnostic tests is used to determine risk and develop a treatment plan. The primary goal of treatment is to improve obesity-related comorbid conditions and reduce the risk of developing future comorbidities. The decision of how aggressively to treat the patient and which modalities to use is determined by the patient's risk status, their expectations, and what resources are available. Therapy for obesity always begins with lifestyle management and may include pharmacotherapy or surgery [35,36]. Setting an initial weight loss goal of 10% over 6 months is a realistic target. Whereas some patients may be successful by working with the physician alone, most require additional support resources, such as a registered dietitian, commercial or Internet weight loss program, or referral to an obesity specialist.

LIFESTYLE MANAGEMENT

Dietary therapy, exercise counseling, and behavioral change are the principal interventions of lifestyle management. The primary intent of lifestyle management is to empower individuals with the knowledge, skills, strategies, resources, and support to choose dietary, physical activity, and coping patterns that are consistent with their lifestyle. These are essential features of obesity care because patient choice and ability to implement change ultimately determine outcome. Lifestyle management has been shown to result in a modest (typically 3–5 kg) weight loss compared with no treatment or usual care [34].

Table 2
Body mass index table

BMI	19	20	21	22	23	24	25	26	27	28	29	30	31	32	33	34	35	36	37	38	39	40	41	42	43	44	45	46	47	48	49	50	51	52	53	54
Height (inches)	Body weight (pounds)																																			
58	91	96	100	105	110	115	119	124	129	134	138	143	148	153	158	162	167	172	177	181	186	191	196	201	205	210	215	220	224	229	234	239	244	248	253	258
59	94	99	104	109	114	119	124	128	133	138	143	148	153	158	163	168	173	178	183	188	193	198	203	208	212	217	222	227	232	237	242	247	252	257	262	267
60	97	102	107	112	118	123	128	133	138	143	148	153	158	163	168	174	179	184	189	194	199	204	209	215	220	225	230	235	240	245	250	255	261	266	271	276
61	100	106	111	116	122	127	132	137	143	148	153	158	164	169	174	180	185	190	195	201	206	211	217	222	227	232	238	243	248	254	259	264	269	275	280	285
62	104	109	115	120	126	131	136	142	147	153	158	164	169	175	180	186	191	196	202	207	213	218	224	229	235	240	246	251	256	262	267	273	278	284	289	295
63	107	113	118	124	130	135	141	146	152	158	163	169	175	180	186	191	197	203	208	214	220	225	231	237	242	248	254	259	265	270	278	282	287	293	299	304
64	110	116	122	128	134	140	145	151	157	163	169	174	180	186	192	197	204	209	215	221	227	232	238	244	250	256	262	267	273	279	285	291	296	302	308	314
65	114	120	126	132	138	144	150	156	162	168	174	180	186	192	198	204	210	216	222	228	234	240	246	252	258	264	270	276	282	288	294	300	306	312	318	324
66	118	124	130	136	142	148	155	161	167	173	179	186	192	198	204	210	216	223	229	235	241	247	253	260	266	272	278	284	291	297	303	309	315	322	328	334
67	121	127	134	140	146	153	159	166	172	178	185	191	198	204	211	217	223	230	236	242	249	255	261	268	274	280	287	293	299	306	312	319	325	331	338	344
68	125	131	138	144	151	158	164	171	177	184	190	197	203	210	216	223	230	236	243	249	256	262	269	276	282	289	295	302	308	315	322	328	335	341	348	354
69	128	135	142	149	155	162	169	176	182	189	196	203	209	216	223	230	236	243	250	257	263	270	277	284	291	297	304	311	318	324	331	338	345	351	358	365
70	132	139	146	153	160	167	174	181	188	195	202	209	216	222	229	236	243	250	257	264	271	278	285	292	299	306	313	320	327	334	341	348	355	362	369	376
71	136	143	150	157	165	172	179	186	193	200	208	215	222	229	236	243	250	257	265	272	279	286	293	301	308	315	322	329	338	343	351	358	365	372	379	386
72	140	147	154	162	169	177	184	191	199	206	213	221	228	235	242	250	258	265	272	279	287	294	302	309	316	324	331	338	346	353	361	368	375	383	390	397
73	144	151	159	166	174	182	189	197	204	212	219	227	235	242	250	257	265	272	280	288	295	302	310	318	325	333	340	348	355	363	371	378	386	393	401	408
74	148	155	163	171	179	186	194	202	210	218	225	233	241	249	256	264	272	280	287	295	303	311	319	326	334	342	350	358	365	373	381	389	396	404	412	420
75	152	160	168	176	184	192	200	208	216	224	232	240	248	256	264	272	279	287	295	303	311	319	327	335	343	351	359	367	375	383	391	399	407	415	423	431
76	156	164	172	180	189	197	205	213	221	230	238	246	254	263	271	279	287	295	304	312	320	328	336	344	353	361	369	377	385	394	402	410	418	426	435	443

Table 3
Classification of weight status

Weight status	Body mass index
Underweight	<18.5
Healthy weight	18.5–24.9
Overweight	25–29.9
Obesity class I	30–34.9
Obesity class II	35–39.9
Obesity class III (extreme obesity)	≥40

Adapted from National Institutes of Health, National Heart, Lung, and Blood Institute. Clinical guidelines on the identification, evaluation, and treatment of overweight and obesity in adults. Washington: US Department of Health and Human Services, Public Health Service; 1998.

Diet Therapy

The primary focus of diet therapy is on reducing overall consumption of calories. The National Heart, Lung, and Blood Institute Guidelines recommend initiating treatment with a diet producing a calorie deficit of 500 to 1000 kcal/d from the patient's habitual diet, with the goal of losing approximately 1 to 2 lb/wk [35]. This often translates into a diet of 1000 to 1200 kcal/d for most women, and a diet between 1200 and 1600 kcal/d for men and heavier women. This goal can be most simply achieved by suggesting substitutions or alternatives to the diet to achieve the desired calorie deficit. Examples include choosing smaller portion sizes, eating more fruits and vegetables, consuming more whole grain cereals, selecting leaner cuts of meat and skimmed dairy products, reducing fried foods and other added fats and oils, and drinking water instead of caloric beverages. It is important that the dietary counseling remains patient-centered and consistent with the patient's cultural preferences.

Macronutrient composition

The macronutrient composition of the diet varies depending on the patient's preference and medical condition. The 2005 US Department of Agriculture Dietary Guidelines for Americans, which focus on health promotion and risk reduction, can be applied to treatment of the overweight and obese patient [40]. The dietary recommendations include maintaining a diet rich in whole grains, fruits, vegetables, and dietary fiber; consuming two servings (8 oz) of fish high in omega-3 fatty acids per week; decreasing sodium to less than 2300 mg/d; consuming three cups of milk (or equivalent low-fat or fat-free dairy products) per day; limiting cholesterol to less than 300 mg/d; and keeping total fat between 20% and 35% of daily calories and saturated fats to less than 10% of daily calories. Application of these guidelines to specific calorie goals can be found on the website www.mypyramid.gov. Additional information for professionals can be accessed at http://www.mypyramid.gov/professionals/index. The revised Dietary Reference Intakes for Macronutrients released by the Institute of Medicine recommends an adult diet that has 45% to 65% of calories from carbohydrates, 20% to 35% from fat, and 10% to 35% from protein [41].

The guidelines also recommend daily fiber intake of 38 g (men) and 25 g (women) for persons over 50, and 30 g (men) and 21 g (women) for those under 50 years of age. The Institute of Medicine report highlights a very important point when it comes to macronutrients: rather than endorsing a fixed ratio of calories from carbohydrates, fat, and protein, one should think in terms of safe and acceptable macronutrient ranges.

Low-carbohydrate diets

A current area of continuing controversy is the use of low-carbohydrate diets for weight loss. Although these diets are typically lumped into one category, they actually represent a continuum of carbohydrate percentage levels and differ slightly in theory. The Institute of Medicine recommends a diet in which 45% to 65% of calories come from carbohydrates. In contrast, most of the popular lower-carbohydrate diets (Southbeach, Zone, and Sugar Busters!) recommend a carbohydrate level of approximately 40% to 46%. The Atkins diet contains 5% to 15% carbohydrate depending on the phase of the diet. Whereas Atkins believes that all carbohydrates are the primary cause of obesity and insulin resistance, the other lower-carbohydrate diets place a greater emphasis on choosing low glycemic index foods to reduce dietary insulin response.

Until recently, the theories and arguments of popular lower-carbohydrate diet books have relied on poorly controlled, non–peer-reviewed studies and anecdotes [42,43]. In recent years, several randomized, controlled trials have demonstrated greater weight loss at 6 months with favorable acute improvement in fasting glucose and insulin levels, reduction of circulating triglyceride levels, and improvement of blood pressure [44–50]. There is no statistically significant difference of weight, however, at 1 year [44,48]. An earlier review on popular diets from a US Department of Agriculture conference [51] concluded that diets that reduce caloric intake result in weight loss regardless of macronutrient composition. A systemic review by Bravata and colleagues [52] concluded that there is insufficient evidence to make recommendations for or against the use of low-carbohydrate diets, and that participant weight loss was principally associated with decreased caloric intake and increased diet duration but not with reduced carbohydrate content. Following this review, Meckling and colleagues [53] confirmed that isocaloric diets that vary only in carbohydrate content result in equal weight loss over a 10-week study period. More recent reviews, however, have attributed a beneficial physiologic effect of higher protein content of the diets [54–57]. Although low-carbohydrate diets can be effective in helping people to lose weight over the short-term, the long-term effects and safety are uncertain [58].

Meal replacements

One of the most effective tools to achieve ideal portions and effectively produce a calorie deficit is incorporation of meal replacements. Meal replacements are foods that are designed to take the place of a meal, while at the same time providing nutrients and good taste within a known caloric limit. Patients who replace one or two meals per day often lose more weight and are more likely to maintain that weight loss than patients who try to count calories on their own [59]. In a meta-analysis of six studies with a study duration ranging from 3 to 51 months, use of partial meal replacements resulted in a 7% to 8% weight loss [60].

Meal replacements consist of shakes, meal bars, or frozen meals. These portion- and calorie-controlled foods typically provide between 200 and 400 calories. Combined with a side of vegetables and fruit, meal replacements help to reduce calories from the total day and provide a nutritionally balance meal. Additional fruits and vegetables are essential to provide adequate fiber and antioxidants. Patients can select from canned vegetable soups; fresh or frozen vegetables; and fresh, frozen, or canned precut fruits. Overall, because meal replacements are convenient and reasonably priced, they provide an effective and healthy option for busy people who make poor food choices because of time constraints.

Energy density

Another dietary approach to consider is the concept of energy density. Dietary studies have demonstrated that people tend to ingest a constant volume of food, regardless of caloric or macronutrient content [61]. The energy density approach to weight loss comes from this observation. Energy density refers to the number of calories (energy) a food contains per unit of weight. This value is affected by the water, macronutrient (fat, carbohydrate, and protein), and fiber content of the food. The theory holds that a smaller number of calories can be consumed for a given weight of food if the food is low in energy density. Adding water or fiber to a food decreases its energy density by increasing weight without affecting caloric content [62]. Examples of foods with low energy density include soups, fruits, vegetables, oatmeal, and lean meats. Dry foods and high-fat foods, such as pretzels, cheese, egg yolks, potato chips, and red meat, have a high energy density. Studies on the topic suggest that diets containing low energy dense foods control hunger and result in decreased caloric intake and weight loss.

Very-low-calorie diets

Very-low-calorie diets are prescribed as a form of more aggressive dietary therapy. The primary purpose of prescribing a very-low-calorie diet is to promote a rapid and significant (13–23 kg) short-term weight loss over a 3- to 6-month period. These propriety formulas typically supply less than or equal to 800 kcal, 50 to 80 g protein, and 100% of the recommended daily allowance for vitamins and minerals. A meta-analysis [63] found that after a weight loss of at least 20 kg, individuals maintained significantly more weight loss than after low-calorie diets or weight loss of less than 10 kg. In contrast, others studies have found no difference in long-term weight loss between very-low-calorie diets and low-calorie diets [64]. According to a review by the National Task Force on the Prevention and Treatment of Obesity [65], indications for initiating a very-low-calorie diet include well-motivated individuals who are moderately to severely obese (BMI >30); have failed at more conservative approaches to weight loss; and have a medical condition that is immediately improved with rapid weight loss. Conditions include poorly controlled type 2 diabetes, hypertriglyceridemia, obstructive sleep apnea, and symptomatic peripheral edema. The risk for gallstone formation increases exponentially at rates of weight loss above 1.5 kg/wk [66]. Prophylaxis against gallstone formation with ursodeoxycholic acid, 600 mg/d, is effective in reducing this risk [67]. Because of the need for close metabolic monitoring, these diets are usually prescribed by physicians specializing in obesity care.

Physical Activity Therapy

Although exercise alone is only moderately effective for weight loss, the combination of dietary modification and exercise is the most effective behavioral approach for treatment of obesity. In contrast, the most important role of exercise seems to be in the maintenance of the weight loss [68]. Currently, the minimum public health recommendation for physical activity is 30 minutes of moderate-intensity physical activity on most, preferably all, days of the week [69,70]. Focusing on simple ways to add physical activity into the normal daily routine through leisure activities, travel, and domestic work should be suggested. Examples include walking, using the stairs, doing home and yard work, and engaging in sport activities. Asking the patient to wear a pedometer to monitor total accumulation of steps as part of the activities of daily living is a useful strategy. Step counts are highly correlated with inactivity (low number of steps) and with activity (high number of steps) [71]. Studies have demonstrated that lifestyle activities are as effective as structured exercise programs in improving cardiorespiratory fitness and weight loss [72,73]. The American College of Sports Medicine recommends that overweight and obese individuals progressively increase to a minimum of 150 minutes of moderate-intensity physical activity per week as a first goal. For long-term weight loss, however, higher amounts of exercise (eg, 200–300 min/wk or ≥2000 kcal/wk) are needed [74]. The Dietary Guidelines for Americans 2005 found compelling evidence that at least 60 to 90 minutes of daily moderate-intensity physical activity (420–630 min/wk) is needed to sustain weight loss [40]. The American College of Sports Medicine also recommends that resistance exercise supplement the endurance exercise program [75]. These recommendations feel daunting to most patients and need to be implemented gradually. Many patients benefit from consultation with an exercise physiologist or personal trainer.

Behavioral Therapy

Implementing sustainable changes in the patient's diet and physical activity patterns is the most challenging feature of obesity care. Multiple behavioral modification theories and techniques have been applied to obesity with mostly modest outcomes. The most commonly used approaches include motivational interviewing [76,77], transtheoretical model and stages of change [78], and cognitive behavioral therapy [79,80]. These techniques can be learned and used by physicians, but they do take time. In the setting of a busy practice, they are probably more reasonably applied by ancillary office staff, such as a nurse clinician or registered dietitian. Nonetheless, a few key behavioral principles should be used when possible. It is important to recognize that increasing knowledge by itself does not seem to be useful in promoting behavioral change.

Cognitive behavioral therapy incorporates various strategies intended to help change and reinforce new dietary and physical activity behaviors [79,80]. Strategies include self-monitoring techniques (eg, journaling, weighing, and measuring food and activity); stress management; stimulus control (eg, using smaller plates, not eating in front of the television or in the car); social support; problem solving; and cognitive restructuring (ie, helping patients develop more positive and realistic thoughts about themselves). When recommending any behavioral lifestyle change, have the patient identify what, when, where, and how the behavioral change will be performed; have the patient and yourself keep a record of the anticipated behavioral change; and follow-up progress at the next office visit.

PHARMACOTHERAPY

Adjuvant pharmacologic treatments should be considered for patients with a BMI greater than or equal to 30 kg/m^2 or with a BMI greater than or equal to 27 kg/m^2 who also have concomitant obesity-related risk factors or diseases and for whom dietary and physical activity therapy has not been successful (Table 4) [35]. The effectiveness of antiobesity drugs is enhanced when they are prescribed with lifestyle modification because of the importance of a drug-behavior interaction. Whether the medication acts centrally to suppress appetite or peripherally to block the absorption of fat, patients must deliberately and consciously alter their behavior for weight loss to occur. For all antiobesity drugs, the pharmacologic action must be translated into behavior change. For anorexiants, a reduced sense of hunger or increased satiety must be translated into choosing smaller healthier meals and reduced snacking. Failure to sense and act on these inhibitory internal signals results in modest or no weight loss. Similarly, if a patient takes an intestinal fat blocking agent and does

Table 4
A guide to selecting treatment

	BMI category				
Treatment	25–26.9	27–29.9	30–35	35–39.9	≥40
Diet, exercise, behavior therapy	With comorbidities	With comorbidities	+	+	+
Pharmacotherapy		With comorbidities	+	+	+
Surgery				With comorbidities	+

From National Institutes of Health, National Heart, Lung, and Blood Institute. The practical guide: identification, evaluation, and treatment of overweight and obesity in adults. Washington: US Department of Health and Human Services, Public Health Service, NIH Publication No. 00-4084; 2000.

not limit the consumption of dietary fat to 30% or less, they will discontinue the medication because of intolerable side effects. Moreover, failure to incorporate physical activity as part of the lifestyle change seriously hinders maintenance of the initial weight loss. There is a bidirectional, mutually beneficial relationship between antiobesity drugs and lifestyle management, each therapy enhancing the efficacy of the other.

In a randomized trial by Wadden and colleagues [81] evaluating the benefits of lifestyle modification in the pharmacologic treatment of obesity, investigators showed that the efficacy of sibutramine-induced mean weight loss at 1 year was significantly enhanced when subjects also attended a lifestyle support group (−10.8%) or lifestyle support group plus portion-controlled diet (−16.5%) versus sibutramine alone (−4.1%). The results of this trial were subsequently confirmed in a follow-up study [82]. When prescribing an antiobesity medication, patients must be actively engaged in a lifestyle program that provides the strategies and skills needed effectively to use the drug.

There are several potential targets of pharmacologic therapy for obesity, all based on the concept of producing a sustained negative energy (calorie) balance. The earliest and most thoroughly explored treatment has been suppression of appetite by centrally active medications that alter monoamine neurotransmitters. A second strategy is to reduce the absorption of selective macronutrients from the gastrointestinal tract, such as fat. These two mechanisms form the basis for all currently prescribed antiobesity agents. A third target, selective blocking of the endocannabinoid system, has recently been identified. Readers are referred to recent comprehensive review articles on the pharmacologic treatment of obesity for more information [83–88].

Centrally Acting Anorexiant Medications

Appetite-suppressing drugs, or anorexiants, effect satiation (the processes involved in the termination of a meal); satiety (the absence of hunger after eating); and hunger (a biologic sensation that initiates eating). By increasing satiation and satiety and decreasing hunger, these agents help patients reduce caloric intake while providing a greater sense of control without deprivation. The target site for the actions of anorexiants is the ventromedial and lateral hypothalamic regions in the central nervous system. Their biologic effect on appetite regulation is produced by variably augmenting the neurotransmission of three monoamines: (1) norepinephrine; (2) serotonin (5-hydroxytryptamine); and (3) to a lesser degree, dopamine. The classical sympathomimetic adrenergic agents (benzphetamine, phendimetrazine, diethylpropion, mazindol, and phentermine) function by either stimulating norepinephrine release or blocking its reuptake. In contrast, sibutramine (Meridia) functions as a serotonin and norepinephrine reuptake inhibitor. Furthermore, unlike other previous Food and Drug Administration–approved anorexiants, sibutramine is not pharmacologically related to amphetamine and has no addictive potential. Sibutramine is the only drug in this class that is approved for long-term use. It produces a dose-dependent weight loss with an average loss of about 5% to 9% of initial body weight at 12 months [88]. The medication has been demonstrated to be useful in maintenance of weight loss for up to 2 years [89,90].

The most commonly reported adverse events of sibutramine are headache, dry mouth, insomnia, and constipation. These are generally mild and well tolerated. The principal concern is a dose-related increase in blood pressure and heart rate that may require discontinuation of the medication. A dose of 10 to 15 mg/day causes an average increase in systolic and diastolic blood pressure of 2 to 4 mm Hg and an increase in heart rate of 4 to 6 beats/min. For this reason, all patients should be monitored closely and seen back in the office within 1 month after initiating therapy. The risk of adverse effects on blood pressure are no greater in patients with controlled hypertension than in those who do not have hypertension, and the drug does not seem to cause cardiac valve dysfunction [91,92]. Contraindications to sibutramine use include uncontrolled hypertension, congestive heart failure, symptomatic coronary heart disease, arrhythmias, or history of stroke. Similar to other antiobesity medications, weight reduction is enhanced when the drug is used along with behavioral therapy and body weight increases once the medication is discontinued.

Peripherally Acting Medication

Orlistat (Xenical) is a synthetic hydrogenated derivative of a naturally occurring lipase inhibitor, lipostatin, produced by the mold *Streptomyces toxytricini*. Orlistat is a potent slowly reversible inhibitor of pancreatic, gastric, and carboxylester lipases and phospholipase A_2, which are required for the hydrolysis of dietary fat in the gastrointestinal tract into fatty acids and monoacylglycerols. The drug's activity takes place in the lumen of the stomach and small intestine by forming a covalent bond with the active serine residue site of these lipases [93]. Taken at a therapeutic dose of 120 mg three times a day, orlistat blocks the digestion and absorption of about 30% of dietary fat. On discontinuation of the drug, fecal fat usually returns to normal concentrations within 48 to 72 hours.

Multiple randomized, 1- to 4-year double-blind, placebo-controlled studies have shown that after 1 year, orlistat produces a weight loss of about 9% to 10% compared with a 4% to 6% weight loss in the placebo-treated groups [94–96]. Because orlistat is minimally (<1%) absorbed from the gastrointestinal tract, it has no systemic side effects. Tolerability to the drug is related to the malabsorption of dietary fat and subsequent passage of fat in the feces. Six gastrointestinal tract adverse effects have been reported to occur in at least 10% of orlistat-treated patients: (1) oily spotting, (2) flatus with discharge, (3) fecal urgency, (4) fatty or oily stool, (5) oily evacuation, and (6) increased defecation. The events are generally experienced early, diminish as patients control their dietary fat intake, and infrequently cause patients to withdraw from clinical trials. Psyllium mucilloid is helpful in controlling the orlistat-induced gastrointestinal side effects when taken concomitantly with the medication [97]. Serum concentrations of the fat-soluble vitamins D and E and betacarotene have been found to be significantly lower in some of the trials, although generally remain within normal ranges. The manufacturer's package insert for orlistat recommends that patients take a vitamin supplement along with the drug to prevent potential deficiencies. Orlistat was approved for over-the-counter use in 2007.

THE ENDOCANNABINOID SYSTEM

Cannabinoid receptors and their endogenous ligands have been implicated in a variety of physiologic functions, including feeding, modulation of pain, emotional behavior, and peripheral lipid metabolism. The cannabinoid receptors, the endocannabinoids, and the enzymes catalyzing their biosynthesis and degradation constitute the endocannabinoid system. Cannabis and its main ingredient, Δ^9-tetrahydrocannabinol, is an exogenous cannabinoid compound. Two endocannabinoids have been identified: anandamide and 2-arachidonyl glyceride. Two cannabinoid receptors have been cloned: CB_1 (abundant in the brain) and CB_2 (present in immune cells). The brain endocannabinoid system is thought to control food intake through reinforcing motivation to find and consume foods with high incentive value and regulating actions of other mediators of appetite. The first selective cannabinoid CB_1 receptor antagonist, called rimonabant, was discovered in 1994. The medication is effective in antagonizing the orexigenic effect of Δ^9-tetrahydrocannabinol and suppressing appetite when given alone in animal models [98].

Several large prospective, randomized controlled trials have demonstrated the effectiveness of rimonabant as a weight loss agent [99–101]. Taken as 20-mg dose, subjects lost an average of approximately 6.5 kg compared with approximately 1.5 kg for placebo at 1 year. Concomitant improvements were seen in waist circumference and cardiovascular risk factors. The most common reported side effects include depression, anxiety, and nausea. Rimonabant is currently under review by the Food and Drug Administration.

SURGERY

Bariatric surgery can be considered for patients with severe obesity (BMI ≥ 40 kg/m^2) or those with moderate obesity (BMI ≥ 35 kg/m^2) associated with a serious medical condition [35]. Surgical weight loss functions by reducing caloric intake and, depending on the procedure, macronutrient absorption. The improvement in comorbid conditions is the result of multiple factors including weight and body fat loss; change in diet; and for the malabsorptive procedures, anatomic changes of the gastrointestinal tract that effect altered responses of glucagon-like peptide-1 and peptide YY_{3-36} , gut hormones involved in glucose regulation and appetite control [102].

Weight loss surgeries fall into one of two categories: restrictive and restrictive malabsorptive (Fig. 1) [103,104]. Restrictive surgeries limit the amount of food the stomach can hold and slow the rate of gastric emptying. The vertical banded gastroplasty is the prototype of this category, but is currently performed on a very limited basis because of lack of effectiveness in long-term trials. Laparoscopic adjustable silicone gastric banding (LASGB) has replaced

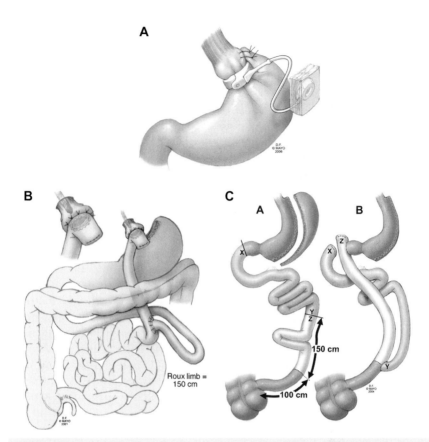

Fig. 1. (A) Laparoscopic adjustable gastric band procedure. (B) Roux-en-Y gastric bypass. (C) Duodenal switch procedure. Greater curvature sleeve gastrectomy has been performed (A). Duodenoileostomy is constructed 250 cm from the ileocecal valve with a common channel of 100 cm (B). (*From* Kendrick ML, Dakin GF. Surgical approaches to obesity. Mayo Clin Proc 2006;81:S19, S21; with permission.)

the vertical banded gastroplasty as the most commonly performed restrictive operation. The first banding device, the LAP-BAND, was approved for use in the United States in 2001. In contrast to previous devices, the diameter of this band is adjustable by way of its connection to a reservoir that is implanted under the skin. Injection or removal of saline into the reservoir tightens or loosens the band's internal diameter, respectively, changing the size of the gastric opening. Because there is no rerouting of the intestine with LASGB, the risk for developing micronutrient deficiencies is entirely dependent on the patient's diet and eating habits.

The three restrictive malabsorptive bypass procedures combine the elements of gastric restriction and selective malabsorption. The Roux-en-Y gastric bypass (RYGB) is the most commonly performed and accepted bypass procedure. It involves formation of a 10- to 30-mL proximal gastric pouch by either surgically separating or stapling the stomach across the fundus. Outflow from the pouch is created by performing a narrow (10 mm) gastrojejunostomy. The distal end of jejunum is then anastomosed 50 to 150 cm below the gastrojejunostomy. "Roux-en-Y" refers to the Y-shaped section of small intestine created by the surgery; the Y is created at the point where the pancreobiliary conduit (afferent limb) and the Roux (efferent) limb are connected. "Bypass" refers to the exclusion or bypassing of the distal stomach, duodenum, and proximal jejunum. RYGB may be performed with an open incision or laparoscopically.

The biliopancreatic diversion is more complicated and less commonly performed than the RYGB. This operation involves a subtotal gastrectomy, leaving a much larger gastric pouch compared with the RYGB. The small bowel is divided 250 cm proximal to the ileocecal valve and connected directly to the gastric pouch, producing a gastroileostomy. The remaining proximal limb (biliopancreatic conduit) is then anastomosed to the side of the distal ileum 50 cm proximal to the ileocecal valve. In this procedure, the distal stomach, duodenum, and entire jejunum are bypassed, leaving only a 50-cm distal ileum common channel for nutrients to mix with pancreatic and biliary secretions.

Biliopancreatic diversion with duodenal switch is a variation of the biliopancreatic diversion, which preserves the first portion of the duodenum. In this procedure, a vertical subtotal gastrectomy is performed and the duodenum is divided just beyond the pylorus. The distal small bowel is connected to the short stump of the duodenum, producing a 75- to 100-cm ileal-duodenal common channel for absorption of nutrients. The other end of the duodenum is closed, and the remaining small bowel connected onto the enteral limb at about 75 to 100 cm from the ileocecal valve.

Although no recent randomized controlled trials compare weight loss after surgical and nonsurgical interventions, available data from meta-analyses and large databases primarily obtained from observational studies suggest that bariatric surgery is the most effective weight loss therapy for those with clinically severe obesity [105,106]. These procedures are generally effective in producing an average weight loss of approximately 30% to 35% of total body weight that is maintained in nearly 60% of patients at 5 years. In general, mean weight loss is greater after the combined restrictive-malabsorptive procedures compared with the restrictive procedures. An abundance of data support the positive impact of bariatric surgery on obesity-related morbid conditions including diabetes mellitus, hypertension, obstructive sleep apnea, dyslipidemia, and nonalcoholic fatty liver disease.

Gastroenterologists often participate in the aftercare of bariatric surgical patients because of postsurgical complications. The most common surgical complications include stomal stenosis or marginal ulcers (occurring in 5%–15% of patients) that present as prolonged nausea and vomiting after eating or inability to advance the diet to solid foods. These complications are typically treated by endoscopic balloon dilatation and acid suppression therapy, respectively. Abdominal and incisional hernias (occurring in approximately 30% of patients with an open surgical approach) necessitate an operative repair, the timing of which is determined by symptoms and stabilization of body weight. For patients who undergo LASGB, there are no intestinal absorptive abnormalities other than mechanical reduction in gastric size and outflow. Selective deficiencies uncommonly occur unless eating habits remain restrictive and unbalanced. In contrast, the restrictive-malabsorptive procedures produce a predictable increased risk for micronutrient deficiencies of vitamin B_{12}, iron, folate, calcium, and vitamin D based on surgical anatomic changes. Patients require lifelong supplementation with these micronutrients [107].

SUMMARY

Obesity is one of the nation's most serious health problems and is expected to increase in prevalence and severity. Health care providers must take an active role in identification, evaluation, and treatment of high-risk individuals. All patients should be provided lifestyle therapy with consideration for pharmacotherapy and bariatric surgery when indicated. Although modest, a 5% to 10% weight loss is achievable and associated with improvement in many co-morbid conditions.

References

[1] Ogden CL, Carroll MD, Curtin LR, et al. Prevalence of overweight and obesity in the United States, 1999–2004. JAMA 2006;295:1549–55.

[2] Kushner RF, Roth JL. Assessment of the obese patient. Endocrinol Metab Clin North Am 2003;32(4):915–34.

[3] Fisher BL, Pennathur A, Mutnick JL, et al. Obesity correlates with gastroesophageal reflux. Dig Dis Sci 1999;44:2290–4.

[4] Locke GR, Talley NJ, Fett SL, et al. Risk factors associated with symptoms of gastroesophageal reflux. Am J Med 1999;106:642–9.

[5] Wajed SA, Streets CG, Bremner CG, et al. Elevated body mass disrupts the barrier to gastroesophageal reflux. Arch Surg 2001;136:1014–9.

[6] Kiljander T, Salomaa ER, Helenius H, et al. Asthma and gastro-oesopheal reflux: can the response to anti-reflux therapy be predicted? Respir Med 2001;95:387–92.

[7] Mayne ST, Navarro SA. Diet, obesity and reflux in the etiology of adenocarcinoma of the esophagus and gastric cardia in humans. J Nutr 2002;132:3467S–70S.

[8] Nilsson M, Johnsen R, Ye W, et al. Obesity and estrogen as risk factors for gastroesophageal reflux symptoms. JAMA 2003;290:66–72.

[9] Pandolfino JE, El-Serag Q, Shah N, et al. Obesity: a challenge to esophagogastric junction integrity. Gastroenterology 2006;130(3):639–49.

[10] Kaltenbach T, Crockett S, Gerson LB. Are lifestyle measures effective in patients with gastroesophageal reflux disease? Arch Intern Med 2006;166:965–71.

[11] Shike M. Body weight and colon cancer. Am J Clin Nutr 1996;63(3 Suppl):442S–4S.

[12] Giacosa A, Franceschi S, La Vecchia C, et al. Energy intake, overweight, physical exercise and colorectal cancer risk. Eur J Cancer Prev 1999;8(Suppl 1):S53–60.

[13] Calle EE, Radriguez C, Walker-Thurmond K, et al. Overweight, obesity, and mortality from cancer in a prospectively studied cohort of U.S. adults. N Engl J Med 2003; 348:1625–38.

[14] Moore LL, Bradlee ML, Singer MR, et al. BMI and waist circumference as predictors of lifetime colon cancer risk in Framingham study adults. Int J Obes Relat Metab Disord 2004;28:559–67.

[15] Marceau P, Biron S, Hould FS, et al. Liver pathology and the metabolic syndrome X in severe obesity. J Clin Endocrinol Metab 1999;84:1513–7.

[16] Ratziu V, Giral P, Charlotte F, et al. Liver fibrosis in overweight patients. Gastroenterology 2000;118:1117–23.

[17] Sheth SG, Gordon FD, Chopra S. Nonalcoholic steatohepatitis. Ann Intern Med 1997;126:137–45.

[18] Diehl AM. Nonalcoholic steatohepatitis. Semin Liver Dis 1999;19:221–9.

[19] Kumar KS, Malet PF. Nonalcoholic steatohepatitis. Mayo Clin Proc 2000;75:733–9.

[20] Clinical Practice Committee. American Gastroenterological Association medical position statement: nonalcoholic fatty liver disease. Gastroenterology 2002;123:1702–4.

[21] Angulo P. Nonalcoholic fatty liver disease. N Engl J Med 2002;346:1221–31.

[22] Clark JM, Diehl AM. Nonalcoholic fatty liver disease: an underrecognized cause of cryptogenic cirrhosis. JAMA 2003;289:3000–4.

[23] Syngal S, Coakley EH, Willet WC, et al. Long-term weight patterns and risk for cholecystectomy in women. Ann Intern Med 1999;130:471–7.

[24] Erlinger S. Gallstones in obesity and weight loss. Eur J Gastroenterol Hepatol 2000;12:1347–52.

[25] Chitturi S, Abeygunasekera S, Farrell GC, et al. NASH and insulin resistance: insulin hypersecretion and specific association with the insulin resistance syndrome. Hepatology 2002;35:373–9.

[26] Eguchi Y, Eguchi Y, Mizuta T, et al. Visceral fat accumulation and insulin resistance are important factors in nonalcoholic fatty liver disease. J Gastroenterol 2006;41(5):462–9.

[27] Church TS, Kuk JL, Ross R, et al. Association of cardiorespiratory fitness, body mass index, and waist circumference to nonalcoholic fatty liver disease. Gastroenterology 2006;130(7):2023–30.

[28] Ruhl CE, Everhart JE. Determinants of the association of overweight with elevated serum alanine aminotransferase activity in the United States. Gastroenterology 2003;124:71–9.

[29] Clark JM, Branacati FL, Diehl AM. The prevalence and etiology of elevated aminotransferase levels in the United States. Am J Gastroenterol 2003;98:960–7.

[30] Bressler BL, Guindi M, Tomlinson G, et al. High body mass index is an independent risk factor for nonresponse to antiviral treatment in chronic hepatitis C. Hepatology 2003;38:639–44.

[31] Lonardo A, Adinolfi LE, Loria P, et al. Steatosis and hepatitis C virus: mechanisms and significance for hepatic and extrahepatic disease. Gastroenterology 2004;126:586–97.

[32] Matos CA, Perez RM, Pacheco MS, et al. Steatosis in chronic hepatitis C: relationship to the virus and host risk factors. J Gastroenterol Hepatol 2006;21(8):1236–9.

[33] Chariton MR, Pockros PJ, Harrison SA. Impact of obesity on treatment of chronic hepatic C. Hepatology 2006;43(6):1177–86.

[34] U.S. Preventive Services Task Force. Screening for obesity in adults: recommendations and rationale. Ann Intern Med 2003;139:930–2.

[35] National Heart, Lung, and Blood Institute (NHLBI). Clinical guidelines on the identification, evaluation, and treatment of overweight and obesity in adults. The evidence report. Obes Res 1998;6(Suppl 2):51S–209S.

[36] National Heart, Lung, Blood Institute (NHLBI) and North American Association for the Study of Obesity (NAASO). Practical guide to on the identification, evaluation, and treatment of overweight and obesity in adults. NIH Publ number 00–4084. Bethesda (MD): National Institutes of Health; Oct. 2000.

[37] Montague CT, O'Rahilly S. The perils of portliness: causes and consequences of visceral adiposity. Diabetes 2000;49:883–8.

[38] Kushner RF. Roadmaps for clinical practice: case studies in disease prevention and health promotion—assessment and management of adult obesity: a primer for physicians. Chicago: American Medical Association; 2003. Available at: www.ama-assn.org/ama/pub/category/10931.html. Accessed December 1, 2006.

[39] Kushner RF, Blatner DJ. Risk Assessment of the overweight and obese patient. J Am Diet Assoc 2005;105(5 Suppl 1):S53–62.

[40] U.S. Department of Health and Human Services and U.S. Department of Agriculture. Dietary guidelines for Americans, 2005. 6th Edition. Washington, DC: U.S. Government Printing Office; 2005.

[41] National Research Council. Dietary reference intakes for energy, carbohydrate, fiber, fat, fatty acids, cholesterol, protein, and amino acids. Washington, DC: National Academy Press; 2002. p. 1–936.

[42] Cheuvront SN. The Zone Diet phenomenon: a closer look at the science behind the claims. J Am Coll Nutr 2003;22:9–17.

[43] Kushner RF. Low-carbohydrate diets, con: the mythical phoenix or credible science? Nutr Clin Pract 2005;20:13–6.

[44] Foster FD, Wyatt HR, Hill JO, et al. A randomized trial of a low-carbohydrate diet for obesity. N Engl J Med 2003;348:2082–90.

[45] Yancy WS, Olsen MK, Guyton JR, et al. A low-carbohydrate, ketogenic diet versus a low-fat diet to treat obesity and hyperlipidemia. Ann Intern Med 2004;140: 769–77.

[46] Brehm BJ, Seeley RJ, Daniels SR, et al. A randomized trial comparing a very low carbohydrate diet and a calorie-restricted low fat diet on body weight and cardiovascular risk factors in healthy women. J Clin Endocrinol Metab 2003;88:1617–23.

[47] Samaha FF, Iqbal N, Seshadri P, et al. A low-carbohydrate as compared with a low-fat diet in severe obesity. N Engl J Med 2003;348:2074–81.

[48] Stern L, Iqbal N, Seshadri P, et al. The effects of low-carbohydrate versus conventional weight loss diets in severely obese adults: one-year follow-up of a randomized trial. Ann Intern Med 2004;140:778–85.

[49] Adam-Perrot A, Clifton P, Brouns F. Low-carbohydrate diets: nutritional and physiological aspects. Obes Rev 2006;7:49–58.

[50] Noble CA, Kushner RF. An update on low-carbohydrate, high-protein diets. Curr Opin Gastroenterol 2006;22:153–9.

[51] Freedman MR, King J, Kennedy E. Popular diets: a scientific review. Obes Res 2001;9(Suppl 1):1S–40S.

[52] Bravata DM, Sanders L, Huang J, et al. Efficacy and safety of low-carbohydrate diets: a scientific review. JAMA 2003;289:1837–50.

[53] Meckling KA, O'Sullivan C, Saari D. Comparison of a low-fat diet to a low-carbohydrate diet on weight loss, body composition, and risk factors for diabetes and cardiovascular disease in free-living, overweight men and women. J Clin Endocrinol Metab 2004;89: 2717–23.

[54] Astrup A. The satiating power of protein- a key to obesity prevention? Am J Clin Nutr 2005;82:1–2.

[55] Anderson GH, Moore SE. Dietary proteins in the regulation of food intake and body weight in humans. J Nutr 2004;134:974S–9S.

[56] Krieger JW, Sitren HS, Daniels MJ, et al. Effects of variation in protein and carbohydrate intake on body mass and composition during energy restriction: a meta-regression. Am J Clin Nutr 2006;83:260–74.

[57] Hu FB. Protein, body weight, and cardiovascular health. Am J Clin Nutr 2005;82(Suppl): 242S–7S.

[58] Nordmann AJ, Nordmann A, Briel M, et al. Effects of low-carbohydrate vs low-fat diets on weight loss and cardiovascular risk factors: a meta-analysis of randomized controlled trials. Arch Intern Med 2006;166:285–93.

[59] Bowerman S. The role of meal replacements in weight control. In: Bessesen DH, Kushner R, editors. Evaluation and management of obesity. Philadelphia: Hanley & Belfus, Inc.; 2002. p. 53–8.

[60] Heymsfield SB, van Mierlo CAJ, van der Knaap HCM, et al. Weight management using meal replacement strategy: meta and pooling analysis from six studies. Int J Obes Relat Metab Disord 2003;27:537–49.

[61] Ello-Martin JA, Ledikwe JH, Rolls RJ. The influence of food portion size and energy density on energy intake: implications for weight management. Am J Clin Nutr 2005;82(Suppl): 236S–41S.

[62] Rolls BJ, Drewnowski A, Ledikwe JH. Changing the energy density of the diet as a strategy for weight management. J Am Diet Assoc 2005;105:S98–S103.

[63] Anderson JW, Kontz EC, Frederich RC, et al. Long-term weight-loss maintenance: a meta-analysis of US studies. Am J Clin Nutr 2001;74:579–84.

[64] Wadden TA, Osei S. The treatment of obesity: an overview. In: Wadden TA, Stunkard AJ, editors. Handbook of obesity treatment. New York: The Guilford Press; 2002. p. 229–48.

[65] National Task Force on the Prevention and Treatment of Obesity. Very low-calorie diets. JAMA 1993;270:967–74.

[66] Weinsier RL, Wilson LJ, Lee J. Medically safe rate of weight loss for the treatment of obesity: a guidelines based on risk of gallstone formation. Am J Med 1995;98:115–7.

[67] Shifman ML, Kaplan GD, Brinkman-Kaplan V, et al. Prophylaxis against gallstone formation with urodeoxycholic acid in patients participating in a very-low-calorie diet program. Ann Intern Med 1995;122:899–905.

[68] Votrubo SB, Horvitz MA, Schoeller DA. The role of exercise in the treatment of obesity. Nutrition 2000;16:179–88.

[69] Pate RR, Pratt M, Blair SN, et al. Physical activity and public health: a recommendation from the centers for disease control and prevention and the American college of sports medicine. JAMA 1995;273:402–7.

[70] Warburton DER, Nicol CW, Bredin SSD. Prescribing exercise as preventive therapy. Can Med Assoc J 2006;174(7):961–74.

[71] Welk GJ, Differding JA, Thompson RW, et al. The utility of the Digi-walker step counter to assess daily physical activity patterns. Med Sci Sports Exerc 2000;32(Suppl): S481–8.

[72] Dunn AL, Marcus BH, Kampert JB, et al. Comparison of lifestyle and structured interventions to increase physical activity and cardiorespiratory fitness: a randomized trial. JAMA 1999;281:327–34.

[73] Anderson RE, Wadden TA, Bartlett SJ, et al. Effects of lifestyle activity vs structured aerobic exercise in obese women: a randomized trial. JAMA 1999;281:335–40.

[74] Jakacic JM, Clark K, Coleman E, et al. Appropriate intervention strategies for weight loss and prevention of weight regain for adults. Med Sci Sports Exerc 2001;33: 2145–56.

[75] Kraemer WJ, Adams K, Cafarelli E, et al. Progression models in resistance training for healthy adults. Med Sci Sports Exerc 2002;34(2):364–80.

[76] Rollnick S, Mason P, Butler C, editors. Health behavior change: a guide for practitioners. Philadelphia: Churchill Livingstone; 2000.

[77] Miller WR, Rollnick S, editors. Motivational interviewing preparing people for change. New York: Guilford Publ; 2002.

[78] Prochaska JO, Velicer WF, Rossi JS, et al. Stages of change and decisional balance for 12 problem behaviors. Health Psychol 1994;13:39–46.

[79] Foreyt JP, Poston WSC. What is the role of cognitive-behavior therapy in patient management? Obes Res 1998;6(Suppl 1):18S–22S.

[80] Wadden TA, Foster GD. Behavioral treatment of obesity. Med Clin North Am 2000;84: 441–62.

[81] Wadden TA, Berkowitz RI, Sarwer DB, et al. Benefits of lifestyle modification in the pharmacologic treatment of obesity: a randomized trial. Arch Intern Med 2001;161: 218–27.

[82] Wadden TA, Berkowitz RI, Womble LG, et al. Randomized trial of lifestyle modification and pharmacotherapy for obesity. N Engl J Med 2005;353:2111–20.

[83] Yanovski S, Yanovski JA. Obesity. N Engl J Med 2002;346:591–602.

[84] Kushner RF, Manzano H. Obesity pharmacology: past, present, and future. Curr Opin Gastroenterol 2002;18:213–20.

[85] Haddock CK, Poston WSC, Dill PL, et al. Pharmacotherapy for obesity: a quantitative analysis of four decades of published randomized clinical trials. Int J Obes Relat Metab Disord 2002;26:262–73.

[86] Padwal R, Li SK, Lau DCW. Long-term pharmacotherapy for overweight and obesity: a systematic review and meta-analysis of randomized controlled trials. Int J Obes Relat Metab Disord 2003;27:1437–46.

[87] Snow V, Barry P, Fitterman N, et al. Pharmacologic and surgical management of obesity in primary care: a clinical practice guideline from the American college of physicians. Ann Intern Med 2005;142:525–31.

[88] Li Z, Maglione M, Tu W, et al. Meta-analysis: pharmacologic treatment of obesity. Ann Intern Med 2005;142(7):532–46.

[89] Arterburn DE, Crane PK, Veenstra DL. The efficacy and safety of sibutramine for weight loss: a systematic review. Arch Intern Med 2004;164:994–1003.

[90] James WPT, Astrup A, Finer N, et al. Effect of sibutramine on weight maintenance after weight loss: a randomized trial. Lancet 2000;356:2119–25.

[91] Hazenberg BP. Randomized, double-blind, placebo-controlled, multicenter study of sibutramine in obese hypertensive patients. Cardiology 2000;94:152–8.

[92] Bach DS, Rissanen AM, Mendel CM, et al. Absence of cardiac valve dysfunction in obese patients treated with sibutramine. Obes Res 1999;4:363–9.

[93] Lucas KH, Kaplan-Machlis B. Orlistat—a novel weight loss therapy. Ann Pharmacother 2001;35:314–28.

[94] Sjostrom L, Rissanen A, Anderson T, et al. Randomised placebo-controlled trial of orlistat for weight loss and prevention of weight regain in obese patients. Lancet 1998;352:167–73.

[95] Davidson MH, Hauptman J, DiGirolamo M, et al. Weight control and risk factor reduction in obese subjects treated for 2 years with orlistat: a randomized trial. JAMA 1999;281:235–42.

[96] Torgerson JS, Hauptman J, Boldrin MN, et al. XENical in the prevention of diabetes in obese patients (XENDOS) study: a randomized study of orlistat as an adjunct to lifestyle changes for the prevention of type 2 diabetes in obese patients. Diabetes Care 2004;27(1):155–61.

[97] Cavaliere H, Floriano I, Medeiros-Neto G. Gastrointestinal side effects of orlistat may be prevented by concomitant prescription of natural fibers (psyllium mucilloid). Int J Obes 2001;25:1095–9.

[98] Cota D, Woods SC. The role of the endocannabinoid system in the regulation of energy homeostasis. Current Opinion in Endocrinology and Diabetes 2005;12:338–51.

[99] Van Gaal LF, Rissanen AM, Scheen AJ, et al. RIO-Europe study group. Effects of the cannabinoid-1 receptor blocker rimonabant on weight reduction and cardiovascular risk factors in overweight patients: 1-year experience from the RIO-Europe study. Lancet 2005;365:1389–97.

[100] Depres JP, Golay A, Sjostrom L, et al. Effects of rimonabant on metabolic risk factors in overweight patients with dyslipidemia. N Engl J Med 2005;353(20):2121–34.

[101] Pi-Sunyer FX, Aronne LJ, Devin J, et al. Effect of rimonabant, a cannabinoid-1 receptor blocker, on weight and cardiometabolic risk factors in overweight or obese patients. RIO-North America: a randomized controlled trial. JAMA 2006;295(7):761–75.

[102] Cummings DE, Overduin J, Foster-Schubert KE. Gastric bypass for obesity: mechanisms of weight loss and diabetes resolution. J Clin Endocrinol Metab 2004;89(6):2608–15.

[103] Kendrick ML, Dakin GF. Surgical approaches to obesity. Mayo Clin Proc 2006;8(Suppl):S18–24.

[104] Crookes PF. Surgical treatment of morbid obesity. Annu Rev Med 2006;57:243–64.

[105] Buchwald H, Avidor Y, Braunwald E, et al. Bariatric surgery: a systematic review and meta-analysis. JAMA 2004;292:1724–37.
[106] Maggard MA, Shugarman LR, Suttorp M, et al. Meta-analysis: surgical treatment of obesity. Ann Intern Med 2005;142:547–59.
[107] Kushner RF. Micronutrient deficiencies and bariatric surgery. Curr Opin Endocrinol Diabetes 2006;13:405–11.

Gastroenterol Clin N Am 36 (2007) 211–218

GASTROENTEROLOGY CLINICS
OF NORTH AMERICA

ELSEVIER
SAUNDERS

INDEX

Note: Page numbers of article titles are in **boldface** type.

Moving?

Make sure your subscription moves with you!

To notify us of your new address, find your **Clinics Account Number** (located on your mailing label above your name), and contact customer service at:

E-mail: elspcs@elsevier.com

800-654-2452 (subscribers in the U.S. & Canada)
407-345-4000 (subscribers outside of the U.S. & Canada)

Fax number: 407-363-9661

Elsevier Periodicals Customer Service
6277 Sea Harbor Drive
Orlando, FL 32887-4800

*To ensure uninterrupted delivery of your subscription, please notify us at least 4 weeks in advance of move.